Macleod's
Clinical Examination

D1460868

Macleod's Clinical Examination

Formerly *Clinical Examination*

Edited by

John Munro

Consultant Physician, Eastern General Hospital, Edinburgh
Consultant Physician, Edenhall Hospital, Musselburgh
Part-time Senior Lecturer, Department of Medicine,
Western General Hospital, Edinburgh

Christopher Edwards

Professor of Clinical Medicine, University of Edinburgh
Chairman of the University Department of Medicine,
Western General Hospital, Edinburgh

EIGHTH EDITION

CHURCHILL LIVINGSTONE
EDINBURGH LONDON MELBOURNE AND NEW YORK 1990

CHURCHILL LIVINGSTONE
Medical Division of Longman Group UK Limited

Distributed in the United States of America by
Churchill Livingstone Inc., 650 Avenue of the Americas, New
York, N.Y. 10011, and by associated companies, branches and
representatives throughout the world.

© E & S Livingstone 1964, 1967
© Longman Group Limited 1973, 1976, 1979, 1983
© Longman Group UK Limited 1986, 1990

All rights reserved. No part of this publication may be
reproduced, stored in a retrieval system, or transmitted in any
form or by any means, electronic, mechanical, photocopying,
recording or otherwise, without either the prior written
permission of the publishers (Churchill Livingstone, Robert
Stevenson House, 1–3 Baxter's Place, Leith Walk, Edinburgh
EH1 3AF), or a license permitting restricted copying in the
United Kingdom issued by the Copyright Licensing Agency
Ltd, 90 Tottenham Court Road, London, W1P 9HE.

First edition 1964
Second edition 1967
Third edition 1973
Fourth edition 1976
Fifth edition 1979
Sixth edition 1983
Seventh edition 1986
Eighth edition 1990
  Reprinted 1991
  Reprinted 1992
  Reprinted 1993

ISBN 0-443-04079-6

British Library Cataloguing in Publication Data
A catalogue record for this book is available from the British
Library

Library of Congress Cataloging in Publication Data
A catalog record is available from the Library of Congress

The
publisher's
policy is to use
**paper manufactured
from sustainable forests**

Printed in Hong Kong
SWT/04

Preface

The practice of medicine is constantly changing as some diseases are controlled or even eradicated while others increase in frequency or significance. New diagnostic techniques are being developed and new therapeutic regimes introduced. This changing pattern demands that medical education must evolve. Accordingly, it has now become apparent that an eighth edition of this textbook is required to ensure that the description and application of clinical methods remains appropriate to the current practice of medicine.

The basic aim of the book is to describe the practical skills the clinician must acquire and develop in order to formulate diagnostic procedures and management plans. Emphasis is placed on the methods of obtaining an accurate history and of performing a physical examination appropriate to the clinical problem. The main chapters in the book conform to a basic pattern. Each chapter starts by emphasizing the importance of careful history taking. The cardinal symptoms are discussed and their significance explained. The method of physical examination is then described and the relevance of positive findings discussed. The type of investigations, their advantages and limitations, are detailed as a logical extension of the clinical examination and an integral part of any management plan. Thereafter, samples are provided of the methods in practice.

The book is intended primarily for undergraduates but it has proved to be of continuing value both to postgraduates in training and to general practitioners. Its international appeal has resulted in its selection by the English Language Book Society for publication in Africa and Asia. The eighth edition of *Clinical Examination* is closely integrated with *Davidson's Principles and Practice of Medicine* in which many of the contributors participate.

Since the first editon was published in 1964, the policy has been that authors who have retired from clinical practice are replaced. On this occasion, there are two new contributors. Mr P. Abernethy has succeeded Mr J. H. S. Scott (locomotor system) and Professor R. E. Kendell takes over the psychiatric examination from Professor H. Walton. The other chapters have also undergone major revision with the introduction of new material and an increased use of figures and diagrams.

This edition is the first in which Dr J. Macleod has not been editor. The present editors suggested to Dr Macleod that the title of the book should be changed to *Macleod's Clinical Examination* to acknowledge his unique contribution, not only to this book but also to medical education. His place on the editorial team has been taken by Professor C. R. W. Edwards who will bring to the book his knowledge, drive and editorial skills.

Edinburgh, 1990   J. F. M

'The aim of medical education is to produce doctors who will promote the health of all people, and that aim is not being realised in many places, despite the enormous progress that has been made during this century in the biomedical sciences. The individual patient should be able to expect a doctor trained as an attentive listener, a careful observer, a sensitive communicator, and an effective clinician; but it is no longer enough only to treat some of the sick. Thousands suffer and die every day from diseases which are preventable, curable, or self-inflicted, and millions have no ready access to health care of any kind.

These defects have been identified for a long time, but efforts to introduce greater social awareness into medical schools have not been notably successful. Such facts have led to mounting concern in medical education about equity in health care, the humane delivery of health services, and the overall costs to society.'

Introduction to the Edinburgh Declaration from the World Conference on Medical Education, 1988

Acknowledgements

We have had generous help from many sources. We are particularly grateful to those students and doctors from all over the world who have provided constructive suggestions. We would like to express our thanks especially to Stephen Braham who produced the new line drawings. The editors are particularly indebted to Dr C. E. Robertson for much helpful advice and to many others for useful comments including Dr M. J. Ford. Dr H. L. Macdonald provided many useful suggestions regarding radiological investigation which have been included in this edition.

Original photographs were kindly supplied by Mr P. J. Abernethy (4.3A), Professor Gavin Arneil (10.4B), Professor J. J. K. Best (8.56), Dr W. A. Copland (7.2), Dr A. A. Donaldson (8.55), Elscint (GB) Ltd (7.5), Dr E. B. French (4.2D and 4.3D), Dr M. C. Grayson (Plate IIIB), Professor Ian Isherwood (7.16), Dr M. V. Merrick (9.53), Dr R. E. Pfaltzgraff (4.3C), Professor C. I. Phillips (Plate IIIA, C and D), Professor Eric Samuel (7.3) and Dr S. R. Wild (7.18). Other acknowledgements are made in the text.

Acknowledgements

Contributors

P. J. Abernethy MB ChB FRCSE
Consultant Orthopaedic Surgeon, Western
General Hospital and Princess Margaret Rose
Orthopaedic Hospital, Edinburgh
The Locomotor system

N. C. Allan MB ChB FRCP(Edin) FRCPath
Consultant Haematologist, Western General
Hospital, Edinburgh
The examination of the blood

G. K. Crompton MB ChB FRCP(Edin)
Consultant Physician Respiratory Diseases Unit,
Northern General Hospital, Edinburgh;
Senior Lecturer, University Department of
Medicine, Western General Hospital, Edinburgh;
Senior Lecturer, University Department of
Respiratory Medicine, City Hospital, Edinburgh
The respiratory system
The analysis of breathlessness

R. E. Cull BSc MB ChB PhD FRCP(Edin)
Consultant Neurologist, Royal Infirmary,
Edinburgh; Senior Lecturer in Neurology,
University of Edinburgh
The nervous system
The use of the ophthalmoscope

D. P. de Bono MD(Cantab) FRCP(Edin)
British Heart Foundation Professor of
Cardiology, University of Leicester
The cardiovascular system
The analysis of blackouts
The analysis of oedema

C. R. W. Edwards MA MD(Cantab),
FRCP(Edin) FRCP(Lond)
Professor of Clinical Medicine and Chairman,
University Department of Medicine,

Western General Hospital, Edinburgh
*The history and the general principles governing
the physical examination*
*The general examination and the external
features of disease*

D. W. Hamer-Hodges MS FRCS(Lond)
FRCS(Edin)
Consultant Surgeon, Western General Hospital,
Edinburgh
The alimentary and genitourinary systems
The examination of the breasts and varicose veins
The examination of swellings

R. E. Kendell MA MD FRCP FRCPsych
Professor of Psychiatry, University of Edinburgh;
Dean of the Faculty of Medicine, University of
Edinburgh
The psychiatric examination

J. F. Munro MB ChB FRCP(Edin)
Consultant Physician, Eastern General Hospital,
Edinburgh and Edenhall Hospital, Musselburgh;
Part-time Senior Lecturer, Department of
Medicine, Western General Hospital, Edinburgh
The alimentary and genitourinary systems
The analysis of pain
The examination of the urine
The appendices

H. Simpson MB ChB MD DCH DObst
RCOG FRCP
Professor and Head of Department of Child
Health, University of Leicester, Leicester Royal
Infirmary, Leicester
The infant and child
*The stages in the development of infants and
children*

Contents

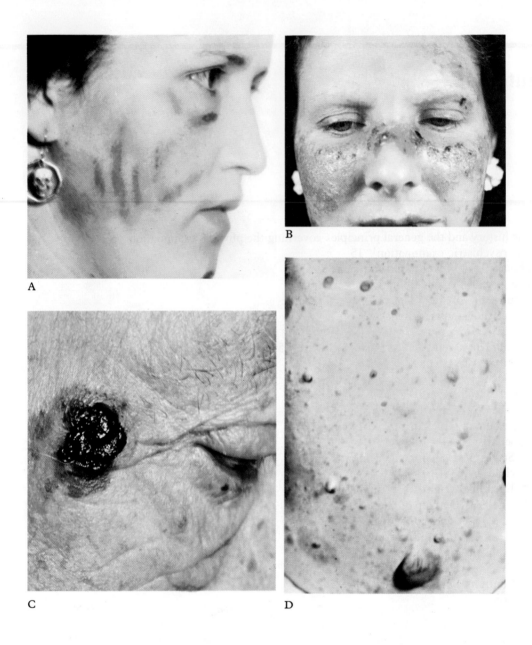

Plate I THE SKIN AS A DIAGNOSTIC AID. A, Dermatitis artefacta; unusual symmetrical lesions with clear-cut margins in an accessible site. The earring is also significant. B, Lupus erythematosus showing characteristic butterfly distribution of facial rash. C, Malignant melanoma. D, Neurofibromatosis; café au lait pigmentation in lower left corner and many nodules.

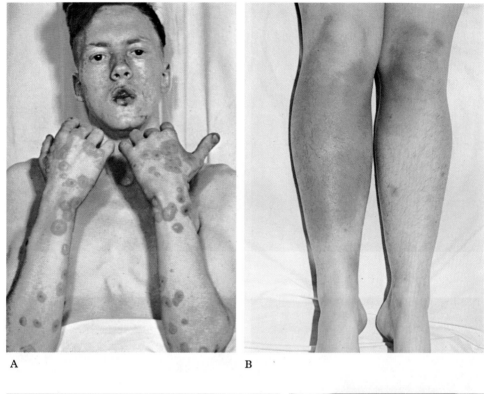

A

B

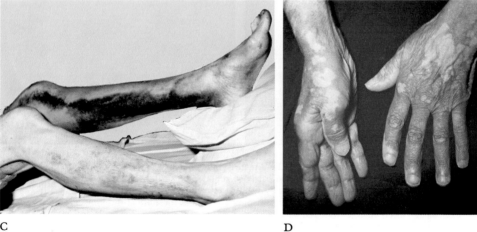

C

D

Plate II THE SKIN AS A DIAGNOSTIC AID. A, Erythema multiforme caused by
sulphonamide. B, Erythema nodosum due to sarcoidosis in a woman aged 30 years; the lesions on
the right leg have become confluent. C, Scurvy in an old man living alone; vitamin deficiency is
often overlooked in the elderly. D, Vitiligo in a patient with autoimmune disease.

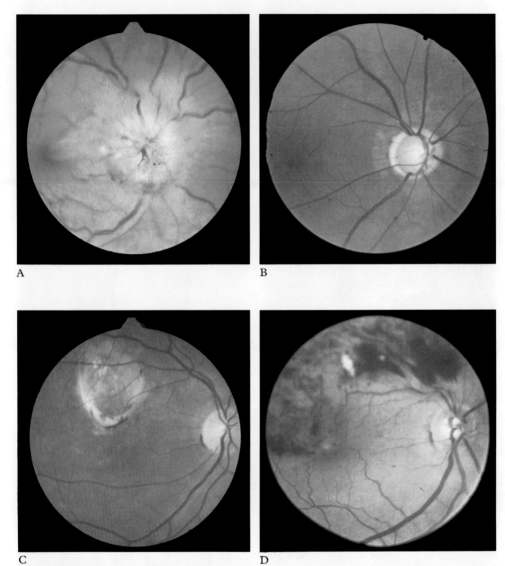

A

B

C

D

Plate III THE FUNDUS AS A DIAGNOSTIC AID. Retinal photographs showing: A, Papilloedema. Edge of optic disc blurred and partly surrounded by small haemorrhages; retinal vessels obscured on and beyond edge of disc by swelling of papilla; small dilated vessels on surface of centre of disc in sharper focus than peripheral vessels as these are at different levels. B, Glaucoma. Vessels emerge from and enter periphery of an atrophic disc over lip of an enormously enlarged and deepened optic cup, in contrast to their level course in primary optic atrophy. C, Disciform degeneration of macula due to ischaemia. Slightly pigmented scar (associated with considerable loss of central vision) above macula; atrophy of temporal third of disc due to loss of macular nerve fibres. Pigment at disc margin is a normal variant. D, Branch vein occlusion. Superior temporal vein has been occluded and has led to haemorrhages and two white patches of oedema. Several small lakes of blood lie in front of retinal vessels in the vitreous and there are some dilated collateral vessels above the macula. It is more usual in this condition for the blood to lie in the nerve fibre layer and to have a flame-shaped arcuate pattern. Disc and lower retina are normal.

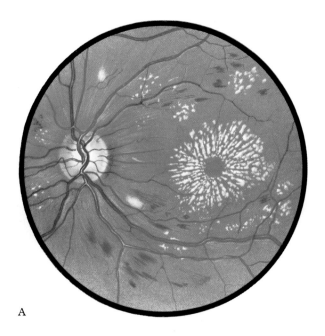

A

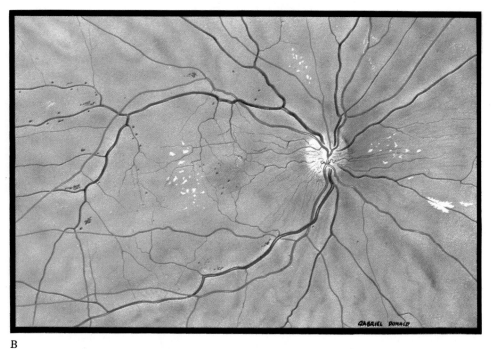

B

Plate IV THE FUNDUS AS A DIAGNOSTIC AID. Retinal painting showing: A, Hypertensive retinopathy. Note haemorrhages, two soft exudates, numerous hard exudates including a mascular star and irregularity of the calibre of the arterioles. B, Diabetic retinopathy. Note microaneurysms and a few hard exudates. From Michaelson, I. C. (1979). *Ballantyne's Textbook of the Fundus of the Eye*. 3rd edition. Edinburgh: Churchill Livingstone.

1. The history and the general principles governing the physical examination

C. R. W. Edwards

The clinical study of disease is founded on two processes, the history of the patient's disability, and the physical examination. 'Clinical Examination' comprises both these components, each of which is based on a methodical and comprehensive routine to which the student should adhere, particularly throughout the junior apprenticeship. This chapter gives an account of the sequence which should normally be followed in the consulting room or at the bedside. Chapter 2 deals with the particular problem of taking a psychiatric history.

THE HISTORY

The full evaluation of the history of a patient's complaints is crucial to making a correct diagnosis. Every medical student is, rightly, taught this — and then spends the remainder of his or her professional life relearning the lesson. The doctor's first task is to listen and observe, not only to obtain information about the current problem but also to understand the patient as a person and that individual's life situation.

The art of obtaining an accurate history expeditiously can be acquired and developed with practice. It has three main stages, the first of which must be a satisfactory approach to the patient. Secondly, adequate opportunity must be given to the patient to tell the story. Thirdly, a competent interrogation must be made by the doctor to clarify the patient's account and, as indicated, to extract further information regarding previous health, family, social and personal matters. The same sequence is followed with almost every patient, the emphasis changing in accordance with the current problem. When the basic

technique has been acquired, skill will improve with experience until an efficient and flexible method has been developed.

1. The approach to the patient

The individual who is ill and who is possibly apprehensive when confronted by a stranger is readily disturbed if first impressions are bad, for example if the doctor appears indifferent or unsympathetic an emotional barrier to effective communication is erected. It is therefore essential that the patient is put at ease by being given a friendly greeting, and made to feel the centre of interest. In the consulting room it is inadvisable to confront the patient across a desk (see Fig. 2.1). It is also important not to acquire the bad habit of completing notes about the previous patient at the crucial moment when the newcomer should be welcomed. It should become second nature for the doctor to have all senses alert, particularly at the outset. The clinical examination begins from the moment of first meeting with the doctor who must not miss the revealing, fleeting gesture, facial expression, intonation, use of eye-to-eye contact, or other body language of non-verbal communication.

Doctors should introduce themselves to the patient by name, and medical students should also explain their status. At the outset the clinician should help the patient to relax. Addressing the patient by his or her name is good for self-esteem and for establishing a less impersonal relationship. It is also wise to be sure whether it is 'Miss','Mrs' or 'Ms'. Initial remarks should be about impersonal matters; a minute or so can be spent with profit in this way to help eliminate any preliminary diffidence. Any impression of hurry on the doctor's part should be avoided. Conversation can readily be round the patient's occupation, past or present, while confidence accrues. A congenial start to the interview creates conditions which should encourage the patient to speak freely.

Students when first taking histories often feel they are imposing upon patients; however the majority of patients enjoy talking to those students whose approach is satisfactory.

2. The patient's account of the current illness

Patients should be given an opportunity to tell their story in their own way, and in order to encourage them to do so the initial question must be of a general nature, e.g. 'Now please tell me about your trouble'. If they have difficulty in starting, ask 'What was the first thing you felt wrong?', followed by 'What happened next?'. 'When were you last well?' or other prompting should encourage patients to talk. Thereafter much can be learned about the symptoms and also about the patient's intellectual capacity and emotional reactions. Attentive listening has, moreover, a therapeutic role, particularly when dealing with a psychiatric problem (p. 15). Wilfred Trotter has described listening in terms of 'the power of attention, of giving one's whole mind to the patient without the interposition of anything of one's self. It sounds simple but only the very greatest doctors ever fully attain it. It is an active process and not merely resigned listening or even politely waiting until you can interrupt. Disease often tells its secrets in a casual parenthesis.'

Patients in hospital often conclude the current history with their admission. They should be encouraged to continue right up to the time of examination.

Medical students (and doctors) frequently make the mistake of interrupting prematurely. Intervention should be based on the initial assessment of the personality of the patient. While the possibilities are innumerable, certain situations commonly recur; for example, there is the intelligent person who gives a clear unemotional account, the 'good witness'. This kind of description often points straight to the diagnosis with little further aid from the doctor. The inarticulate

person will require help by the posing of very simple questions, whereas the verbose individual, giving irrelevant details, will need guidance to direct attention to essentials; even so, there is still a danger of interrupting too soon. The individual with some medical knowledge tends to give a diagnosis rather than an account of symptoms and speaks in terms of 'flu', 'gastritis', 'rheumatism', 'migraine', etc. Such statements must not be accepted without reviewing their basis. The patient who is worried by illness or frightened in a doctor's presence, must be handled sympathetically, but the doctor must distinguish such an individual from those whose primary problem is one of psychological stress. Deafness or early dementia may create misunderstanding, particularly if the doctor has failed to appreciate that the patient's mental functions are impaired. Timidity, guilt or fear of disease may lead to information being suppressed. In contrast, symptoms, may be exaggerated in an attempt to ensure attention. Another problem is that a patient's memory may be very fallible because of emotional stress at the time of examination. Wilful deceit is rare except by alcoholics and drug addicts; the latter are often expert at faking symptoms, as are patients with Munchausen's disease whose motive is to gain admission to one hospital after another on the basis of a convincing but mendacious tale of illness. In Trousseau's words, '*Il n'y a pas de maladies; il n'y a que les malades.*'

3. Interrogation by the doctor

(a) The current illness

It is first necessary to clarify the patient's account to ensure that all the symptoms have been elicited and to evaluate them. The art of interrogation develops with practice, provided certain principles are observed. Questions should be formulated simply and clearly. When a satisfactory answer has been obtained, the same question should not be repeated later. This usually results from inattention and gives a justifiably poor impression of the carefulness of the examiner.

Many individuals are very open to suggestion and unintentionally provide erroneous information if a certain answer would appear to be expected.

Biased and premature questioning of a perplexed patient anxious to help the doctor may result in a very distorted history. It is therefore important, not to ask leading questions while the basic facts are being elicited. Later in the proceedings, however, use may be made of such questions to elucidate the patient's account provided that the potential fallacies involved are kept in mind. It is good policy to indicate in the case notes any information obtained by asking leading questions.

The principal symptoms must be thoroughly analysed. Examples of this process are given in Chapter 3, but the doctor must be satisfied that accurate information has been obtained regarding the time and mode of onset of any important symptom, the circumstances in which it occurred, its duration and the existence of any ameliorating or aggravating factors. The relationship to other symptoms must be defined and a chronological account obtained of the development of the illness

Table 1.1 Systemic enquiry: standard questions

1. Cardiovascular system
   ankle swelling
   palpitations
   breathlessness when lying flat (orthopnoea)
   attacks of noctural breathlessness (paroxysmal nocturnal dyspnoea)
   chest pain on exertion
   pain in legs on exertion

2. Respiratory system
   shortness of breath: exercise tolerance
   wheezing
   cough
   sputum production (colour, amount)
   chest pain isolated to respiration or coughing
   blood in sputum (haemoptysis)

3. Central nervous system
   headaches
   visual symptoms (e.g double vision, loss of acuity or visual field)
   fits
   faints
   tingling (paraesthesiae)
   numbness
   muscle weakness
   hearing symptoms (e.g.deafness, tinnitus)
   excessive thirst
   sleep patterns

4. Urogenital
   pain on passing urine (dysuria)
   frequency of passing urine (nocturia?)
   abnormal colour of urine (e.g. blood)

number of sexual partners
males:
if appropriate age ask for prostatic symptoms such as difficulty in starting to pass urine, poor stream, terminal dribbling
if appropriate ask for mental attitude to sex (libido), morning erections, frequency of intercourse, ability to maintain erections, ejaculation, urethral discharge
female:
if premenopausal, age of onset of periods (menarche), regularity of periods (e.g. 28-day cycle), length of period, blood loss (e.g. clots, flooding), note of last period, contraception if relevant, presence of vaginal discharge
stress and/or urge incontinence
pain during intercouse (dyspareunia)
post-menopausal bleeding where relevant

5. Alimentary
   condition of mouth (infected tongue or bleeding gums)
   difficulty with swallowing (dysphagia)
   indigestion
   heartburn
   abdominal pain
   weight loss
   change in bowel habit
   colour of motion (e.g. pale, dark, black, fresh blood)

6. Locomotor
   joint pain or stiffness
   muscle pain or weakness

7. Endocrine
   heat intolerance
   cold intolerance
   change in sweating
   prominence of eyes
   swelling in neck

from the first symptom to the date of interview. If possible, exact dates should be recorded rather than vague statements such as 'last Saturday' or 'a few weeks ago'. It may be helpful to observe what happens when the symptom is reproduced. For example the patient who complains of breathlessness on exertion may be studied walking up stairs. If there is difficulty in describing a recurrent symptom of varying severity, the position may be clarified by asking for an account of the first and of the most severe attacks. It is important to record negative findings, e.g. cough but no sputum, or breathlessness but no cough.

Elderly or ill patients easily tire during the initial history taking which should then be curtailed and completed later.

Systemic enquiry. When a clear record has been obtained of the current complaint specific enquiries should be made about the presence or absence of cardinal symptoms suggestive of involvement of various systems. The student should compile a list of standard questions about the cardiovascular, respiratory, urogenital, alimentary, locomotor, endocrine and central nervous systems. If a positive response is elicited then further questions will need to be asked, e.g. radiation of pain, and its severity, duration, frequency and relief with medication. Such questions can be asked very quickly and enable a comprehensive systemic history to be taken and often reveal crucial information necessary for making a diagnosis or point to the presence of pathology unrelated to the presenting complaint. This and other information can also be elicited by questionnaires and analysed by computers but such techniques will not detect any emotional reactions which would be apparent to the alert clinician. Questionnaires, however, can usefully be exploited in selected circumstances (p. 357).

Information from a third party. It is necessary to obtain information from a relative or friend when the patient is unable to supply it because of immaturity, illness, senility or mental disturbance or if there is any suspicion of drug or alcohol abuse. Corroboration is often helpful when the patient is a poor historian. Every effort should be made to procure an account from an eye-witness in the case of a person who has been unconscious or who may be suffering from a condition in which knowledge of the patient's behaviour or appearance may be useful. Some patients wear necklaces or carry cards or other documents which give details of the diagnosis and current drug treatment, — e.g. special cards are provided to patients taking steroids, anticoagulants or anticonvulsants. In patients who are unconscious or unable to provide details, a search of the patient's clothing and personal belongings may provide vital information. In the acutely ill, it may be necessary to contact the patient's own general practitioner to obtain the relevant information.

Patients give information to medical students or to nurses which has not been previously divulged, perhaps because they were unsure of its relevance or were afraid of wasting the time of a busy doctor. Social workers often obtain crucial evidence from patients or their relatives or in the course of a home visit. Other hospital staff can also be the source of useful knowledge. All these sources of information are available to a well organised clinical team.

(b) Previous illness and state of health

Information should be obtained about previous illnesses, operations and accidents and recorded in chronological order. Patients may be reminded about past illness by being asked if they have ever been in hospital or been confined to bed at home. It should be borne in mind, however, that the diagnosis supplied by the patient may not be correct. If medical records are not available, the examiner may have to decide about past episodes on the patient's description of symptoms and circumstances at the time, but it is salutary to realise that what may now be obvious because of the progress of the disease may have been impossible to diagnose previously. Frequently patients hold an accident responsible for subsequent troubles; any claim of this kind must be considered critically. A history of sexually transmitted disease may be suppressed, because of a feeling of guilt, and when it is suspected the individual must be asked about their sexual activity (p. 165). It is important to remember HIV infection may remain asymptomatic for years.

Residence or travel abroad and any illness which occurred there may be relevant; a puzzling fever may prove to be due to malaria or amoebiasis contracted outside Britain. Air transport enables vast distances to be covered within the shortest of incubation periods so that infection may be transmitted to an area where it is not normally encountered. Patients may not necessarily mention their journeyings unless specifically asked if they have been abroad. The onus is on the doctor to make the relevant enquiry. It is also important to ask details about prophylactic medication, for example for malaria, and about immunisation.

Previous health. Just as knowledge of previous illness may be necessary in assessing a clinical problem, so also may information about past health. A medical examination for insurance or employment purposes would give a good basis for comparison with the present findings. Family planning clinics often record the blood pressure and such measurements can be invaluable in a woman on an oral contraceptive who has been found to be hypertensive. In all cases it is most helpful to know the date and result of any previous radiological examination. The films should be reviewed if there is any doubt about the result.

Drug history

It is essential to know about any drugs that are being taken on medical advice or otherwise and sometimes, it is important to know what drugs have been taken previously. A drug treatment history can be of value because it may provide a diagnosis, such as analgesic nephropathy, warn about possible drug interactions or previous adverse effects, or indicate how effective, or ineffective, previous treatments have been in the management of a chronic disorder. Specific enquiry should be directed to determine what medicines the patient is currently taking or has previously received from their own doctor or from a hospital clinic. This is particularly important if the patient has received previous treatment with corticosteroids. It is important not to overlook treatments provided by 'alternative' practitioners including herbal remedies or by the patients themselves with self-medication using potentially harmful preparations such as laxatives, analgesics or oral contraceptives. Any previous adverse experience with medicines must be clearly recorded, preferably on the outside of the case notes.

Direct questions are sometimes useful in reminding patients about medications they may have forgotten, e.g. 'Do you ever take anything for headaches, to help yourself to sleep, to prevent constipation, for indigestion or as a tonic?' Those who have travelled abroad should be asked specifically about timing of chemoprophylaxis. Patients who take medicines should be asked either to identify them by name or to bring them to the clinician so that they can be identified. Where patients are on multiple drug therapy the possibility of drug interactions must always be considered.

Self abuse with drugs is becoming a major problem in some societies. Not only may some drugs produce life-threatening addiction but also their usage may be associated with fatal infections including hepatitis B and HIV. The clinician must be prepared to ask patients if they are taking or have previously taken such drugs of addiction. Direct questions rarely cause offence but may only be understood if the clinician uses the local colloquim, e.g. 'Have you ever used pot?', or 'Do you mainline?'.

(d) Family history

Information regarding the age and health, or the cause of death of patients' relatives is often valuable. Are both parents still alive? Does, or did, the patient get on with them in the recent past and during childhood? How many siblings are there and where did the patient come in the family? What are the siblings doing now and how does the patient get on with them now and in the past? In certain conditions such as polycystic kidneys or Huntington's chorea there is a well defined mode of inheritance. In others such as the autoimmune diseases there appears to be a genetic and an environmental component. However, regardless of aetiology the knowledge that there is a family history of diabetes, coronary artery disease, hypertension, gout or an infectious disease such as tuberculosis, should increase the doctor's awareness of the possibility of that condition in the patient. The symbols used in the construction of a family tree (pedigree chart) are illustrated in Figure 1.1 (p. 6).

Often there is unwarranted anxiety: for example that a patient may develop a crippling disease affecting a close relative. Considerable tact must be deployed when asking about problems such as alcoholism or mental disorder in a close relative. Overall, however, a display of interest in the welfare of the family usually helps to secure rapport.

At this stage it is usually possible to obtain at least an impression of the individual's personal relationships but enquiry about more intimate matters, if deemed necessary, is often best postponed until after the physical examination. However, if the patient wishes to speak about emotional disturbances at any phase of the proceedings the opportunity to do so should be taken as it may not occur again. An unhappy childhood, sexual difficulties, a broken marriage and problems with children, adolescents or elderly relatives are all very potent influences on an individual's well-

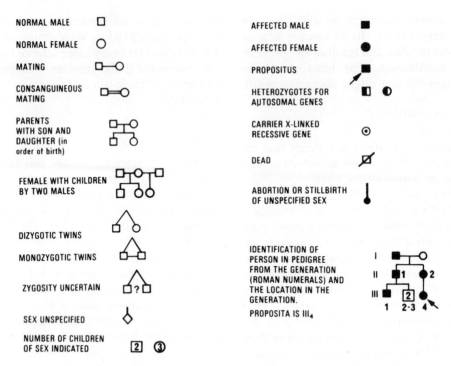

Fig. 1.1 Symbols used in pedigree charts. Drawing up a family tree begins with the affected person first found to have the trait (propositus if male, proposita if female). Thereafter relevant information regarding siblings and all maternal and paternal relatives is included. (Reproduced with permission from Emery A E H 1983 Elements of medical genetics, 6th edn. Churchill Livingstone, Edinburgh.)

being. On the other hand, the family may constitute a united group able to give substantial support to any member in difficulty.

(e) Social history

Patients' occupational and social environments may, like family influences, have profound repercussions on their health. Illness may ensue directly as in the case of coalworkers' pneumoconiosis or indirectly as in malnutrition; social problems may arise as a result of illness. Much of this information may be known to the general practitioner. In contrast the doctor working in hospital sees the patient in an artificial setting and must acquire some knowledge of the individual's normal background, not only in relation to diagnosis, but also in the planning of rehabilitation. A description ('profile') of how the patient spends an average day may be helpful in determining realistic therapeutic goals. The patient's functional capacity must be assessed and related to the employ-

ment; for example in cases of heart or lung disease return to heavy work or to a polluted atmosphere may be contraindicated. Enquiry should, therefore, be made about home, occupation, personal interests and habits.

The home. It may be necessary to know about the other occupants, the number of rooms, the sanitary arrangements, the heating or lack of it, the state of repair of the house and the financial obligations of the residents. The number of steps leading up to or inside the home will be relevant when planning to rehabilitate patients with severe cardiac or lung disease. Neighbours may create problems or may be very helpful in times of stress. A social worker or occupational therapist can often obtain essential information by visiting and reporting on home conditions.

Occupation. It is desirable to know the patient's employment and what this involves. It is good practice to encourage conversation about this and allied topics; useful information is obtained, the anxious patient is diverted and the doctor's interest is usually appreciated. It may be helpful to find out if women with family commitments work because of economic necessity, boredom at home or job satisfaction. Attention should be paid to the congeniality or tedium of the employment, to any occupational hazards, and to stresses imposed by others or by the individual's own ambitions. Unemployment or job insecurity may have an adverse effect on the patient's health. It is necessary to have some appreciation of the patient's overall economic position particularly in situations such as one parent families.

Personal interest. The doctor should also be aware of the patient's leisure pursuits, such as the amount of physical exercise undertaken, and intellectual activities. Such questions do not only relate to the promotion of mental and physical health. Excessive physical exercise, for example, is a common cause of oligomenorrhoea or amenorrhoea.

Habits. Tobacco, alcohol and food may have important implications in relation to nutritional problems, cardiorespiratory disease and psychological instability. A dietary history should be obtained if there is an obvious nutritional abnormality. In most instances an approximate assessment of the patient's food and vitamin intake will suffice but the doctor should not accept the corpulent patient's claim to eat nothing or the statement by the girl with anorexia nervosa that she eats everything. Deficiencies of substances such as folate or vitamins C or D may occur in elderly patients whose accounts of their eating habits may not be corroborated by a neighbour or by evidence obtained from a brief inspection of the kitchen. Occasionally a precise evaluation by a trained dietician is necessary.

Accurate histories of tobacco and alcohol intake are often difficult to obtain. Direct questioning may be met by denial. In some patients, measurement of carboxyhaemoglobin or blood alcohol is necessary to refute this. Most patients will underestimate their intake. It may be useful to get patients to talk about their normal working and leisure days. Such accounts will usually give a much more accurate picture of their smoking and drinking habits. In certain situations it will be necessary to retake the history either after the physical examination or further investigation. The findings of the stigmata of chronic liver disease or

of an elevated mean corpuscular volume in the absence of vitamin B_{12} or folate deficiency, or unexplained abnormal liver function tests should alert the clinician to the possibility of concealed alcohol abuse.

Where alcohol dependence is suspected, the clinician should enquire about the quantity of alcohol consumed per day or per week, whether alcohol is drunk daily or in bouts, the amount of money spent on alcohol, the age at which the patient started to drink, the time of day when the first drink is taken and whether or not the patient has ever experienced the 'shakes' of D.Ts. Further information should be obtained from a close relative.

At this stage in the history taking, a picture should have been obtained of the individual as a whole in relation to his or her background and with experience the details can be elaborated as required by the current problem.

(f) The psychological assessment

In all illness it is necessary to evaluate the part played by psychological factors. The account of the history and the manner in which it is delivered usually reveal much about the patient's personality. The reaction of the individual to distressing situations in the past is also relevant, as similar patterns of behaviour tend to recur. Frequently emotional reactions during the history taking, supplemented by negative findings on physical examination, will direct attention to the need for a more detailed psychological assessment by the clinician (see Ch. 2). In the course of the general clinical examination the doctor should have recognised any traumatic events, such as bereavement, separation or rejection and these should now be further explored. For example, grief may be intermingled with anger, resentment or guilt. It is usually possible to start the patient talking about emotionally disturbing topics by such remarks as, 'You had begun to tell me about a disagreement with —', or 'Tell me more about your mother who died last year'. If no obvious opening presents, a more direct approach is necessary: 'Do you feel guilty about your mother's death?' Patients should be asked if they are worriers by nature and if anything particular is concerning them now. Thereafter any factor of possible significance must be further explored. Often specific questions must be posed about the existence of anxieties regarding financial, occupational, domestic, sexual or religious matters. Frequently fear of disease, such as cancer, is a potent source of stress, and the same fear may inhibit disclosure of what is in the individual's mind. It may help to explain that one aspect of medical care comprises an opportunity to reassure a patient of specific health worries. Many individuals have some insight into their own personalities and it may be profitable to know how they evaluate themselves, with reservations about the opinion offered.

Patients should be encouraged to talk freely about problems, and about current difficulties with people important to them, as self-disclosure to an understanding listener is of therapeutic as well as diagnostic value. It may become apparent to the doctor and to the patient that the presenting symptom, apparently physical in origin, is in fact a manifestation of a psychological difficulty. Frank, discussion in privacy can be time-consuming but is time well spent, as many emotional problems are resolved when they are brought to the surface. When emotional distress persists or when significant abnormalities are suspected in the patient's personality or mental processes, a formal psychiatric examination is required. The interview technique used for this purpose is described in Chapter 2.

The doctor-patient relationship. The interactions between the patient and the doctor are complex and the interplay betweeen different personalities may result in anything from harmony to antagonism. The patient may 'transfer' to the doctor habitual modes of behaviour, some of these learned from parents and deeply ingrained. Thus an aggressive attitude to the doctor may represent the patient's normal reaction to people regarded as uncompliant, in this case a doctor who does not speedily relieve painful or frustrating symptoms. An overdependent attitude is also common. The patient with hysterical symptoms characteristically masks distress by a show of 'smiling unconcern'. Other defence mechanisms include the repression of unpleasant matters, the projection of faults on to others, rationalisation and over-compensation.

Inappropriate and troublesome relationships can develop between the patient and the clinician, the best known being erotic transference. This involves a patient believing that he or she is in love with the doctor and conveying their feelings by gesture or statement. Occasionally, and sometimes disastrously, a clinician reacts by responding to this suppposed sexual invitation. Erotic transference however is really indicative of a longing to be accepted without at the same time being exploited. The clinician is not called on to react to the overtly seductive statements but rather to the basically childlike behaviour of the patient. Thus, far from responding either on a similar level, or by rejection of the patient, the doctor can properly view the declaration of love as an aspect to be assessed as methodically and calmly as any other highly emotional communication.

The clinician should not depart from a professional position as a non-judgemental observer but should be prepared to ask some patients why they feel angry or are critical. In contrast, some patients strive to manipulate by flattery or other manoeuvres and the doctor should avoid going to undue lengths to meet their demands. Yet other patients cause the doctor to feel helpless and inadequate; in contrast the clinician may make the mistake of treating adult patients like children. By observation of their own feelings — i.e. the effect the patient has on them — clinicians often gain a much clearer perception of what the patient is trying to achieve. The management of a situation can be improved when the feelings aroused by the patient are carefully assessed, but not acted upon. It is seldom that the doctor loses control of the position when a conscious effort is made to create an effective relationship with the patient.

The adaptation of medical students to their patients will be facilitated if they give consideration to interpersonal factors of this kind and discuss problems with their teachers. Poise will come with understanding, self-awareness and self-control.

The taking of notes

The human memory is far from reliable and its efficiency deteriorates with ageing and with time. It is, therefore, essential that a record be made without delay. The history should be written down as it is given; with practice this can be done with little or no interruption of the patient's narrative. Some doctors develop a form of shorthand which may serve their own purposes, but notes should be legible and comprehensible if others have to use them. The importance of this will be clear to any doctor called upon to give evidence in a court of law.

It is not necessary to write down all that is said as much may be irrelevant, but the recording of the patient's own words is particularly valuable in psychiatric illness (p. 17). However, note taking may have an inhibitory effect when personal matters are being discussed; it may be advisable to lay the pen aside and later record an appropriate account. An anxious patient often jumps from one topic to another and then it is best to jot down headings and elucidate the sequence and details later. In some circumstances, for example if the history is very complicated, it may be good policy to make rough notes at the time and later elaborate these into an orderly account. This should commence by stating the presenting symptoms and their duration and be followed by a description of the development of the illness. Students will inevitably make mistakes at first, but with practice they will learn to sift the evidence, select the facts which merit prominence and record them in a coherent form.

Conclusions on completion of history

When the history has been obtained to the doctor's satisfaction the first step has been taken towards diagnosis. The relevant facts must be separated from the irrelevant and evaluated objectively. The logical analysis and interpretation of the evidence will usually lead to a provisional diagnosis or suggest a differential diagnosis. While the physical examination will be influenced accordingly, the doctor should remain unbiased and proceed to attempt to elicit further objective evidence which may confirm the interpretation of the history or which may point in a wholly different direction.

THE PHYSICAL EXAMINATION

During any clinical examination attention is fre-

quently concentrated on one or more systems. Indeed, a review of a patient's complaints too closely restricted to a single system can lead to errors in diagnosis as important disease elsewhere may be missed. It is not always possible to make a single diagnosis to embrace all the features encountered, particularly in the elderly in whom multiple unrelated pathological processes, are commonly present.

The doctor carrying out a physical examination is entirely responsible for seeking out the features of disease and must not expect the patient to draw attention to them. Failure to recognise these signs is due to careless or inadequate examination. Shortage of time may be a contributing cause. More commonly, the critical factor is the failure either to recognise the obvious or to remain sufficiently alert when performing repetitive tasks. This emphasises the value of assessing the history before undertaking the physical examination.

It is not practicable to carry out all the minutiae of examination in every patient, and some degree of compromise must be accepted. The undergraduate must not hurry or attempt any short-cuts, but follow a careful routine until thoroughly acquainted with the procedure. It is essential for the student to become familiar with the range of normal signs before abnormalities can be confidently recognised. Discrimination comes with practice.

Environment and equipment

Consideration has to be given to the conditions under which the physical examination is conducted. Privacy is essential and this usually constitutes no problem in the home or in the consulting-room. In some families relatives may feel it is their duty to be present in numbers which may embarrass the patient and the doctor. The tactful request that all, or all but one, leave is desirable. In a hospital ward, screens must be drawn round the bed before the examination begins. When necessary, steps should be provided for easy access to a high couch in the consulting-room. Comfort is important and encourages adequate relaxation. The examination couch should have an adjustable back-rest as it is easier for the patient in the semi-reclining position to converse, and not feel at a disadvatage as when lying supine. A back support is essential for the patient with heart failure who becomes breathless when lying flat. Illumination must be good. Exposure of the area to be examined must be adequate but not to an extent that might unnecessarily embarrass or chill. Both patient and doctor should be warm; auscultation of the chest of a shivering subject and palpation of the abdomen with cold hands are common faults. Apart from the discomfort, the consequent muscle sounds and the resistance of the abdominal wall impair the efficiency of the examination. Patients have, with good reason, complained about such practices since the first century, when Martial wrote:

I'm ill. I send for Symmachus; he's here,
An hundred pupils following the rear;
All feel my pulse, with hands as cold as snow;
I had no fever then — I have it now.

It is imperative to ask about pain so that the handling of any painful area is gentle. Exhaustion, as a result of a prolonged examination, must be avoided; the risk of this is greatest in the frail or elderly. While privacy is important, sometimes the presence of a nurse or relative is essential, particularly when a rectal or vaginal examination is performed.

It is convenient for the doctor to carry a stethoscope, a torch and a measuring tape. A sphygmomanometer, an ophthalmoscope with auriscope attachment, a pin and cottonwool, a tendon hammer, a tuning fork, a clinical thermometer, disposable wooden tongue-depressors, disposable gloves, lubricant and a proctoscope should be available. The consulting-room should also have a weighing machine, a height scale and facilities for procedures such as the testing of the urine (Ch. 12).

A method of examination

While the doctor records the findings in terms of systems, the actual sequence of examination should be conducted with the comfort of the patient in mind. After a general inspection, the hands, upper limbs, head, neck, chest, abdomen and lower limbs are usually dealt with in turn.

Thus information about the heart, lungs, breasts, axillary lymph nodes and spine is obtained while dealing with thorax, whereas facts relating to the nervous system are usually acquired piecemeal. This compromise presents difficulties to students. At the outset of their training they should concentrate on the individual systems in turn and, later, learn to integrate their techniques. Practice may be obtained, at an early stage, by examining, and being examined by a student colleague. This will help to attain proficiency and will also give some insight into the patient's point of view. A routine is gradually acquired which should be both methodical and flexible. The experienced doctor varies the emphasis as a result of information obtained from the history. In some cases a comprehensive examination of all systems is indicated, while in other instances one system may require special attention. A word of explanation to the patient may be advisable if the examination commences at a point remote from the site of the complaint. Procedure will vary with individuals and circumstances and the method which is outlined here is intended to provide only a working basis; it should be adapted as the occasion demands.

1. General inspection of the patient (demeanour, colour, physique, etc.) and surroundings, e.g. the temperature chart in hospital
2. Feel pulse and examine hands and arms
3. Examine head and neck.
4. Proceed now either to area mainly affected or to anterior chest (heart, lungs, breasts and axillae) and then to back (lungs and spine)
5. Examine abdomen, groins and external genitalia
6. Examine lower limbs
7. Record blood pressure
8. Ophthalmoscopic examination
9. Rectal or vaginal examination if indicated
10. The temperature, weight and height can be recorded and a specimen of urine obtained either at the outset or at the end of the examination.

If unexpected abnormalities are elicited, a change in emphasis in the examination may be required and it may be advisable to reassess some of the earlier findings.

Observer error

All doctors must be constantly critical of their clinical abilities. The scientific training of the preclinical years should have engendered an objective approach but preconceived ideas may lead to mistakes. This is illustrated in Figure 1.2; when first seen most people read the legends incorrectly as 'Paris in the spring' 'Once in a lifetime', and 'Bird in the hand'. We tend to see largely what we expect to see. We also tend to pay attention to findings which we consider significant and to ignore those which we judge unimportant.

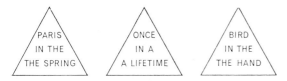

Fig. 1.2   The three triangles

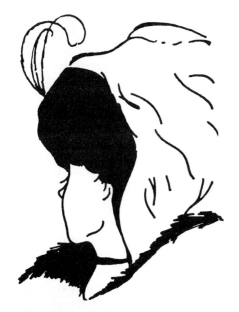

Fig. 1.3   How old is she? Some observers see a young woman, others an old one. The chin and neck of the former become the nose and mouth of the latter and vice versa. Thus different observers, confronted by the same evidence, can reach different conclusions.

Varying interpretations of the same material are also possible as shown in Figure 1.3. Location of an apex beat or assessment of jugular venous pressure by experienced physicians often differ. Disagreements also occur in the interpretation of radiographs and electrocardiograms. Furthermore when the same evidence is reviewed at a later date by the same individuals the second reports often differ significantly from the first. The range of observer variation and error is wide but mistakes should be fewer when there is a constant awareness of one's limitations, and a testing of conclusions against other findings. If, for example, the pulse is thought to be collapsing in nature then this should be confirmed by measuring the blood pressure. If bronchial breathing is suspected, then whispering pectoriloquy should also be present. When errors do occur the reasons for them should be analysed in order to learn how they may be avoided.

CASE RECORDING

Whatever sequence the physical examination may follow, it is essential that the findings are recorded systematically. When acquiring clinical experience, undergraduates should take every opportunity of examining patients in detail and of writing a comprehensive report of their findings. Later they will learn how the account may be adapted to meet the needs of the individual patient; in many circumstances quite brief notes will suffice. With most hospital patients, however, a detailed systematic report is recommended. Records of normal or negative findings often prove very helpful when comparison has to be made at a later date.

Case notes should be precise and free from any irrelevant or facetious comment which might cause embarrassment in more formal circumstances elsewhere. It is as well to remember that courts of law are empowered to demand a view of official records. The value of adequate notes, accurately and promptly recorded at the time of the illness or injury, has repeatedly been emphasised by medical defence societies. It is also important that notes are signed by the doctor who has made them.

The record must be legible, written in ink, and easily understood. Incomprehensible abbreviations and symbols must be avoided, but simple diagrams of the site and extent of abnormal findings are useful (p. 37). The abdomen in particular lends itself to the graphic illustration of areas of tenderness, palpable masses and enlargements of the viscera or lymph nodes (p. 169 and p. 171). Diagrams of neurological abnormalities (p. 266) and the effects of trauma (p. 267) are also highly informative. When a patient is found to be hypersensitive to a drug the fact should be recorded prominently on the front of the case notes. Serious repercussions and even fatalities may be prevented if, for example, *penicillin allergy* is clearly recorded.

Systems of case recording

A traditional system of case recording is given on page 358; it also outlines the main features dealt with in this and later chapters.

Problem orientated case records are discussed on page 361.

FURTHER INVESTIGATION

At the conclusion of the clinical examination it may be possible to offer either a final or a provisional diagnosis. In the latter event consideration should be given to the further investigations which may be indicated. The nature of these should be regarded as a logical extension of the clinical examination. The number of investigations carried out varies greatly between one doctor and another depending upon knowledge, experience or philosophy. Some are insufficiently critical of the deficiencies of clinical methods, whereas others employ a large number of routine tests and special investigations, many of which may be irrelevant to the problem under consideration. This latter practice has been possible in Britain where the National Health Service involves no increase in expense to the individual patient, but unnecessary investigations can never be justified and are becoming increasingly unacceptable as medical audit becomes established. Even the simplest test costs money; laboratories are apt to be overloaded with work and inaccuracies tend to occur; the patient may suffer unnecessary discomfort, and the doctor's clinical acumen does not develop in proportion to increasing experience.

Many pitfalls are avoided if a full clinical assessment is always made before instituting any investigation, and then only those selected for a specific purpose. If in doubt it is helpful to ask oneself — 'What is the benefit of this test to the patient?'.

The range of investigation is ever widening. Direct visual examination may, by means of instruments, be extended to the optic fundus, tympanic membrane, nasal passages, larynx, trachea, bronchi, oesophagus, stomach, duodenum, pleura, peritoneum, lower gut, urinary bladder, vagina and joints. Biopsies may be obtained directly from many sites and also by aspiration methods, blindly, from the small intestine, pleura, lymph nodes, liver, spleen, kidney and other organs. Information may be obtained by recording electrical activity in the body by electrocardiography, electroencephalography and electromyography. Much help comes from the radiologist where the range of investigation is now extended by the non-invasive techniques of computed tomography, ultrasonic and magnetic resonance imaging. In the laboratory area there are contributions from the biochemist, microbiologist, pathologist, physicist and the pharmacologist with whom discussion of the problem is often most rewarding. However, all tests are prone to errors of measurement or interpretation and it should be the doctor in charge of the patient who finally weighs up all the evidence before deciding on the diagnosis and prescribing treatment.

THE METHODS IN PRACTICE

Diagnosis is an intellectual process requiring the integration of information derived from many sources. The medical student must learn first how to collect the facts and then, by analysing them, how to reach a diagnosis. With increasing experience it becomes possible at an early stage in the clinical encounter to decide on a provisional explanation. This is an hypothesis which is formulated to account for the symptoms and signs. This hypothesis is then tested systematically by further physical examination and by special investigation if necessary; these lead to the confirmation or adjustment of the hypothesis or sometimes to its rejection. If this occurs alternative hypotheses are selected and analysed in turn as further data are collected until the presenting problem is solved. The student, trained in scientific method, will recognise that this attitude conforms to the contemporary scientific approach in studying a biological phenomenon whereby explanatory hypotheses are tested and are given up when refuted by new evidence.

Making and testing diagnostic judgements constitutes a strict but rewarding discipline of continuous educational value; but, in addition to the intellectual approach required to reach a diagnosis, decisions made by scientific methods must then be applied effectively and compassionately to meet the needs of the individual patient.

2. The psychiatric examination

R. E. Kendell

THE PSYCHIATRIC HISTORY

There is no fundamental difference between a psychiatric history and any other medical history, but for various reasons taking a psychiatric history often places greater demands on the interviewing skills of the clinician.

In the first place, psychiatric histories need to be more detailed, and therefore take longer, than in most other disciplines because more information is needed about the patient's personal life and background. This is partly because laboratory tests and other investigations contribute so little to diagnosis that the history is, *faute de mieux*, all important. A more fundamental reason is that many of the stresses which contribute to the genesis of psychiatric disorders are highly personal. The clinician can only understand why one patient was so devastated by his failure to obtain promotion, or why another was already at the end of her tether when her daughter announced that she was pregnant, by knowing about their previous lives — their upbringing, their careers and their marriages.

Another important issue is that the symptoms which have led to the consultation often themselves interfere with the conduct of the interview. The patient may be abnormally anxious, or suspicious, or deeply depressed or retarded. Indeed, some patients are so psychotic, or so badly demented, that they are virtually incapable of giving a history. Even if they are able to sustain a conversation they simply do not realise how abnormal or alarming their recent behaviour has been. Others deliberately conceal vital information. People with drinking problems habitually minimise both their drinking and its ill effects and the information provided by those who are abusing illegal drugs is even more unreliable. Others may conceal vital information because they are too embarrassed to talk, too ashamed to confess or too loyal to other members of their family to divulge. It is therefore frequently advisable and sometimes essential to obtain a second independent history from someone else, usually a relative.

For these reasons psychiatrists and others involved in the care of patients with psychiatric disorders have to make more deliberate attempts to develop interviewing skills and to think more deeply about what happens in their interviews than members of other medical disciplines. *Psychiatric interviewing is rather like skiing in powder snow. You can't get away with poor technique in the way that you can in less demanding settings.*

It is important to recognise at the outset that in taking a history a clinician is usually trying to combine two objectives which are not readily compatible. On the one hand it is important to put patients at ease, to allow them to describe their own problems in their own way, to appear interested in them as individuals and not merely be concerned with symptoms or diagnoses, and to win their confidence and trust. On the other hand it is necessary to end up with a coherent written account with different categories of information in a set order for ease of reference afterwards, and with answers to all the questions that seem relevant to the patients' presenting complaints and their own evolving formulation of the problem. The art of history taking is to come as close as possible to both these objectives in the limited time available.

Students often try to resolve this dilemma by giving the patient their undivided attention and then writing their notes from memory afterwards. Although this is reasonable at an early stage of training it is a bad habit to get into for two reasons. First it is impracticable: there is never enough time. Secondly, it has repeatedly been shown that histories which are only written up in retrospect are inaccurate. The interviewer forgets some things and distorts others, and tends to end up with a history which 'fits' the (possibly incorrect) provisional diagnosis and omits or distorts those elements which do not fit but which may be vital clues to the real diagnosis.

Although the setting in which the interview takes place is usually constrained by the furniture and space available it is always worth a few moments reflection, for its influence will be considerable. Curtains drawn round a bed may provide an adequate visual barrier but they do not prevent the occupants of neighbouring beds or cubicles from hearing every word that is said and it is naive to expect anyone to talk openly in such circumstances. Obtaining a reasonably soundproof room is only the beginning, however. If doctors talk to their patients across a desk, or even from a higher chair, they emphasise their 'magisterial role', and perhaps remind patients of uncomfortable occasions when the figure on the other side of the desk was their headmaster, a government official or a police officer (Fig. 2.1A). This makes it unnecessarily difficult for them to relax and to talk openly. Doctors, on the other hand, find their desks very useful. Many clinicians resolve the dilemma by seating the patient at the side of their desk, which creates a rather more friendly and personal atmosphere without depriving them of their writing surface, drawers and stationery (Fig. 2.1B or C). For relatively brief consultations this is quite appropriate but for longer and more important interviews it is probably better for doctor and patient to be seated on similar comfortable chairs at an oblique angle to one another and for the latter to write on a clipboard rather than a desk (Fig. 2.1D). The advantage of this arrangement is that it puts doctors and their patients on a more equal footing, creates the aura of an informal discussion rather than a formal interview, and allows interviewers to shift their gaze to and fro between the patient's face (which they want to be looking at as much as possible) and their notes (which they need to look at while writing) without having to turn their heads.

Initially patients should be given almost total

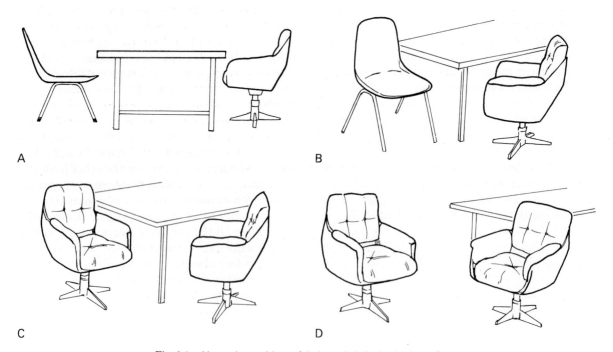

A

B

C

D

Fig. 2.1   Alternative positions of desks and chairs in the doctor/patient interview

freedom to say what they want in their own way and at their own pace. Interviewers will need to ask questions or comment from time to time but these interruptions should be kept to a minimum, and be designed to encourage the speaker to elaborate on or clarify something just said rather than changing the topic. 'When was that?', 'How did you feel about that?' for example. As time goes on, however, interviewers must slowly take control, so that in the later stages they are asking a series of specific questions to fill gaps in the story which have not been covered by the patient's spontaneous account. The underlying intention is to allow patients to feel that they are telling their own story, saying what they want to say in their own way, while at the same time allowing the interviewer to end up with a coherent and reasonably comprehensive written account with information recorded under a series of standard headings in a set order. This is rarely achieved in full, but with practice it is possible to learn how to change from one sheet of notes to another as the topic changes and so end up with the information in the appropriate order even though this is not the order in which it was provided.

The conventional categories into which the history is divided, and the order they are normally recorded in case notes, are set out below. How much information is obtained, and the relative emphasis on different aspects of the history, will obviously depend on the time available and the nature of the clinical problem, though basic information should be obtained, and recorded, under every heading. Detailed information about childhood and schooling, for example, is more likely to be important in a young woman with anorexia nervosa than in an elderly man with a dementing illness.

The presenting complaint

The patient's complaint, or complaints, should be elicited at the outset, in some detail, and then recorded verbatim, together with a brief note of their duration, e.g.:
'I just can't seem to pull myself together . .'
'Irritable with the children for no reason . . .' for 3–4 months
'Sleeping badly even with tablets'   last 2 weeks.

There is no ideal, all purpose, question for eliciting presenting complaints. The appropriate wording will depend on the setting, whether the patient is already known to the doctor, and to some extent on the latter's personality. Something like 'What is the most important problem, the main trouble, that's bringing you to see me?' will usually serve. It is crucial, though, that the interviewer should not put words into the patient's mouth by asking such questions as 'Your depression's come back, has it?' or 'Your GP tells me you've been getting panic attacks'. It is also well worth encouraging patients to add to their original list by asking 'Has anything else been going wrong?' or 'Are there any other ways in which you haven't been your normal self recently?' This is because one can always place more credence in complaints which are volunteered than in those which are only elicited by direct questions. The spontaneous comment about sleeping badly, for example, would be more significant than a similar statement which was only elicited by a question about insomnia.

History of the presenting illness

Although logically this comes immediately after the presenting complaint it is often preferable to obtain the personal history first so that you have some understanding of who it is that has developed this illness, and can make sense of such casual references as 'that was before Peter went to Australia' and 'when my man got his cards'.

What the interviewer requires is a clear account of the development of the patient's symptoms, and the stresses which preceded them, in chronological order. Some patients can provide this but many cannot and, of course, many episodes of illness do not have a clearly defined onset. Asking patients when they were last really well, or felt their normal selves, may help to elicit an anchor point from which to start. As well as obtaining a description of the patients' symptoms and their evolution in time it is important to understand what impact these have had on their lives. One way of doing this is to ask patients to describe a typical day both before they became ill and in the recent past. It is also important to obtain details of any treatment they have already received and their response to this.

Family history

It is essential to find out the past, or present, occupation of the patient's parents, because of the many social implications involved. It is also necessary to ask if any relative has ever had a psychiatric illness of any kind, or committed suicide, or been conspicuously 'nervy' because there is an important genetic component to many psychiatric disorders. If there is time many other questions can be asked. Are both parents still alive? How does or did the patient get on with them, including during childhood? How many siblings are there and where did the patient come in the family?

Personal history

This is basically a chronological account of the salient facts in the patient's life, starting with the date and place of birth and always containing at least some information under the following subheadings:

1. Early childhood
2. Schooling — age of leaving, academic prowess, relationships with teachers and peers
3. Occupations
4. Marital history including a description of the emotional and sexual relationship with the present partner (and other sexual partners if relevant)
5. Children
6. Previous physical health
7. Previous psychiatric health
8. Friendships, leisure activities, drinking habits.

   The patient's relationship with his·wife, or her husband, is particularly important and should be explored in some detail. Questions like 'Do you love him?' 'Do you think he loves you?' 'Do you think you married the right man?' will usually elicit frank and informative replies. So will questions about the patient's sexual relationships if the clinician asks them in a sympathetic but matter of fact way. Patients are usually only upset by questions about their sexual lives if the interviewer is embarrassed, or if they feel that the doctor is prying unnecessarily.

   The patient's previous psychiatric health is another crucial area, partly because many psychiatric disorders tend to recur at intervals throughout life, which makes it likely that the present episode is related to past episodes. The duration of these and their response, or lack of response, to treatment may also provide valuable clues to the likely prognosis of the current episode.

   Particular attention should also be paid to drinking habits, for many psychiatric problems are the result of excessive drinking and patients with depressions or anxiety states often attempt to control their symptoms by drinking. Never accept the bland assurance 'Oh, I'm just a social drinker' at face value. Try instead to establish how many drinks the patient has in an average week, now and in the past (p. 7).

Personality

It is important to try to assess this. A few patients, if asked to describe their normal selves as they think other people would describe them, can provide four or five appropriate adjectives or phrases, but most cannot. The task is obviously easier if an independent informant is available, but even in the absence of any informant the plain facts of the patient's life — occupational history, sexual relationships, friendships and leisure activities — will usually make it possible for an experienced clinician to draw a few valid inferences about his or her personality.

Current social status

Where is the patient living at present and with whom? Likewise, it is important to know if the patient is still working, unemployed or off sick or in debt. Such facts should always be recorded as they often constrain treatment options.

Finale

At the end of the interview, but before starting to discuss the diagnosis and treatment plans, it is sometimes a good idea to say 'Now, is there anything else that might be important which we haven't yet talked about?' If simultaneously the clinician puts aside notes and pen, this emphasises to patients that they have the doctor's undivided attention, and also that this is their last chance.

Sometimes patients will use this opportunity to mention something they have previously been unable to talk about, and when they do it is often of crucial importance.

THE MENTAL STATE EXAMINATION

Examination of the patient's mental state is the psychiatric equivalent of the physical examination, though this must not be taken to imply that patients whose symptoms are primarily psychiatric do not also need to be examined physically.

It cannot be emphasised too strongly that the ability to carry out a mental state examination and to draw appropriate conclusions from it should be within the competence of all practising clinicians. Physical and psychiatric disorders commonly coexist. Indeed, it is an important epidemiological fact that they coexist more commonly than can be accounted for by chance. Depressions and phobic anxiety states are extremely common and all doctors should be able to diagnose them (and in the case of depressions to treat them). Dementing illnesses are common in old age and anyone dealing with the elderly must be able to decide whether or not they show evidence of early dementia. Organic mental disorders (delirium and confusional states) may complicate a wide range of illnesses from ischaemic heart disease to pneumonia, as well as states of drug intoxication or withdrawal of varied kinds. It is important that these be recognised, and that the doctor concerned is able to distinguish the acute hallucinosis of delirium from schizophrenia.

As with physical examination, the amount of time and attention devoted to the patient's mental state will vary considerably depending on the range of diagnostic possibilities raised by the patient's presenting complaints and history. In many cases no formal examination of the mental state is needed. The nature of the patient's symptoms do not suggest psychiatric illness, the process of history taking has not raised the possibility of memory impairment or disorientation and the patient's behaviour has been unremarkable throughout the consultation. When a mental state examination is required the time devoted to different components of the examination should depend on the range of diagnostic possibilities under consideration. Just as there is usually little

point in carrying out a detailed neurological examination in a man whose history suggests that he has a duodenal ulcer, so there is little point in asking detailed questions about orientation and memory in a young woman whose presenting symptoms suggest that she has a depressive illness. Making the best use of the limited time available is one of the most important of clinical skills and can only be achieved by focusing on relevant topics and possibilities. Even so, it is important for students and other trainees to conduct a comprehensive mental state examination as often as possible, partly to become fluent in the administration of simple tests of concentration, orientation and memory and to become familiar with the wide range of normal responses to these.

Although the mental state examination need not be conducted in any set order it is traditional to record information in the patient's notes in the sequence, and under the headings, listed below.

Mental state

General behaviour

The interviewer should note, and record, anything about the patient's behaviour, demeanour or dress which seems unusual, or may have diagnostic significance, either during the consultation itself or in any other setting (e.g. on the ward or in the outpatient waiting area) in which the clinician has the opportunity to observe the patient. The range of possiblities is extremely wide. The patient may weep, or their eyes may fill with tears at some crucial stage in the interview. They may be restless and incapable of sitting still for longer than a few minutes. They may be agitated, sitting in a tense posture on the edge of their chair and twisting a handkerchief in their hands or constantly adjusting their rings or some article of clothing. They may be shy or sullen, deferential or overfamiliar, flirtatious or aggressive. Clinicians need to be thoroughly familiar with the cultural setting in which they are working in order to know what is abnormal and therefore potentially significant. Claims to hear the voice of God or the Devil would be strong presumptive evidence of a psychotic illness in a native born Scot but would probably have little psychiatric significance in a member of some religious sects. A willingness to discuss sexual matters which would be unremarkable in a young Englishwoman might be very unusual, and evidence of pathological disinhibition, in a woman from a Muslim country or community.

Technical terms are best avoided, despite their convenient brevity. It is more informative to describe someone as 'sitting woodenly with almost no facial expression or gestures' than as 'being retarded,' and more informative to describe a woman as 'wearing a low cut dress, and describing her life story and symptoms in rather sensational terms' than as being 'attention seeking' or 'histrionic'.

Talk

The patient's style of speech is simply one aspect of their behaviour but its importance is so great that it is convenient to treat it separately. Some patients are so garrulous that the interviewer is forced to interrupt them repeatedly. Others seem almost incapable of giving straightforward replies to simple questions; others reply to questions with monosyllables and almost never make spontaneous remarks. Quite apart from the difficulties such verbal behaviours may pose for the interviewer they may provide important clues to diagnosis. Pressure of speech may suggest hypomania, monosyllabic replies may be a manifestation of retardation or resentment and remarks which are consistently vague and off the point may suggest schizophrenic thought disorder. A sudden change in the patient's verbal style may indicate an emotionally sensitive topic that may need further exploration.

Any particularly striking features, particularly those which may indicate aphasia or other disorders of the form of speech, should also be recorded.

Mood

Mood is a subjective state, and information about it can only be obtained by questioning patients, or noting their spontaneous comments. People who are depressed or anxious or perplexed often have characteristic facial expressions or behave in characteristic ways, but these observable concomitants of mood should be recorded as part of the subject's general behaviour. They are evidence of a fundamentally different kind and it is important not to confuse subjective description and observed behaviour, particularly if the two are in conflict.

Mood states are extremely variable and our language has a great range of adjectives to describe them — happy, sad, dejected, miserable, anxious, panic stricken, ecstatic, euphoric, suspicious, perplexed, and so on. Depression — which may vary from mild despondency to black despair — and anxiety — which may range from a vague feeling of being ill at ease to uncontrolled terror — are the commonest abnormal mood states and should always be enquired about. This is best done by asking an open-ended question like — 'How have your spirits been recently?' or 'How have you been feeling in yourself?' and recording the answer verbatim. If the patient admits feeling anxious or miserable further questions should be asked to determine how severe and how consistent this feeling is and how long it has lasted.

Anyone who admits to being badly depressed should be asked whether life still seems worth living and whether they have had thoughts of suicide. The belief that one may thereby put into the patient's mind ideas that had not previously occurred is wholly mistaken. Anyone who is deeply depressed has almost invariably had transient thoughts of suicide and it is often a relief to be able to talk about these. More importantly, the management of a depressive illness is strongly influenced by the clinician's assessment of the risk of suicide and direct questions are needed to establish how serious this is. Fleeting thoughts are of little consequence, but the risk should be taken seriously in anyone who is preoccupied with thoughts of suicide, is planning how to kill themselves, or frightened that they might do so.

Anyone who admits to bouts of anxiety, or episodic physical symptoms like palpitations or dizziness which commonly accompany anxiety, should be questioned closely about where they are when their attacks occur, and whether they habitually avoid particular places or situations in case these symptoms develop. Any unpleasant sensations, subjective or somatic, which only occur in crowded or enclosed places, or when the subject is alone, are highly likely to be manifestations of phobic anxiety. More widespread recognition of this simple fact would save many patients complaining of palpitations, or bouts of dizziness, nausea or other unpleasant symptoms of varied kinds from many tedious and unnecessary investigations.

It is often valuable to record the patient's replies to key questions verbatim in the case notes. It is traditional to record the questions on the left and the patient's replies, or the key phrases in these, on the right. For example:

How feeling recently?	'Pretty low, I'm afraid'
Every day the same?	'More or less, yes'
Life worth living nowadays?	'Well, sometimes I've wondered if it really is, recently'
Thought of suicide?	'Well, I've thought about it, but I don't think I'd ever have the courage'.

Thought content

This is usually the most appropriate stage to elicit and record the patient's main, or most significant, preoccupations. Often the history will already have revealed what these are and questions like 'What is your biggest worry?' may reveal others.

Some people are troubled by *obsessional symptoms*, stereotyped ideas or impulses which they strive unsuccessfully to resist. Obsessional thoughts are invariably distressing to the subject, because they are frightening, obscene, blasphemous, or simply because they are so obviously pointless. That is why they are resisted, albeit unsuccessfully. Obsessional rituals are behavioural rather than purely mental (e.g. repetitive checking or handwashing) and usually represent a symbolic defence against an underlying idea (e.g. I am dirty or guilty and must wash to cleanse myself).

Only a small minority of patients are deluded but if they are it is important to establish the fact. A *delusion* is a private, firmly held belief which is erroneous, often but not necessarily absurd, and uninfluenced by logical argument. It must be distinguished from an *over-valued* idea, an unusual and sometimes bizarre conviction which the patient shares with other people and has acquired from them under comprehensible circumstances (e.g. belief in witchcraft, or a conviction that animal foods poison the bloodstream). The dis-

tinction matters because a delusion implies that the patient has a psychotic illness whereas overvalued ideas are evidence only of eccentricity.

Some delusional ideas emerge spontaneously at various stages in the interview, others have to be sought. It is, of course, no good asking patients if they are deluded. The clinician has to know from experience what kinds of delusions particular patients are likely to have and enquire tactfully. If delusions of persecution are suspected, for example, one might ask 'Are other people ganging up against you?' or 'Are you in any danger at present?' As before, it is important to record verbatim the patient's replies to key questions and to explore in detail any abnormal phenomena elicited. It is an important general principle to start with questions which are as non-specific as possible, like 'Has anything strange been happening to you recently? Or going on around you?' because one can be much more confident about the presence of phenomena which the patient mentions spontaneously or in response to general questions. Often it is eventually necessary to ask very specific questions like, 'Have you felt as though someone was trying to hypnotise you?' in an attempt to detect schizophrenic passivity experiences, for example, but in these circumstances mere assent means little. The patient must volunteer a convincing description of the experience in question before any confidence can be placed in their reply.

Perceptual abnormalities

Hallucinations are perceptions occurring in the absence of any sensory stimulus which are indistinguishable to the subject from normal perceptions. They may involve any of the five senses — vision, hearing, touch, taste and smell. *Pseudohallucinations* are similar except that the subject is able to recognise them as false perceptions and therefore responds quite differently. (A man who hears a voice threatening to kill him may attack and even kill his neighbour, but if he recognises that he is 'hearing voices' he is more likely to consult his doctor.) *Illusions* are misinterpretations of genuine perceptual stimuli e.g. insisting that a pyjama cord on the floor is a snake.

The commonest hallucinations are visual or auditory, the latter usually, though not necessarily,

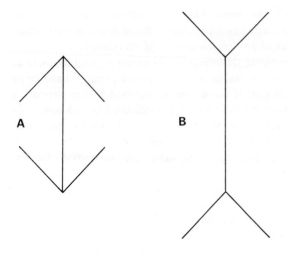

Fig. 2.2   Normal illusion

taking the form of human voices. Visual hallucinations occurring in the absence of auditory
hallucinations are nearly always organic in origin,
particularly if they are nocturnal. Delirium
tremens, in which patients are characteristically
terrified by imaginary insects or reptiles crawling
around their rooms, is the classical example. Such
hallucinations often start as illusions e.g. as a
misinterpretation of the pattern on the wallpaper.
Other illusions, like the conviction that line B
above is longer than line A, are normal phenomena
(Fig. 2.2).

Attention and concentration

Although it also occurs in confusional states impairment of concentration is a characteristic
depressive symptom and depressed patients often
complain, or admit, that they are no longer able
to read a novel, or even a newspaper. They read
a paragraph and don't take it in, so they read it
again but with no more success and eventually give
up. On this basis they often conclude, quite
wrongly, that they have lost their memory and are
dementing. A simple and widely used test of concentration is to ask the patient to subtract 7 from
100 serially and see how far they get and how
many errors they make in 60 seconds. Patients
who cannot subtract, or panic when asked to do
mental arithmetic, can be asked instead to list the

days of the week in alphabetical order. It is important to practice both these tests in order to find
out the range of normal response. The latter is
surprisingly hard.

Orientation

There are three aspects to orientation — in place,
in time and in person (meaning the ability to
identify other people and oneself correctly). Any
or all of the three may be disturbed in organic
mental states. Indeed, disorientation is a cardinal
feature of confusional states and dementias and has
considerable diagnostic significance. Orientation in
time and place is tested by asking a few simple
questions about the day, the month, the year and
the time of day, and in which building and city
the patient now is. Obviously, the patient's replies
have to be interpreted in the light of recent events.
Somebody who has been taken to hospital by ambulance in the middle of the night may well not
know the name of the hospital, but should be in
no doubt about being in a hospital. Disorientation
in person is commonly revealed by the patient
misidentifying a nurse as their daughter, or a visiting grandson or nephew as their son or husband.

Memory

There are many aspects to memory but the most
important clinically is a loss of recent memory with
a relative preservation of distant memory.
Dementing patients often have a remarkably
detailed memory of their early lives but very little
memory for the last few years. For this reason they
characteristically make statements that were true
some years ago but are no longer e.g. that Harold
Wilson is Prime Minister, or that it is 1979. A
simple and widely used test of recent memory is
to give patients a fictitious name and address to
remember, preferably in writing, and ask them to
repeat it five minutes later. Distant memory can
be tested by asking the dates and salient facts of
the second world war or some other well known
but distant public event. It is important, of course,
only to ask patients questions to which it can be
assumed they once knew the answers, and to
which the replies can be validated. It is surprising
how often physicians attempt to assess their

patients' memories by asking questions about date or place of birth, or what was eaten for breakfast that morning, when they have no immediate means of knowing whether the answers are true or false.

General knowledge

Questions like 'Who is the Prime Minister?', 'Who preceded her?', 'Who is the president of the USA?', 'What has been in the news recently?', 'What is the cost of a 1st class stamp?' may reveal important deficiencies, though it is sometimes difficult to distinguish between failing memory and loss of interest. It is important to learn the range of normal responses to such questions before drawing conclusions about impairments from the replies.

Other cognitive tests

Patients suspected of brain damage or localised brain disease of some kind may need to be given a variety of tests to establish whether they have an expressive or a receptive aphasia, and whether they have dysgraphia, dyslexia, or apraxias or agnosias of various kinds (see Ch. 8). Different components of memory (e.g. visual v. auditory, short term v. long term, retention v. recall) may also need testing individually. Although the tests involved are quite simple and require little elaborate apparatus they only need to be used by neurologists, psychiatrists and clinical psychologists.

Formal tests of intelligence or personality are similarly best left to specialists, particularly as it is only rarely that they make a vital contribution to diagnostic assessment.

FURTHER READING

Gelder M, Gath D, Mayou R 1989 Oxford textbook of psychiatry, 2nd edn. Oxford University Press, Oxford

Insight

Patients can be asked if they regard themselves as ill, and if so, whether they consider the illness to be physical or mental and whether they think they need to be in hospital. The replies to such questions have some diagnostic significance and may also place important constraints on treatment. For example, patients who don't believe they are ill, or can't accept that their illness is psychiatric, are rarely willing to take psychotropic medication regularly.

THE FORMULATION

When the history has been obtained, the mental state examination completed and other relevant information collected it is a valuable discipline, both for students and experienced clinicians, to write a brief formulation. This should consist of a summary statement of the essence of the clinical problem followed by a diagnosis or differential diagnosis, a brief discussion of the likely aetiology and likely prognosis, and a provisional treatment plan. For example:

Recently married woman of 24 with 10 month history of attacks of palpitations, usually on buses or in supermarket. No significant depressive symptoms. Diagnosis agoraphobia. Probably precipitated by separation from mother (who seems to have had similar symptoms herself). Worth trial of amitriptyline. Behaviour therapy if no response. Prognosis probably not good — always been nervous and dependent. But husband seems sympathetic and understanding. See them jointly in future.

One of many reasons for writing a formulation is to learn how frequently assumptions about prognosis turn out to be wrong!

Kendell R E, Zeally A K 1988 Companion to psychiatric studies, 4th edn. Churchill Livingstone, Edinburgh

3. The analysis of symptoms and signs

J. F. Munro

The object of this chapter is to demonstrate by a few examples how to obtain in full and to analyse in detail the information which may be derived from a symptom or sign. Three common symptoms have been selected which illustrate different points. *Pain* is a purely subjective complaint. *'Black-outs'* show among other things the importance of the interrogation of eyewitnesses. *Breathlessness* is often associated with objective findings and can, if necessary, be reproduced.

Three signs have been chosen: *swellings* require systematic examination and may be encountered in almost any part of the body; *oedema* provides a simple example of the clinical application of physiological and pathological knowledge; and *shock* is a clinical state.

PAIN

General considerations

The importance of pain in diagnosis cannot be overestimated. Sudden or severe pain may be accompanied by objective signs such as the withdrawal of a limb when the skin is pricked or the muscle spasm which accompanies deep pain. Examples of the latter are the sudden fixation of the lumbar spine in flexion at the onset of lumbago, the catching of the breath due to pleurisy or the rigidity of the abdominal wall in the presence of peritoneal inflammation. Other signs may include pallor, sweating, vomiting or fainting, an involuntary shout evoked by pain of abrupt onset, screaming attacks due to intestinal colic in children, and groaning due to protracted pain. It is very unusual for an adult to weep with pain for which there is an organic explanation. Relief may

be sought by characteristic actions such as the adoption of specific postures, the application of heat to the affected area or the use of appropriate medicines such as aspirin or alkalis.

The solution of a clinical problem may demand that every aspect of a pain is elicited from the history. There will be many occasions when the cause of a pain is obvious without entering into details, but even then it is good practice, when time permits, to make a full enquiry. The experience gained through the variations which are encountered will improve diagnostic accuracy in atypical cases.

The analysis of a pain

The patient should be encouraged to describe the features of the pain in detail without interruption. Thereafter further information should be obtained by a system of analysis of pain based upon questions about the undernoted 10 features:

1. Main site
2. Radiation
3. Character
4. Severity
5. Duration
6. Frequency and periodicity
7. Special times of occurrence
8. Aggravating factors
9. Relieving factors
10. Associated phenomena.

1. Main site of pain

With the eyes shut, it is possible to point precisely to the site of a pinprick on a finger-tip, yet on the skin of the back a spot several centimetres away from the point pricked may be indicated. Localisation is proportionately less accurate in structures from which sensory stimuli rarely reach consciousness. For example, pain arising in the lower thoracic spine may be felt in the hypogastrium, whereas a kick on the shin bone is correctly localised. Normal viscera rarely give rise to conscious sensation, and pain localisation is poor. The oesophagus is, however, sensitive to extremes of temperature, and the bladder and rectum arouse characteristic sensations when they are full. To some extent therefore we are trained in the knowledge of the position of these organs, and pain arising in them tends to be correctly orientated. Localisation of pain originating in other viscera is far less accurate or specific. However, a useful principle is that midline pain arises from single structures while paired organs never cause symmetrical midline pain. Unpaired structures such as the heart, pericardium, alimentary tract, liver, biliary system, pancreas, bladder and uterus tend to give pain deep in the midline anteriorly. Such mal-localisation could well be called referred pain, but this term is usually reserved for spread beyond the main site. Paired structures such as muscles, bones and joints, eyes, pleura and renal tracts cause unilateral pain on the affected side. The localisation of pain in limb joints is usually accurate, but a notable exception is the frequency with which pain from a disorder of the hip is 'referred' to the knee, through mutual innervation by the obturator nerve.

It may help to find out if the main site of pain is localised or diffuse, and at the same time to note any gesture made by the patient. For example, the epigastric pain of peptic ulcer is often indicated by one, or more, finger localising the affected area. The palm of the hand rubbed diffusely over the epigastrium may be used to indicate the pain of biliary colic or acute hepatitis. Characteristic gestures are also used to describe angina pectoris (p. 82).

The common sites of pain arising from the various organs and structures of the body are mentioned in the appropriate chapters.

2. Radiation of pain

Two main aspects of the radiation of pain from the site of the initial lesion must be considered, namely referred pain and spread of pain due to extension of disease.

Referred pain. Deep pain may sometimes be felt in or may spread to areas remote from the main site or point of origin, and the distribution of such a referred pain may be highly characteristic. Diaphragmatic pain caused by pleurisy or peritonitis may be referred, through the phrenic nerve, to an area of skin over the shoulder-tip. Local lesions of the skin or of the fourth cervical root may give pain in a similar distribution, while in a few patients with biliary colic or acute cholecystitis pain may similarly be referred to the tip of the right shoulder through involvement of some twigs of the phrenic nerve supplying the gall bladder.

The distribution of referred pain may be more complicated and less readily explained. Sometimes referred pain may be felt without the main pain, and diagnosis then depends on other features. Thus pain in the left forearm could be due to cervical spondylosis, the carpal tunnel syndrome or perhaps even a hiatus hernia, but regular induction by exercise and relief by rest would point to myocardial ischaemia as the cause (p. 82).

Pain due to pressure upon a nerve root or to sensory nerve involvement by a disease (e.g. herpes zoster) is referred to the corresponding dermatome. For example, compression of the fifth lumbar nerve root by a prolapsed intervertebral disc may cause pain in the buttock, the posterolateral aspect of the thigh, the anterolateral aspect of the leg and the dorsum of the foot. However, the pain may be felt only in the buttock, leg or foot, or there may be a pain-free gap. In fact, nerve root pains may be indistinguishable from pains originating in the viscera or other deep structures.

Spread of pain due to extension of disease. The pain of appendicitis is usually first felt in the umbilical area. After some hours, extension of the inflammation to the serous surface of the appendix and involvement of the overlying parietal peritoneum may occur. The pain will then move into the right iliac fossa or occasionally elsewhere, according to the position of the appendix.

Pain due to extension may be the first indication of a latent disease. For instance, peptic ulceration may be symptomless with pain only occurring following an acute perforation. Diagnostic difficulties and errors will result unless such possibilities are borne in mind.

3. *Character of pain*

It has been shown that all pain arising in the skin has a pricking quality if brief or a burning quality if protracted. However, it is common experience that pains due to a pinprick, burn, cut, pinch or wasp sting can be distinguished, mostly by the context in which they occur, but also by the intensity, duration and distribution of the pain, and by various associated sensations such as heat or traction.

Deep pain is a diffuse aching sensation such as that reproduced by squeezing the tendo achilles; yet its site and duration lead to variations which are detailed in comparable terms by different patients. Headaches of organic origin are described as an intermittent pain, felt mostly over the frontal, occipital or occasionally temporal regions and usually relieved by suitable analgesics. By contrast, psychogenic headaches are described in terms of a pressure or perhaps a tightness or lightness, are continuous and the patient may frequently resort to an analgesic in spite of the fact that it has little or no effect upon the headache. Sometimes descriptions are highly imaginative, and such expressions as 'like being in a vice', or 'like an iron band round the chest' frequently replace the common terms 'tight', 'heavy', 'crushing', 'pressing', or 'like a weight' which are used for the retrosternal pain of myocardial ischaemia. Yet when myocardial pain is felt in areas of reference elsewhere it does not have this special quality. It appears to be the retrosternal site which determines the character of this pain. A similar crushing pain may be due to pericarditis, dissecting aneurysm of the aorta, pulmonary embolism, collapsed thoracic vertebra, fractured sternum, peptic ulcer or hiatus hernia.

The epigastric pain of peptic ulcer on the other hand is not described in these terms, but is usually said to have a gnawing, aching or dull quality. Pain across the epigastrium which is described as burning should lead to suspicion of a psychogenic disorder.

The behaviour of the patient in pain may be characteristic. In biliary and renal colic, patients are usually restless and, having unsuccessfully sought relief by lying down in all sorts of positions, they try sitting, standing or walking. By contrast, the perforation of a peptic ulcer tends to make the patient lie still. Hysteria or acute anxiety may lead to restlessness and groaning, but diversion by conversation may immediately calm the patient.

4. *Severity of pain*

With experience, a reasonably accurate judgement of the true intensity of the pain may be made, particularly if the patient is witnessed during its occurrence. In some diseases pain is characteristically severe, while in others it is mild or may vary in severity. Thus in most cases of perforated peptic ulcer, acute pancreatitis, biliary and renal colic, and dissecting aneurysm of the aorta, the pain is normally so bad that is unusual to obtain a description of quality. Pain due to trigeminal neuralgia, glaucoma, toothache, earache, pleurisy and myocardial infarction is often severe. However, individuals vary so much in their tolerance to pain that a mere statement of severity is insufficient; it is the doctor's responsibility to form a reasoned judgement on the evidence available. In doing so it must be remembered that the intensity of a pain depends greatly upon the patient's state of mind. Thus a remarkable indifference to pain may be observed in states of mania, religious fervour and hypnosis or after prefrontal leucotomy. Endorphins, opiate-like substances which are present in the brain, play a part in the neural transmission of pain. Fluctuations in the concentration of these may be one explanation of variations in the appreciation of pain. Pain suffered on the sports field is apt to be borne much more easily than that due to an injury of similar severity inflicted in the home. On the other hand, depression, anxiety and introspection tend to aggravate the severity of pain. Similar influences affect the appreciation of all subjective symptoms. For example, the tick of an alarm clock may irritate some to the extent of interfering with sleep, yet others may not hear either the tick or the alarm! Similarly the incessant sounds (tinnitus)

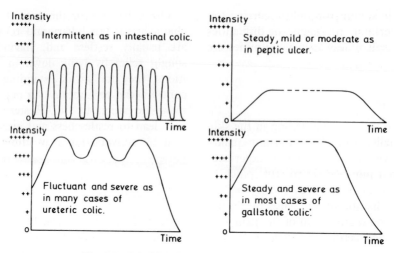

Fig. 3.1   Pain. Examples of time-intensity graphs

which may accompany disorders of the cochlea and its connections may make life miserable for some patients, yet others can ignore these noises so successfully that they are no longer aware of them without consciously trying to hear them.

5. Duration of pain

Estimations of time without actual measurement are often very inaccurate. Yet the duration of pains of various origins may range from less than a second to several days, so that even approximations may be helpful. Thus the excruciating jabs of trigeminal neuralgia last for less than a second at a time. Each of the griping pains of intestinal colic is felt for less than a minute. The pain of angina of effort ceases within five minutes of resting whereas that of a myocardial infarct may continue for hours. The head pain of migraine may be relieved in an hour or so, or it may persist for days.

6. Frequency and periodicity of pain

Some pains may occur at regular intervals every few minutes as in labour or intestinal colic. Other pains may be unpredictable as in biliary colic, which may return more than once in a day, though an interval of days, weeks, months or even years may elapse between two attacks. On the other hand, the symptoms of peptic ulcer recur in

episodes lasting for one to several weeks, interspersed with pain-free intervals of weeks or months. During an attack the pain usually appears at predictable times on more than one occasion during the 24 hours. Trigeminal neuralgia is another example of a disease with spontaneous remissions. These may last for months and naturally the last remedy given often gets the credit.

The information about the severity, duration and frequency of a pain may be usefully summarised in the form of a time-intensity diagram (Fig. 3.1).

7. Special times of occurrence

It is important to ask if the pain recurs at any special times. Are symptoms present on wakening? Do they occur in the forenoon, afternoon, evening or night? The results of such interrogation may lead to the recognition of a rhythm which can then be related to activity, meals, posture, etc.

Migraine, for example, may occur especially in the morning, or every weekend, or at the menses. Most other headaches are intermittent but some occur at special times. That associated with arterial hypertension is often present on wakening, whereas the headache of frontal sinusitis is usually at its peak a few hours after rising. The pain of duodenal ulcer may waken the patient in the early hours of the morning, yet is very rarely present at the ordinary hour of wakening, although it may reappear at predictable times in the forenoon, afternoon and evening. Pain due to bone disease is commonly worse when the patient is warm in bed.

8. Aggravating factors

The patient should first be asked if any aggravating factors are known. Positive replies must then be assessed for reliability. For example, if bending is alleged to bring on a pain, some specific examples should be sought. It may have happened once only and position may have been incorrectly blamed. On the other hand, if bending to tie shoelaces brings on a pain regularly, then posture is an acceptable cause. Indeed, the patient may take to putting the foot up on a chair to tie the laces. If no aggravating factors have been noticed, a few suitable questions should be asked. These should be framed so as to avoid directly mentioning the possible association. For instance, 'Does posture make any difference?' is preferable to 'Does bending make the pain worse?' Sometimes, however, it may be necessary to resort to leading questions to clarify a vague history. It is important to obtain further information as an extra check when a positive association has been elicited. For example, a housewife might spend a vigorous week cleaning her home and then incidentally develop biliary colic. With a natural tendency to rationalise symptoms, a clear statement might be made that unusual exercise involving repeated bending has been the cause of the pain. Such misleading assumptions can be eliminated by enquiry into the precise time relationships.

9. Relieving factors

Similar caution must be exercised before accepting patients' statements about relieving factors. Many pains subside spontaneously, and the evidence upon which the patient's belief is based must be obtained in detail and carefully considered. For example, epigastric pain due to peptic ulcer is relieved by alkali in 5 to 15 minutes, but never immediately nor in an hour or more, and even half an hour is a suspiciously long time. A combination of faith and gratitude may convince a patient that

the condition has improved as a result of treatment which has in fact had no effect.

10. Associated phenomena

Severe pain is commonly associated with pallor, sweating, vomiting, an increase in the pulse rate and blood pressure and a leucocytosis. Some pains may be accompanied by other manifestations which are of diagnostic value. Migraine, for example, is often preceded by visual disturbances and accompanied by vomiting, thus giving rise to the lay terms 'blinding headache' or 'bilious attack'. Rarely, premonitory symptoms such as hunger, an unusual sense of well-being or depression, may precede the attack by a day or so. Added to these characteristics there are usually other members of the family who suffer from recurrent headaches. Further examples are the rigors of acute pyelonephritis, the haematuria which may accompany renal colic, or the brown urine, pale stools and yellow sclerae which may follow a bout of pain due to gallstones.

Conclusion

Almost any pain can be analysed in relation to these 10 features. Examples are given of the application of the method in the assessment of chest pain (p. 82) and of abdominal pain (p. 155). When these principles are employed not only will progress be made towards a solution of the problem but the clinician's store of knowledge will often be increased.

BLACKOUTS

The complaint of blackouts is common, and presents a challenging diagnostic exercise since the causes range from the trivial to the serious. Although the term 'blackout' is most frequently used to describe some from of lapse of consciousness, it is also sometimes employed to denote attacks of vertigo, of weakness and of psychiatric disturbances such as fugue-like states.

The nature of episodes wherein consciousness is lost is best diagnosed by a trained observer who has witnessed such an attack. However this is not often possible and the interpretation has to be inferred from the patient's accounts of the events which precede and succeed the attack, supplemented whenever possible by the history from a witness of the incident.

Most blackouts are due either to a reduction of blood flow to the brain or to epilepsy. There are a number of miscellaneous causes, but these are quantitatively far less important.

1. Reduction of blood flow to the brain

Syncope is defined as loss of consciousness which is due to a reduction of blood flow to the brain. Loss of vision often precedes unconsciousness because the extravascular pressure in the eye, averaging +18 mmHg, contrasts with that in the skull (in the erect posture) of about −20 mmHg. Loss of consciousness may sometimes be averted by putting the head well down. Syncope may result from a fall in cardiac output, from excess peripheral vasodilatation, or a combination of the two.

Simple faints (vasovagal attacks) are so common as to be within the experience of most people, particularly in adolescence. Precipitating factors include intense emotional stimulation, prolonged standing especially in a hot crowded atmosphere, pain, fright or anxiety. Fainting may also be provoked by procedures such as venepuncture or cardiac catheterisation. Spontaneous fainting is uncommon in the sitting position and very rare when lying. Faints do not occur during exercise, but may happen when exercise is suddenly stopped. There is usually a prodromal period which lasts for up to several minutes during which the patient may complain of weakness, nausea, sensations of heat or coldness or buzzing in the ears. The sufferer rarely falls precipitately, but rather sinks to the ground. During the attack the patient is limp and pale, and the pallor persists after recovery. The period of unconsciousness rarely lasts longer than a minute, unless the patient is prevented from lying down, in which case prolonged unconsciousness and even epileptic fits may result.

The 'fainting reflex' is triggered by receptors in the left ventricle which are activated when left ventricular volume falls below a critical level. Loss of blood, or pooling of blood in inactive muscles will reduce left ventricular filling pressure, and sympathetic stimulation reduces left ventricular volume as well as sensitising the receptors. The reflex consists of sudden vagally-mediated cardiac slowing together with vasodilatation in skeletal muscle. The combination of reduced cardiac output and reduced peripheral resistance causes the fall in blood pressure which results in syncope. Sweating is due to sympathetic activation, and the prolonged pallor is due to cutaneous vasoconstriction mediated by release of vasopressin from the pituitary.

Postural syncope occurs on standing up and is a feature of impairment of the vasomotor reflexes. It can occur when arterial hypertension is overtreated, in the elderly and in autonomic neuropathy (e.g. diabetic). Postural syncope is readily overlooked unless the blood pressure is measured with the patient standing as well as lying flat. Those who are liable to this symptom suffer more severely after being confined to bed; indeed it is a fairly common complaint at any age, on rising from bed after prolonged illness.

Syncope associated with movements of the head suggests either a hypersensitive carotid sinus reflex or insufficiency of the vertebro-basilar arterial flow. In the former, confirmation should be obtained by observing whether a brief pressure on one or other carotid sinus (p. 89) causes extreme bradycardia. Lapses of consciousness due to insufficient blood flow in the vertebro-basilar arteries are often attended by other features of brain stem ischaemia such as double vision or vertigo. Syncope is apt to occur on turning the head or on looking upwards.

Cough syncope refers to a transient loss of consciousness at the end of a purple-faced paroxysm of coughing in some patients with chronic bronchitis and is particularly liable to occur in obese, thick-set men, overindulgent in tobacco and alcohol.

Micturition syncope is rare and occurs in the male who leaves a warm bed at night; the upright position and straining are contributory factors.

Syncope on exertion is found in some patients with extreme limitation of cardiac output due to severe obstruction at the aortic or pulmonary valve, the signs of which would usually be evident; it may also occur in patients under treatment with drugs which block the sympathetic nervous system.

Syncope resulting from cardiac arrhythmias. Syncope may result from either excessively slow or excessively fast cardiac rates. Patients may notice palpitation before losing consciousness, but this is not constant. If the tachycardia is very rapid, a pulse may not be palpable during the attack. Frequent extrasystoles or short bursts of tachycardia may be noted on examination of the patient between attacks, but these findings are increasingly common with advancing age even in a 'normal' population. Tachycardia-associated syncope is sometimes precipitated by exercise, and recording an electrocardiogram (ECG) during exertion may be helpful.

Syncope resulting from excessive bradycardia or asystole characteristically occurs without premonitory symptoms. The patient collapses suddenly, is pale and pulseless, and may seem dead. There may be grand mal fits. Recovery is often rapid, and may be accompanied by a pink flushing of the skin. Examination of patients between attacks may reveal a degree of heart block, or the features of the sick sinus syndrome. In many patients no abnormalities can be detected but the diagnosis of syncope resulting from cardiac arrhythmias has been greatly helped by continuous ambulatory ECG (Holter) monitoring.

2. Epileptic attacks

An epileptic fit is a transient disturbance (not necessarily a loss) of consciousness due to a brief, excessive electrical discharge of cerebral neurones. The abnormal electrical discharge may remain localised to a small area of the brain, or it may become generalised.

Fits may occur at any time and in any situation. Sometimes, however, in an individual they run to a pattern; some epileptics have fits only during sleep, or when they are pyrexial or during menstruation. A minority of patients develop seizures in response to specific stimuli such as flashing lights or noise. It is important to ask about such relationships during the taking of the history.

Characteristically an epileptic fit is of abrupt onset. The features of a *grand mal* fit with its tonic

phase ushered in by a cry or groan followed by the jerking movements of the clonic phase, are so distinctive that most people can diagnose such an attack. During the tonic phase the eyes remain open and deviated to one side. The arms are flexed, the legs extended and the face becomes congested and cyanosed. In the absence of an observer the patient's history will often be indicative as the fall may cause an injury and there is frequently incontinence of urine, or tongue biting during the attack.

The very short lived 'absences' of *petit mal* when clearly described by an observer present an easily recognisable pattern. The sufferer, almost always a child, is described as looking vacant or blank for a few seconds. Petit mal seizures are usually very frequent; scores of attacks may occur daily.

In some varieties of *focal epilepsy* consciousness is not entirely lost and the clinical features may be unusual or bizarre. Seizures which originate in the temporal lobe (the commonest type of focal epilepsy) may give rise to diverse manifestations, depending on the site of the initial electrical abnormality and the extent to which it spreads. In the most characteristic variety the onset is associated with a hallucination of smell which is almost always unpleasant. On occasion the prodromal features of a temporal lobe fit are manifest by the patient developing an intense feeling of familiarity with the surroundings — the 'déjà vu' phenomenon. Visual hallucinations of a specific organised nature occur; miniscule men or animals may be seen in part of the patient's visual field. Less commonly the patient may describe auditory hallucinations hearing voices or music.

These and allied phenomena will be accompanied by variable or commonly complete loss of consciousness. When consciousness is retained patients may carry out motor acts of a bizarre or even antisocial nature. They may appear to the outside observer to be in control of their actions, but patients afterwards have no memory of their behaviour. Sometimes this form of *automatism* also occurs after the major events of a fit are over.

In *Jacksonian attacks* patients can retain contact with their environment. They may be able to describe involuntary movements beginning in one area and spreading. The fit may then cease or consciousness may be lost and the features of a grand mal seizure supervene. Occasionally after a Jacksonian fit the affected parts of the body exhibit a temporary paresis, rarely lasting for more than a few hours.

The cause of epilepsy

The recognition that a patient's blackouts are epileptic is the first stage in the diagnostic process. The underlying cause of the fits must then be determined. Epilepsy may be due to genetically determined factors of unknown nature, to any intracranial injury or disease, or to a variety of systemic illnesses or metabolic disturbances. Close attention should be paid to the age of onset of the fits, the family history, the previous medical history, including details of the birth, associated symptoms and the results of neurological as well as the general systematic examination. It is particularly important to identify those epileptics whose fits arise from a potentially curable cause.

A history of generalised fits which began in childhood and which have been present for many years in a patient who knows of relatives similarly affected, strongly suggests that there is no underlying structural lesion. Fits of recent onset and focal nature, developing for the first time in an adult raise the possibility of a primary cause such as an intracranial tumour. Associated features such as headache or focal neurological signs would reinforce this suspicion. Fits which occur only in the early morning before breakfast or after prolonged fasting should evoke consideration of an insulin-secreting tumour resulting in periodic hypoglycaemic fits. Clinical features of renal or hepatic failure may point to the underlying cause.

It is becoming increasingly important always to explore the possibility that fits may be drug induced. Some drugs such as LSD, are epileptogenic. The sudden withdrawal of many hypnotic drugs, including alcohol, after their long continued and regular ingestion may result in epileptic fits.

3. Miscellaneous causes of blackouts

Narcolepsy and cataplexy may sometimes mimic epileptic attacks. *Narcolepsy* is characterised by attacks wherein the patient has an irresistible desire to sleep. These episodes often occur in situations which normally produce drowsiness such as sitting in front of a fire, watching television, or sitting for long periods in a lecture theatre. But they occur too in most inappropriate circumstances as when eating a meal, or driving a motor car. Sometimes narcolepsy may be accompanied by *cataplexy* wherein the patient suddenly becomes intensely weak and may fall to the ground but throughout remains fully conscious.

Hysterical attacks are often bizarre in their manifestations. They may be mistaken for epileptic fits but are rarely accompanied by the stigmata of tongue biting or incontinence of urine. Interviewing an eye witness would reveal none of the features observed in epileptic attacks such as deviation of the eyes or cyanosis. Hysterical seizures usually take place in the presence of others, and create maximal disturbance. Movements of the limbs often occur in hysterical episodes but these are coordinated and may be aggressively directed towards other people.

Conclusion

The approach of blackouts exemplifies how a clinical problem may be clarified by the analysis of a single symptom in meticulous detail, seeking evidence from diverse sources, notably in this instance from the interrogation of eye witnesses.

BREATHLESSNESS

A complaint of shortness of breath (dyspnoea) implies that the act of breathing has become a conscious effort. Although many dyspnoeic patients breathe rapidly, there is no direct correlation between the observed rate of breathing and the subjective sensation of dyspnoea. Patients with acute pneumonia, especially children, may take as many as 60 breaths per minute without experiencing respiratory discomfort, while in other conditions, such as respiratory paralysis, a feeling of breathlessness may not be accompanied by any increase in the rate of breathing. There is considerable variation in what might be called the 'dyspnoea threshold'. Some patients with objective evidence of gravely impaired respiratory function may complain of relatively mild breathlessness

Table 3.1 Increased work of breathing

Airflow obstruction	Decreased pulmonary compliance	Restricted chest expansion
Bronchial asthma	Pulmonary oedema	Kyphoscoliosis
Chronic bronchitis	Diffuse pulmonary fibrosis	Ankylosing spondylitis
Emphysema	Fibrosing and allergic alveolitis	Obesity
Stridor		Respiratory muscle weakness

while others with only slight disturbance of function may experience quite severe respiratory distress.

Factors contributing to the production of breathlessness

While *hypoxaemia* and dyspnoea frequently co-exist, hypoxia *per se*, unless it is severe, plays a relatively minor part in the production of dyspnoea. Many patients with severe breathlessness are not hypoxaemic, while in hypoxaemic patients dyspnoea is not always a conspicuous symptom. There is a similar lack of direct correlation between breathlessness and *hypercapnia*. Although a rise in the carbon dioxide tension of arterial blood immediately causes hyperventilation and dyspnoea in normal subjects, it may not do so in patients with chronic ventilatory inadequacy in whom the respiratory centre may have become unresponsive to carbon dioxide or to an increase in hydrogen ion concentration. Stimulation of peripheral receptors in the lung thought to be situated in alveolar capillary walls (juxtapulmonary-capillary receptors or J receptors) is thought to contribute to the sensation of dyspnoea in disorders such as pulmonary oedema and thrombo-embolism.

The disturbances of respiratory function which may contribute to the production of breathlessness are now well recognised. The most important of these are an increase in the work of breathing, increased pulmonary ventilation, and weakness of the respiratory muscles. Each of these disturbances has a variety of causes, and there are thus many factors which may operate, singly or in combination, to produce dyspnoea in an individual case.

1. Breathlessness associated with an increase in the work of breathing

Airways obstruction, decreased pulmonary compliance ('stiff lungs') and restricted chest expansion all increase the work of breathing (Table 3.1).

2. Breathlessness associated with increased pulmonary ventilation

An increase in the respiratory dead space, severe hypoxaemia and metabolic acidosis, may all be responsible for an increase in pulmonary ventilation. Hyperventilation may also be a manifestation of hysteria.

An *increase in the volume of the physiological dead space* occurs in massive pulmonary embolism as a result of a drastic reduction in blood flow through capillaries perfusing well ventilated alveoli. Patients who survive a massive embolism for a few hours may exhibit striking hyperventilation ('air hunger'), but this is usually overshadowed by the effects of a sudden severe reduction of cardiac output, such as hypotension and syncope.

Severe hypoxaemia, in conditions such as pneumonia, pulmonary oedema and interstitial lung disease, increases pulmonary ventilation by reflex stimulation of the respiratory centre via the aortic and carotid chemoreceptors.

In *metabolic acidosis*, caused for example by diabetic ketoacidosis or renal failure, the respiratory centre is stimulated by the increased hydrogen ion concentration in the blood, and the resultant hyperventilation may produce the sensation of breathlessness.

Hyperventilation syndrome is also accompanied by a sensation of breathlessness. Breathing is often irregular, and may be sighing. If the hyperventilation is sufficiently severe and prolonged, it may lead to tetany, or even to an epileptic fit.

3. Breathlessness associated with weakness of the muscles of respiration

Neuromuscular lesions, such as high spinal cord

injuries, poliomyelitis, polyneuropathy and myasthenia gravis, may cause partial or complete paralysis of the muscles of respiration, with the result that the patient is no longer able to meet the ventilatory requirements.

4.   Breathlessness associated with multiple factors

In some cases a single factor may be chiefly or even entirely responsible for the breathlessness, as for example in patients with airflow limitation or with respiratory paralysis. In most conditions, however, the mechanisms responsible for the production of dyspnoea are more complex. Two examples are given:

a. In *pneumonia* the restriction of chest expansion by pleural pain is probably the chief cause of dyspnoea in the early stages of the illness; later, if the lungs become extensively consolidated, dyspnoea is mainly due to a combination of decreased pulmonary compliance and increased pulmonary ventilation caused by stimulation of J receptors and hypoxaemia.

b. *Pulmonary oedema* of cardiac origin begins in the alveolar walls and causes dyspnoea by stimulating pulmonary receptors and reducing pulmonary compliance thereby increasing the work of breathing. Later, intra-alveolar transudate aggravates the dyspnoea, at first by increasing pulmonary ventilation in response to hypoxaemia, and then by producing airways obstruction.

Clinical forms of breathlessness

The sensation of dyspnoea is apparently the same, whatever its cause, but its mode of presentation varies considerably (Table 3.2). There are, however, two main patterns, which may occur either independently or together, namely *acute onset* breathlessness and exertional breathlessness.

1.   Acute onset breathlessness

This usually develops when the patient is at rest, but in some conditions is provoked by exertion. An acute attack of dyspnoea is usually due to the rapid development either of airflow limitation or of a restrictive lesion of lungs or pleura. Rarely, as in massive pulmonary embolism, it may be associated with a sudden increase in the volume of the physiological dead space. Four major causes are: (a) Bronchial asthma (b) Left heart failure (c) Massive pulmonary embolism (d) Spontaneous pneumothorax.

History. A carefully taken history is often of great help in identifying the cause of an acute attack of dyspnoea.

a. Bronchial asthma. Usually an attack of bronchial asthma is readily recognised. As airways obstruction in this condition is maximal during expiration, the latter is slow and laboured while inspiration is relatively rapid but restricted because the lungs may already be almost fully inflated. Wheeze and rhonchi are commonly present and predominantly expiratory. In severe attacks of asthma, however, there may be insufficient airflow to generate these noises and the chest will be paradoxically 'silent'. Often there have been previous episodes which will probably have responded promptly to a bronchodilator drug. It may be difficult to recognise a patient's first attack of asthma from the history. This is particularly a problem in the child, as anxious parents are often unable to give an accurate account. The diagnosis usually becomes obvious, however, when a subsequent attack is witnessed by a trained observer.

Table 3.2   Onset of breathlessness

Sudden (within minutes)	Rapid (hours — days)	Gradual (days — weeks — months)	Slow (months — years)
Pneumothorax	Haemothorax	Pleural effusion	Pleural fibrosis
Severe acute asthma	Acute asthma	Chronic asthma	Emphysema
Pulmonary oedema	Pulmonary oedema	Fibrosing alveolitis	Pneumoconiosis
Pulmonary embolism	Pneumonia	Tuberculosis	Sarcoidosis
Laryngeal oedema	Acute bronchitis	Chronic bronchitis	Chronic bronchitis
Foreign body inhalation	Allergic alveolitis	Bronchial carcinoma	Ankylosing spondylitis
Hyperventilation syndrome			

b. Left heart failure. Attacks of breathlessness occurring during the night (paroxysmal nocturnal dyspnoea) may be due to bronchial asthma, but in middle-aged and elderly patients pulmonary oedema secondary to left heart failure is the likely cause. In such patients a previous history of exertional dyspnoea can usually be elicited and they often state that they sleep more comfortably in the upright position, supported by several pillows. The attack usually develops in the early hours of the morning as a result of sliding into the recumbent position during deep sleep. They then waken with intense breathlessness, which often produces feelings of suffocation and panic. The usual reaction is to sit upright and legs over the side of the bed or even struggle to an open window in the hope that cool fresh air will ease their breathing. In most cases the attack subsides spontaneously in about half an hour, but acute pulmonary oedema (p. 82) may occasionally be fatal.

In the later stages of left heart failure paroxysms of breathlessness may develop whenever the patient lies down. Such intolerance of the recumbent position is known as *orthopnoea*. In left heart failure the recumbent position is avoided because the increase in venous return is liable to compromise cardiac function and induce pulmonary oedema (p. 81). In emphysema, on the other hand, the upright position is more comfortable because it improves pulmonary ventilation by facilitating the range of movements of the thoracic cage and allowing the use of the accessory muscles of inspiration.

Paroxysmal dyspnoea may also be experienced during the phase of overventilation in Cheyne-Stokes breathing (p. 138).

c. Massive pulmonary embolism. The dyspnoea which follows massive pulmonary embolism produces a sensation of suffocation in which the patient feels desperately short of air, although, in fact, breathing may be deep ('air hunger'). It is accompanied by acute circulatory failure caused by a fall in left ventricular output. The differential diagnosis from myocardial infarction may be very difficult or even impossible by clinical methods, particularly in the elderly who may experience similar pain in the two conditions. However, the character of the breathlessness and the absence of crepitations heard on auscultation favour the possibility of pulmonary embolism.

d. Spontaneous pneumothorax. Dyspnoea due to this cause usually develops suddenly and is distressing. In other cases the dyspnoea is slight at first but becomes more severe following exertion or a bout of coughing. Unilateral chest pain or 'tightness' typically precedes or accompanies the onset of breathlessness.

e. Other causes of acute onset breathlessness. These include the very rapid accumulation of fluid in the pleural space. Massive intrapleural haemorrhage is probably the only condition in which this occurs and can usually be recognised without difficulty, as the dyspnoea is accompanied by features of acute blood loss.

In children the possibility of a foreign body in the larynx or of membranous exudate obstructing the air passages should not be forgotten. In adults unable to cough effectively because of weakness of the respiratory muscles, the retention of secretions may produce acute breathlessness, as may the inhalation, during coma or anaesthesia, of acid gastric secretions, with the production of a chemical pneumonia.

Physical examination. The following findings are of particular value in the differential diagnosis of acute breathlessness. These are described in detail in Chapters 5 and 6 but are summarised here for convenience.

a. Clinical features indicating a possible cause for left heart failure, e.g. arterial hypertension, myocardial infarction, aortic or mitral valve disease.

b. An increase in jugular venous pressure (p. 95) which is usually raised in massive pulmonary embolism and in some cases of dyspnoea of cardiac origin.

c. Central cyanosis (p. 88) which is a relatively late feature in acute dyspnoea of cardiac origin but develops at an early stage in severe airflow limitation of all types. In massive pulmonary embolism cyanosis is both central and peripheral (p. 87) which, in combination with intense cutaneous vasoconstriction, imparts a slate-grey colour to the lips and cheeks.

d. Hypotension, which occurs in massive pulmonary embolism and also in extensive myocardial infarction, and may be associated with acute dyspnoea in both conditions.

e. Physical signs indicating either a primary abnormality in bronchi, lungs or pleura, or a pulmonary abnormality secondary to a cardiac lesion:

(i) Expiratory rhonchi which, if the sole clinical abnormality, strongly suggest a diagnosis of bronchial asthma.

(ii) Markedly diminished or absent breath sounds on one side of the chest, accompanied by hyperresonance on percussion in spontaneous pneumothorax and by stony dullness in pleural effusion or haemorrhage.

(iii) Basal crepitations produced by pulmonary oedema, are very common in acute dyspnoea of cardiac origin.

2. *Exertional breathlessness*

When breathlessness on exertion is the dominant complaint it is usually due to heart failure or chronic lung disease, although it may be aggravated, or even caused, by obesity, anaemia or hyperthyroidism. Its severity can be assessed and graded only by reference to the level of physical activity at which it is induced.

History. Patients with sustained exertional dyspnoea should be asked whether it is increasing or improving in severity. If it varies spontaneously in degree, this may provide a lead to its cause, as in the case of chronic asthma, while an improvement following treatment with a diuretic will suggest a cardiac origin. The nature of the patient's other symptoms may also be of value in identifying the cause of exertional breathlessness.

Physical examination. The clinical investigation of exertional dyspnoea calls, in particular, for a detailed examination of the cardiovascular and respiratory systems. Amongst the abnormalities which should be looked for are, in the cardiovascular system, increased jugular venous pressure, peripheral oedema, cardiac enlargement, the heart rate and rhythm, left ventricular hypertrophy, hypertension, valve lesions, added heart sounds and pericardial effusion, and in the respiratory system, severe chest deformities, airways obstruction and emphysema, interstitial lung disease, pulmonary oedema, pleural effusion and pneumothorax.

Conclusion

Breathlessness may be the presenting complaint in a large number of important cardiovascular and respiratory diseases. A correct assessment of its significance requires a clear understanding of the disturbances in physiology with which it is associated, and of the pathological processes by which these disturbances are created. By taking a careful history the possible causes of dyspnoea in an individual patient can usually be narrowed down to two or three conditions, and a final diagnosis can often be made from the physical signs. In some cases, however, special investigations such as radiological examination of the chest, ECG or tests of respiratory function (including arterial blood gas studies) may be required.

THE EXAMINATION OF SWELLINGS

In reporting the discovery of a lump, a patient often assumes that it has appeared suddenly because nothing had been noticed previously. Physical examination may reveal a lump whose presence is unknown to the patient. An open mind must always be kept about the apparent duration of a lump or errors will be made.

The local findings should give some indication of the tissue of origin and the pathological nature of the swelling — whether this is due to trauma, inflammation or neoplasm.

Inspection may show the position, size and shape, and any discolouration. By palpation, tenderness may be elicited, the mobility, consistency, surface texture, and type of edge of the mass determined, and any enlargement of the regional lymph nodes detected. The examination of a goitre (p. 66) provides a good example of the methods in practice.

Inspection and palpation

Position

The anatomical situation of a mass must be defined accurately. The site of swellings such as those in the breast, the thyroid or the parotid glands, will present no difficulty. In others, the ease with which the lump can be localised will vary especially in the abdomen. Other features such as shape or mobility will help to identify the anatomical origin.

Size

The size of a swelling should always be measured. A diagram, indicating the dimensions, position and shape of the swelling should be recorded and dated (Fig. 3.2). In this way, significant changes, which may occur later, can be recognised. In contrast, vague statements about size, such as large, medium or small, or comparisons with fruit, eggs or vegetables, are inaccurate and misleading.

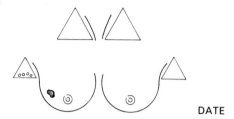

DATE

Fig. 3.2 The use of diagrams in case recording. Hard irregular mobile mass size 3 × 2 cm, not fixed in the right breast with metastases in the right axilla but not in the neck.

Shape

The characteristic outline of a mass in the appropriate position should signify its origin. Examples in the abdomen include an enlarged spleen or liver, a distended bladder or the fundus of the uterus in later pregnancy. Sometimes additional evidence is required such as the disappearance, after catheterisation, of a full bladder.

Colour and temperature

The skin over acute inflammatory lesions is usually red and this will be accompanied by a rise in temperature. A vascular skin tumour may range in colour from red to blue or purple according to the proportions of reduced haemoglobin present and the depth of the layer of skin through which it is seen. In haematomas the pigment from extravasated blood may produce the range of colours caused by various breakdown products of haemoglobin so familiar in a bruise. A brown or black colour is common in melanomas, though

some are not pigmented. A xanthoma is a small skin nodule which may be identified by its yellow colour due to the lipids it contains.

Tenderness

Inflammatory swellings are characterised by tenderness and palpation should be gentle. Many large tumours, in contrast, are entirely free from pain or tenderness, partly because they carry no nerve supply and also because they may have developed in an area where tissue tension is low and where a mass can be accommodated without subjecting any structure to undue stretching. Tumours eroding bone or growing into nerve roots and plexuses are capable of causing severe persistent pain of a most intractable type, and this is often worse at night.

Movement

A mass must be tested to determine whether it is part of, attached to, or free from adjacent structures, such as skin or bone. Skin fixation may be tested by attempting to pick up a fold of skin over the swelling and comparing this with the mobility of the skin over other structures in the vicinity. Fixation of the skin may be associated with a fine dimpling at the opening of the hair follicles resembling 'pigskin' or 'orange skin' when there is lymphatic obstruction. Such a change is most commonly due to malignant disease.

Fixation to deeper structures will be recognised by attempting to move the swelling in different planes relative to the surrounding tissues. For example, with a tumour in the breast, the patient is asked to press the hand firmly on the hip of the affected side. The mobility of the mass may then be tested in relation to the contracted and immobilised pectoral muscle. Again it may be difficult to decide whether a mass is situated in the abdominal wall or within the abdominal cavity. This distinction is made by noting the effect of contraction of the rectus and other muscles on the accessibility of the swelling, as described on page 170. In the case of the thyroid, most goitres will move up and down on swallowing.

Adherence to a blood vessel will cause pulsation which will readily be appreciated if the palpating hand is kept still for a few moments. It is then necessary to determine whether this is the expansile pulsation of an aneurysm or a vascular tumour, or whether the movement is transmitted from the nearby artery.

An impulse on coughing is characteristically felt in certain swellings within which a rise in pressure may occur because their contents communicate with the thoracic or abdominal cavity. The commonest example is an inguinal hernia.

Consistency

The consistency of a swelling may vary from soft and fluctuant through increasing degrees of firmness until this may be so striking as to merit the term 'stony hard'. Very hard swellings are usually malignant or calcified, or consist largely of dense fibrous tissue.

Fluctuation indicates a fluid-containing swelling, such as an abscess or a cyst. Soft tumours such as lipomas may also show some degree of fluctuation. The sign is elicited by detecting with one finger the bulge created by compressing the swelling suddenly with another finger placed at a distance. Fluctuation should be detectable in two planes before the sign is regarded as positive.

Surface texture

The surface of a swelling may vary widely from the uniformly smooth to the grossly irregular. The surface of a simple goitre and of some primary toxic goitres is usually uniformly smooth, whereas other goitres may be so irregular in outline that they are described as nodular. A similar variety of texture may be noted on palpation of the liver, ranging from the smooth surface found in acute right ventricular failure, to the gross degree of nodular change in some cases of metastatic tumour. A thick abdominal wall may make it impossible to appreciate variations with confidence.

Ulceration

Lesions which arise within the skin, such as squamous or basal cell carcinomas, or lesions which lie close to the skin, such as breast cancer or malignancy in axillary lymph nodes, may ulcerate. The character of the edge, the size and shape of the ulcer and the nature of its base should all be noted. Similar observations should be made of visible or palpable ulcers in the mouth or rectum.

Margin

The edge or margin may be well delineated or ill-defined, regular or irregular, sharp or rounded. The margins of enlarged organs such as the thyroid gland, liver, spleen or kidney can usually be defined more clearly than those of inflammatory or malignant masses. The indefinite margin of a mass is sometimes a valuable indication of an infiltrating malignant growth as opposed to the clearly defined edge of a localised benign tumour.

Associated swellings

Conditions in which multiple swellings occur include neurofibromatosis (Plate I), lipomatosis, metastases in the skin, lymph nodes in the lymphomas, and fibrocystic changes in the breast. The suspicion that a tumour is malignant should invariably lead to a thorough examination for evidence of involvement of the lymph nodes draining the area concerned.

Additional methods of examination

Percussion

This is of limited value but occasionally may be helpful in defining an abdominal mass (p. 173).

Auscultation

Vascular sounds. If the blood flow through a tumour is large, a systolic murmur (bruit) may be audible over the swelling and, if it is sufficiently marked, a thrill may also be palpable. Systolic murmurs may also be heard over arterial aneurysms, while over the very rare swelling due to an arteriovenous fistula there is a continuous murmur, often accompanied by a thrill, similar to the bruit of a persistent ductus arteriosus (p. 111).

Fetal heart sounds. These may be audible over

the pregnant uterus after the 30th week. The noise of blood flowing through the extensive vascular formation in the pregnant uterus may also be audible (uterine souffle).

Bowel sounds (p. 174). These may be heard over a hernia which contains intestine.

Friction. This may sometimes be heard over an enlarged spleen or liver when fibrinous perisplenitis or perihepatitis is present.

Transillumination

This is a useful test in distinguishing between a swelling composed of solid tissue and one consisting of transparent or semi-transparent liquid. The sign is sought in darkened surroundings by pressing the lighted end of an electric torch into one side of the swelling. A cystic swelling will light up if the fluid within it is translucent provided that the covering tissues are not too thick. The sign is useful in helping to distinguish a hydrocele from other scrotal swellings though it must be borne in mind that a testicular tumour may lie within hydrocele (p. 175).

Further investigation

Radiographs may define a mass either directly or by the use of various contrast media and *ultrasonography* distinguishes between a solid and a cystic swelling (Fig. 7.18, p. 180).

Biopsy is required if there is any suspicion of malignancy.

OEDEMA

Oedema means swelling of the tissues due to an increase in interstitial fluid. It may be generalised due to a disorder of the heart, kidneys, liver, gut, or diet, or it may be local from venous or lymphatic obstruction, allergy or inflammation. Sometimes, oedema may be postural and relatively unimportant or it may be idiopathic (p. 51). (See Fig. 3.3.)

Clinical manifestation of oedema

The doctor may be consulted because of swelling of the ankles, face or abdomen, breathlessness or a rapid gain of weight. When oedema is due to generalised fluid retention, for whatever reason, its distribution is determined by gravity. Thus it is usually observed in the legs, back of the thighs and the lumbosacral area as in cardiac failure in the semi-recumbent patient. If a patient can lie flat quite comfortably, it may be seen in the face and hands as in children with acute glomerulonephritis. Regional rises in venous pressure also determine the distribution of oedema fluid as exemplified by pulmonary oedema in left heart failure or by ascites when there is portal hypertension.

The cardinal sign of subcutaneous oedema is the indentation or *pitting* made in the skin by firm pressure maintained for a few seconds by the examiner's fingers or thumb. The pitting may persist for several minutes until it is obliterated by the slow reaccumulation of the displaced fluid. However, pitting on pressure may not be demonstrable until an increase in body weight of as much as 10 or 15% has occurred. Day to day alterations in weight usually provide much the most reliable index of progress or response to treatment.

Myxoedema, in contrast to oedema, is characterised by swelling which does not pit on pressure and which is due to infiltration of the tissues by a firm mucinous material. Chronic lymphoedema may also fail to pit on pressure.

The genesis of oedema

Generalised oedema is bound to occur if, after allowing for water loss through the skin, the breath, the stools or discharges, the fluid intake exceeds the renal excretory capacity. The latter may be reduced by disease of the kidneys or renal function may be altered by extrarenal factors. For example, a fall in renal blood flow leads to a reduction in glomerular filtration rate and an increase in obligatory water absorption by the proximal tubule in the early stages of cardiac failure. Renal tubular reabsorption of water may be greater when a rise in circulating aldosterone enhances the reabsorption of sodium as occurs in some patients with hepatic cirrhosis, the nephrotic syndrome or cardiac failure. The retained fluid dilutes the plasma and so causes a drop in the osmotic pressure of the proteins and consequent oedema (Fig. 3.4). How-

ask about:

cardiac causes
e.g. past history or rheumatic fever,
breathlessness, palpitations
malabsorption
(e.g. stool odour,
bulk and colour)
malnutrition
liver disease
renal disease
(e.g. diabetes, sore throat
colour of urine,
frothing of urine)

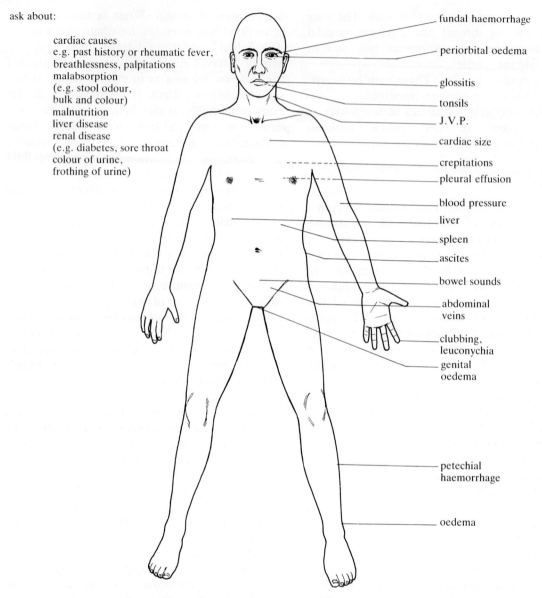

fundal haemorrhage
periorbital oedema
glossitis
tonsils
J.V.P.
cardiac size
crepitations
pleural effusion
blood pressure
liver
spleen
ascites
bowel sounds
abdominal veins
clubbing, leuconychia
genital oedema
petechial haemorrhage
oedema

Fig. 3.3   Generalised oedema check list.

ever, many instances of generalised oedema and all forms of local oedema are due to alterations in the factors which control the formation and disposal of interstitial fluid at capillary level. In some types of oedema, such as that due to advanced cardiac failure, the genesis is multifactorial.

The formation and disposal of interstitial fluid

Interstitial fluid is formed as the result of filtration through the capillary walls, and it is removed partly by reabsorption into the capillaries and partly by drainage along the lymphatic channels. It is convenient to regard the capillary wall as a semipermeable membrane although the full explanation of the transport of water and solutes across it is much more complicated. The main force causing filtration is the hydrostatic pressure within the vessels; in addition, there is the osmotic pressure of the proteins in the interstitial fluid.

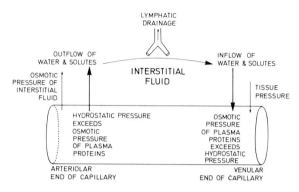

Fig. 3.4 The formation and disposal of interstitial fluid

The latter is normally very low as albumin in a concentration of not more than 20 mg % escapes through the intact capillary. In inflammatory, allergic and lymphatic oedema, on the other hand, there is a high concentration of protein which retains tissue fluid by its osmotic effect. Reabsorption of the fluid is determined by the osmotic pressure of the plasma proteins (oncotic pressure) with an additional effect from tissue pressure depending upon site and position. These factors are shown diagrammatically in Figure 3.4.

The hydrostatic pressure within the capillaries varies widely at different sites. For example, the mean pressure in the pulmonary capillaries during recumbency is less than 10 mmHg, while that in the glomerular capillaries is about 75 mmHg. Thus the lungs are well protected from oedema in spite of the low tissue pressures, while the kidneys are adapted to a high filtration pressure. Another example, is the effect of gravity on assuming the erect posture when the pressure in the capillaries of the scalp falls, while that in the feet rises. The theoretical mean capillary pressure in the feet of a person of average height during quiet standing is at least 110 mmHg. It is not surprising that some swelling of the feet at the end of a day's work may be normal. This swelling would be much greater were it not for the muscle contractions which pump the venous blood and lymph towards the heart and because of the valves in the veins which normally prevent the capillary venous pressure from rising above 20 mmHg. Similarly the puffiness under the eyes for a short time after rising in the morning is due to the rise in capillary pressure during recumbency in areas where the tissue is lax.

The types and causes of oedema

Oedema may be generalised or localised and it results from factors disturbing the physiological control of body fluid.

Generalised oedema

The causes of generalised oedema (anasarca) may conveniently be considered under three headings, namely, hypoproteinaemia, cardiac failure and renal causes. Several factors may contribute in some instances.

1. Hypoproteinaemia. The oncotic pressure is mostly due to the serum albumin so that a fall in the concentration of this protein in particular predisposes to oedema. Hypoproteinaemia may arise for a variety of reasons:

a. Inadequate intake of protein may be responsible as in kwashiorkor, the most important nutritional disorder in the world. Famine conditions, the diet of food faddists, or pyloric obstruction with vomiting, may also impair the protein intake.

b. Failure of digestion of dietary protein results from impairment of the exocrine secretion of the pancreas, as in chronic pancreatitis.

c. Failure of absorption of the products of digestion may occur after resection of considerable lengths of small intestine or in conditions such as Crohn's disease or gluten enteropathy.

d. Reduced synthesis of albumin is found in diseases of the liver, such as cirrhosis. When the portal venous pressure is high, ascites is a more prominent feature than dependent oedema.

e. Excessive loss of protein may occur, especially in the urine in the nephrotic syndrome. Protein may also be lost into the gut in a variety of disorders from the stomach to the colon. Although in gastric lesions the protein lost is digested and reabsorbed, the rate of loss exceeds hepatic synthesis. The syndromes are grouped as protein losing enteropathy. The repeated removal of ascitic fluid by paracentesis or drainage of an empyema or other discharge will also cause depletion of protein.

In any one patient several of these reasons may co-exist. In addition a low intravascular volume may itself cause secondary hyperaldosteronism via the renin-angiotension system, promoting sodium retention and an increase in the oedema.

2. Cardiac failure. The causes of oedema in cardiac failure are multiple and are not fully understood. Significant factors are:

a. Impairment of renal blood flow. In cardiac failure the coronary and cerebral circulations are maintained at the expense of other organs. Reduction in renal blood flow, alteration in the pulsatile pattern of renal perfusion, and possibly alteration in the distribution of blood flow within the kidney promote excessive reabsorption of salt and water — this is the main cause of 'cardiac' oedema.

b. Increased venous pressure. In cardiac failure there is a rise in venous pressure proximal to the failing chamber. Thus in right-sided failure the increase in venous pressure can be detected by inspection of the neck (p. 95). In left-sided failure, pulmonary venous congestion is inferred from the symptoms of dyspnoea and cough and from the auscultatory findings of crepitations in the lungs. However, the heights of these rises in venous pressure do not correlate with the degrees of oedema and it is clear that the hydrostatic effect does not account for the major part of the fluid retention.

c. The effect of aldosterone. In some cases of cardiac failure secondary hyperaldosteronism occurs and contributes to the oedema.

d. Antidiuretic hormone. There is evidence of an increase in antidiuretic substances in the urine of some patients with cardiac failure.

e. Lymphatic factors. Lymphangiectasis, incompetent valves, and poor lymph drainage have been demonstrated in cardiac failure.

f. Oncotic pressures. A combination of chronic passive congestion of the liver reducing albumin synthesis, a poor appetite, and loss of protein into the oedema fluid and the urine may account for a significant drop in the concentration of the serum albumin in some cases.

At the same time there is an increase in the protein content of the interstitial fluid which may rise to as much as 1 g % compared with only 0.02 g % in normal interstitial fluid. This change has sometimes been interpreted as evidence for an increase in capillary permeability supposedly due to ischaemia, but it is likely to be mainly due to lymphatic failure.

3. Renal causes. The oedema of the nephrotic syndrome has been discussed under hypoproteinaemia. In acute glomerulonephritis the cause of the fluid retention is not fully understood. There is an expansion of the circulating fluid volume as well as the extracellular space due at least in part to increased tubular reabsorption of sodium and consequent reduction in urine volume. Should normal fluid intake be maintained, oedema results. This also applies to any condition in which urine production is diminished (oliguria) or negligible (anuria).

Localised oedema

This may be due to venous, lymphatic, inflammatory, or allergic causes.

1. Venous causes. External pressure upon a vein, venous thrombosis or incompetence of the valves due to varicose veins may each contribute to a rise in capillary pressure in the areas of drainage. A common example is thrombosis in a leg vein complicating an operation, pregnancy, or an illness which confines a patient to bed. Venous return will also be impaired if the normal pumping action of the muscles is diminished or absent, and accordingly oedema (with or without thrombosis) may occur in an immobile bedridden patient, in a paralysed limb, or even in a normal person sitting still for long periods as, for example, during air travel.

2. Lymphatic causes. The small quantity of albumin filtered at the capillary is normally removed through the lymphatics. In the presence of lymphatic obstruction, the water and solutes are reabsorbed into the capillaries as the tissue pressure rises, but the protein remains until its concentration approaches that in the blood. Ultimately, fibrous tissues proliferate in the interstitial spaces and the whole part becomes hard and no longer pits on pressure.

Lymphatic oedema (*lymphoedema*) is common in some tropical countries due to obstruction by filarial worms. One or both legs, the female breast, or the external genitalia in either sex, are the parts most frequently involved. The skin of the affected area may eventually become very thick and rough — elephantiasis. Lymphoedema is comparatively rare in Britain. It may be due to congenital lymphangiectasis or hypoplasia of the lymph vessels of the legs (Milroy's disease) or may affect an arm after radical mastectomy and irradiation for carcinoma of the breast.

3. Inflammatory causes. As a result of damage to tissues by injury, infection, ischaemia, or chemicals such as uric acid, there is liberation of histamine, bradykinin, and other factors which cause vasodilatation and an increase of capillary permeability; the inflammatory exudate, therefore, has a high protein content which upsets the normal balance of forces. The resulting oedema is accompanied by the classical signs of inflammation, namely, redness, heat and pain. Testing for pitting on pressure in inflammatory oedema causes pain and should be avoided.

4. Allergic causes. Increased capillary permeability also occurs in allergic conditions but, in contrast to inflammation, there is no pain, there is less redness, and eosinophil cells rather than polymorphs and red cells make their way into the exudate, which has a high protein content. Angiooedema is a specific example of allergic oedema; it is particularly prone to affect the face and lips. The swelling develops rapidly, and it is pale or faintly pink in colour. The condition may constitute a serious threat to life by suffocation if the tongue and glottis are affected.

Conclusion

In analysing the pathogenesis of oedema, it is desirable to think particularly in terms of disturbance at the capillary level, where the fluid exchanges are taking place. Elevation of the jugular venous pressure is a sign of fluid overload and suggests either a cardiac cause or acute glomerulonephritis. Thereafter, further evidence should be sought from the associated clinical features in order to determine the primary cause. Physiological principles can be applied along similar lines to the interpretation of many other clinical signs.

SHOCK

Although commonly used by lay persons, the term 'shock' has a specific medical connotation. Shock is a purely clinical term indicating an acute systemic disorder characterised by hypoperfusion resulting in the dysfunction of vital organs. The three organ systems most commonly affected in the shock state are the central nervous system, the cardiovascular system and the renal system.

Central nervous system hypoperfusion is characterised by an altered state of consciousness. In the earliest stages, features of anxiety, agitation or apathy occur followed by clouding of consciousness which, if the state is not reversed, will lead to coma and eventually death.

In the cardiovascular system, arterial hypotension is one of the cardinal features. There is, however, no absolute level of systolic or mean arterial pressure at which shock is said to develop. For previously fit patients, a systolic blood pressure of below 100 mm of mercury is commonly associated with other features of the shocked state, but patients with pre-existing hypertension may be shocked with an apparently normal blood pressure. In association with the fall in blood pressure, there is frequently a reduction in the pulse pressure and a coexistent tachycardia. Peripheral vasoconstriction with resulting features of pale, cool, clammy skin may be seen, although in some forms of shock the peripheral circulation may be relatively undisturbed and cutaneous features alone are poor indicators of the shock state.

The renal features of oliguria or anuria occur as a direct result of renal hypoperfusion. Other commonly seen features of shock include tachypnoea, thirst and occasionally nausea or vomiting.

A multitude of clinical conditions can result in shock, but for practical purposes these may be classified under 3 headings.

Hypovolaemic shock

In clinical practice, hypovolaemia is the single commonest cause of shock, and blood loss is the major cause of acute hypovolaemia. This may be obvious, as in external blood loss related to trauma or gastrointestinal haemorrhage. However, blood losses in trauma are frequently underestimated. In penetrating injuries the degree of external blood loss bears no relationship to actual losses, and similarly in blunt injury to the chest or abdomen occult haemorrhage of major proportions can occur with little in the way of external signs.

Other common causes of hypovolaemia are related to loss of fluid and electrolytes such as occurs from the gastrointestinal tract in diarrhoea or prolonged vomiting, and conditions where there is loss of plasma such as burns and pancreatitis. The severity of hypovolaemia matches the exhibition of the early features of shock. With acute circulating blood loss of less than 10% of the normal volume (up to 500 ml in a 70 kg individual) there will not usually be any abnormal clinical features. With greater losses (up to 1.5 l) a tachycardia will usually be present together with postural hypotension, a reduced pulse pressure and early features of peripheral vasoconstriction. With losses up to 2.5 l, these features are exacerbated and the patients commonly have arterial hypotension together with tachypnoea and evidence of central nervous system dysfunction such as confusion and agitation. Acute blood volume deficits greater than 2.5 l are associated with severe hypotension, coma and oliguria or anuria.

It must be stressed that these changes will vary from individual to individual and may be modified by any preexisting medical condition, especially those involving impaired cardiorespiratory function. In addition, the development of the clinical features of shock depends upon the rate of blood or circulating volume loss together with changes in relation to the medical management of such a patient.

Cardiogenic shock

Any condition which produces a reduction in the pumping mechanism of the heart can produce shock. Most commonly this results from a failure of normal cardiac contractility such as occurs following acute myocardial infarction. Impedence to ventricular filling occurring in tension pneumothorax, cardiac tamponade or, rarely,

atrial myxoma produces a similar effect. Cardiac output is also compromised by any cause of ventricular outflow obstruction such as severe aortic stenosis or massive pulmonary embolism and if severe may be accompanied by shock. Finally, any extremes of cardiac rhythm producing a profound brady- or tachycardia can cause a reduction in cardiac output which, if maintained, will lead to the development of shock.

Distributive shock

Shock may result from conditions producing alterations in the normal vascular capacity and resistance. Common clinical conditions in this group include systemic sepsis, anaphylactoid states, spinal cord injury and some forms of drug overdose. In these conditions, there are marked alterations in the blood flow to vital tissues as a result of the condition itself, although cardiogenic and hypovolaemic components frequently coexist and exacerbate the problem.

Septic shock is seen in patients with systemic infection from Gram negative, Gram positive and fungal organisms with the resulting activation of a complex series of mediators including complement components, kinins, histamine and leukotrienes. These lead to arteriolar and venular smooth muscle relaxation with resultant vasodilatation and a relative loss in circulating blood volume. Associated with this are direct effects increasing the degree of capillary permeability and subsequent escape from the circulation of fluid, electrolytes and plasma proteins producing further loss of circulating blood volume. To aggravate the situation further, normal cardiac and pulmonary functions are disturbed by systemic infection preventing the normal physiological responses to hypovolaemia and hypoperfusion and leading to the vicious circle of hypoperfusion and dysfunction being established.

Septic shock occurs in up to 50% of patients with bacteraemia and has a high mortality.

REFERENCES

Campbell E J et al 1984 Clinical physiology, 5th edn, Blackwells Publications, Oxford
Culter P 1985 Problem solving in clinical medicine: from data to diagnosis, 2nd edn. Williams and Wilkins, Baltimore

4. The general examination and the external features of disease

C. R. W. Edwards

The object of this chapter is to describe those aspects of clinical examination which it would be inappropriate to assign to any single system. These include the observations made on first meeting the patient, while the history is being taken. Several other important elements of a general examination are also described, for example, study of the hands, the head and neck, the lymphatic system, the breasts and the skin. During this phase of the examination much useful information can be gathered about the endocrine system including the function of the pituitary, thyroid and adrenal glands. Cushing's syndrome, acromegaly, hypopituitarism, hyperthyroidism, hypothyroidism and Addison's disease may be obvious to the alert clinician; indeed if the diagnosis is not made at this stage it is often not made at all.

The general examination begins as soon as the patient enters the consulting room or the doctor approaches the bedside. Early impressions will be formed while taking the patient's history and all the doctor's faculties should be on the alert from the outset. At the start of the formal examination an analysis is made of the patient's demeanour, complexion, physique and the other features which together constitute the individual's appearance. Thereafter the hands, head and neck are examined in turn. With constant practice this part of the examination can be dealt with expeditiously. At first students must be prepared to take their time and develop a methodical routine. With increasing experience, facility and speed will be acquired as well as the ability to discriminate between the details of examination that are vital in one case and superfluous in another. To compromise too early in this respect is to invite disaster.

GENERAL OBSERVATIONS

Demeanour

Early impressions of the patient's condition are compounded from many factors including the greeting, mobility and facial expression. The handshake of a patient with acromegaly, for example, may arouse suspicion because of the size of the hand (Fig 4.3) and the excessive palmar sweating. The gait may indicate neurological or locomotor disturbances (p. 258). The posture of the patient in bed can be informative. Can the position be adjusted spontaneously or is help required? Does the patient sit up or lift the head when addressed or have to be supported or propped up on several pillows? Does the patient tend to slip helplessly into some awkward position and seem to disregard the associated discomfort?

Facial expression may serve as an initial guide to physical or mental disorder. A look of pain, fear, excitement, anxiety or grief does not require a medical training for its recognition. More subtle, however, may be the appreciation of such features as the agitation of hyperthyroidism or hypomania, the apathy of hypothyroidism and of some types of depression and the poverty of facial movement in parkinsonism. Without intending to deceive, the more intelligent patients may manage to conceal their apprehension, or cloak their feelings in an air of feigned cheerfulness. They may occasionally make light of their symptoms or signs, or deal facetiously with features about which they feel the most anxiety; the doctor should avoid adopting the patient's light-hearted attitude, but on the other hand should not be too ponderous. The inexperienced clinician will do well to behave naturally and so eliminate risks of misunderstanding.

Complexion

Everyday experience leads to familiarity with the wide variety of the physical characteristics of the face. Among these, abnormalities of complexion may be the first to be noticed by patients or by their friends or relations. When these simple observations are reinforced by medical training, complexion may become a remarkably sensitive index of disease. It must be remembered, however, that lighting conditions affect the appreciation of colour. This is well known to shoppers when choosing clothes and cosmetics, but the effect of light on the complexion is not so widely appreciated. For instance, jaundice deep enough to be obvious to anyone in daylight, may be undetectable in artificial light.

The colour of the face depends upon variations in oxyhaemoglobin, reduced haemoglobin, melanin and, to a lesser extent, carotene. Unusual colours, excluding those which have been applied externally, are due also to abnormal pigments such as sulphaemoglobin and methaemoglobin (bluish tinge), bile pigments (yellow or greenish), and uraemia (sallow with a brownish tinge).

Haemoglobin. The contribution of haemoglobin to the normal complexion is largely determined by the amount which is present in the subpapillary venous plexuses and the proportion which is oxygenated or reduced. Abnormal pallor may be due to vasoconstriction as in fright or when the upright subject faints, or it may be due to anaemia. The observation by relatives or friends of increasing pallor may be an early feature of progressive anaemia. Although it is common knowledge that a sallow face is not necessarily an indication of anaemia, it is not so widely recognised that vasodilatation may produce a deceptively pink complexion in spite of a severe degree of anaemia. An unduly plethoric complexion may be seen in some chronic alcoholics (alcohol may produce a pseudo-Cushing's syndrome), in Cushing's syndrome itself or in polycythaemia. The presence of plethora in Cushing's syndrome (p. 50) relates to thinning of the skin with enhanced visibility of superficial blood vessels rather than true polycythaemia (i.e. increase in red cell mass).

Cyanosis is discussed on page 87.

Melanin. This pigment is normally formed in the deepest layer of the epidermis and colours the skin brown or even black according to the amount present. The colour is largely determined by hereditary influences but may be modified by a number of factors. The pigment diminishes or increases in amount with withdrawal from or exposure to ultra-violet light. Absence of melanin from the skin may occur in patches, described as vitiligo (Plate II) which may be associated with autoimmune disease. Total absence of pigmentation occurs in albinism as a result of a genetically determined failure to form tyrosinase in the melanocytes, and this may occur in any race. An acquired form of failure to synthesise pigment is largely responsible for the pallor which is a characteristic feature of hypopituitarism in the white races.

In Addison's disease reduction in the output of adrenocortical hormones is associated with excessive production of adrenocorticotrophin, β-lipotrophin and N-terminal pro-opiocortin by the pituitary gland. These peptides all contain a melanotropin core sequence and their overproduction is accompanied by the development of brown pigmentation of the skin particularly in creases, in recent scars, overlying prominent bones and on areas exposed to pressure from belts, braces and tight clothing. Melanin may also be deposited in the mucous membranes of the lips and of the mouth where it results in a slaty grey pigmentation (Plate II). In both Addison's disease and hypopituitarism vasoconstriction occurs in the skin, so that pigmentation and pallor respectively are accentuated by the absence of the normal red background. Pregnancy is also commonly associated with a blotchy pigmentation of the face, the so-called pregnancy mask — chloasma gravidarum — and melanin is also formed in the areolae, the linea alba and around the genitalia. Increased melanin formation can be induced by heavy metals deposited in the skin, as for example, iron in haemochromatosis. Local over-production of melanin is responsible for freckles and for the pigmentation of moles.

Carotene. Hypercarotenaemia occasionally occurs in vegetarians or in food faddists, particularly in those who elect to eat excessive quantities of raw carrot. The yellow pigment carotene is unevenly distributed and is seen particularly in the face, palms and soles but not in the sclerae. A distinct yellow colour of the face may appear in hypothyroidism because of impaired metabolism of carotene in the liver.

Bilirubin. In haemolytic (acholuric) jaundice, the sclerae and the skin are a lemon-yellow colour. The stools are dark and the urine looks normal, but contains an excess of urobilinogen (p. 341). This form of jaundice is due to an increase in circulating unconjugated bilirubin which is not excreted in the urine.

In hepatocellular and obstructive jaundice bilirubin has been dissociated from plasma albumin and is conjugated with glucuronic acid by the liver. It is water soluble and readily passes through the renal glomerular filter (p. 341). The urine is brown like beer and the stools tend to be pale in colour like putty, because of the reduction in the amount of bile in the faeces. If the jaundice is deep and of long standing a distinct greenish colour becomes evident in the sclerae and in the skin due to the development of appreciable quantities of biliverdin. Scratch marks may be prominent on the skin in obstructive jaundice as a result of the pruritus which is believed to be due to the retention of bile acids.

Abnormal movements

Involuntary movements may be due to organic disease of the central nervous system, particularly when the extrapyramidal system is involved (p. 224). Disorders of movement may also result from primary disease elsewhere. Beta adrenergic stimulants such as Ephedrine and Salbutamol, can aggravate the normal physiological tremor. This also occurs in thyrotoxicosis when the patient is often very restless or fidgety, a state of affairs sometimes described as hyperkinetic. The 'flapping tremor' of encephalopathy due to hepatic failure may not be apparent by inspecting the outstretched arms except with the hands dorsiflexed. The sign consists of jerky movements of the hands due to flexion and extension of the wrists and fingers in a manner somewhat resembling the action of a bird's wing, though less regular and rhythmical. Similar twitching movements may occur in renal failure ('uraemic twitchings') and in

respiratory failure with carbon dioxide retention. Other causes of tremor are described on page 217.

Abnormal sounds

Sounds which are heard either by the doctor or the patient or another witness, may be of considerable value in diagnosis. Foremost amongst such is the information to be gained by attention to peculiarities of voice and speech.

The factors which contribute to the production of the voice include the ability to expel sufficient air from the lungs as well as the integrity of the mucosa, muscles and nerve supply of the larynx. Normal speech depends also upon the tongue, lips, palate and nose. The neurological abnormalities which cause disturbances of voice and speech are described on page 189. Many of the other causes can be recognised by inspection, for example a cleft palate, nasal obstruction, loose dentures, or a dry mouth. Hoarseness of the voice, again excluding neurological causes, may be due to laryngitis of infective origin, or it may result from excessive smoking. The chronic alcoholic is frequently hoarse, but in such cases there are probably several factors concerned, including cigarette smoking.

The voice in myxoedema may be so characteristic that the diagnosis can be made without seeing the patient, perhaps even over the telephone. The normal inflections of tone disappear, speech is low-pitched, slow and deliberate, and seems to require more effort than normal; it sounds 'thick', in that it flows less freely than normal, and the patient may stumble over individual syllables. Many of these changes are due to myxoedematous infiltration of the tissues concerned in voice production and the diagnosis may be suspected by the alert otolaryngologist when looking at the vocal cords by indirect laryngoscopy.

Several other types of sound may be heard, especially in connection with the respiratory system. Wheezing, rattling or stridor may help in the differentiation of dyspnoea. The character of a cough may be revealing (p. 126). Witnesses may give an account of a whoop suggestive of pertussis or the cry of an epileptic fit. Audible noises of cardiovascular origin and various sounds arising from the alimentary tract are described in the appropriate chapters.

Abnormal odours

Though the olfactory sense is poorly developed in man, there are occasions when the smell is so offensive that it is tempting to give the patient a wide berth. One of the major sources of malodour, apart from dirty clothing and general soiling, is the skin, particularly of the axillae, the external genitalia, the feet and under the breast. Some odours are sufficiently characteristic as to be diagnostic, like the sickly 'fetor hepaticus' of liver failure, or the sweetness of the breath in diabetic ketoacidosis, which is obvious to some observers but is not appreciated at all by others. The source of smells is usually easy to identify if the cause is excessive sweating, gangrene, chronic suppuration, necrotic tumours or some skin disorders. In communities with access to the usual amenities, odour due to dirt should not occur, except in the very young, the elderly infirm and the mentally defective who are incapable of looking after themselves and their toilet needs. Nevertheless, from time to time one comes across patients who have access to the necessary facilities but who are too lazy or incompetent to take the trouble to keep themselves clean, and who show little if any embarrassment at the filthy state of their skin, and particularly of their feet.

Halitosis is an affliction which is less readily avoided. Malodorous breath often passes unrecognised by the patient but may be particularly offensive to others. Some individuals are afflicted with halitosis for which no adequate explanation can be found. In others it may be associated with decomposing food wedged between the teeth, carious teeth, gingivitis, stomatitis, atrophic rhinitis, and tumours of the nasal passages, as well as pulmonary suppuration. Bronchiectasis may be associated with offensive breath, and in some cases the patient may notice that expectorated sputum tastes foul. In patients with gastric outlet obstruction from scarring or carcinoma of the stomach, foul-smelling eructations may occur, but probably the most offensive odour of this type is associated with a gastro-colic fistula, due to the faecal contents of the stomach.

The *smell of alcohol* may prompt the doctor to ask appropriate questions about the patient's habits, but it should also be remembered that a comatose patient may have been given whisky or brandy as a remedy by a well-intentioned layman, and that alcohol may not be responsible for the patient's condition.

Anthropometry

A routine examination should include the measurement of *weight* and *height*, both for their immediate value and for future reference. Other measurements such as *span, sitting height* and *pubis to ground height* are made occasionally when a more precise evaluation of growth and development is required. The special measurements applicable to infants and young children are given on page 352.

The *weight* of an adult patient taken in the outpatient department or consulting-room should include normal indoor clothing without shoes. Patients in hospital should be weighed in pyjamas and dressing-gown, again without shoes. The *height* should be recorded with a suitable rigid arm sliding on a vertical scale, and with the patient standing on an even floor surface, so that the heels, calves, buttocks, shoulders and occiput can be aligned against the vertical plane. Under certain circumstances, such as when children with short stature are being measured, a more accurate device is required; one such is called a stadiometer.

Increase in height. Gigantism as a feature of hyperpituitarism is very uncommon, but the appearance of some patients with hypogonadism and of patients with Marfan's syndrome may give the impression that they are disproportionately tall. In hypogonadism the limbs continue to grow for longer than is appropriate because of the absence of sex hormones which normally serve to close the epiphyses after puberty. Thus the sitting height of the patient (head, neck and trunk) will be considerably less than half the height of the patient measured standing. Alternatively, the height from the top of the symphysis pubis to the ground can be recorded and this measure of the length of the lower limbs will be found to exceed the sitting height. The span of the arms measured fully extended will be found to exceed the height standing or, more significantly, twice the sitting height, thus once more emphasising the disproportionate length of the limbs in contrast to the trunk.

In Marfan's syndrome the appearance of the patient is rather similar, that is to say, the limbs are longer than appropriate to the length of the trunk. As a rule there are additional features to distinguish the patient with Marfan's syndrome, in particular long slender hands (arachnodactyly Fig. 4.1) and narrow feet, a high arched palate, dislocation of the lens or dilatation of the aorta causing aortic regurgitation.

Short stature may be due to many causes such as growth hormone deficiency, hypothyroidism, chronic subnutrition, intestinal malabsorption, severe congenital heart disease and various chronic respiratory and renal conditions. In achondroplasia, gross shortening of all four limbs with a normal trunk length is a constant and characteristic finding. The stunted growth of rickets is usually associated with some limb deformity, particularly genu valgum (knock knee) or varum (bow leg). If cretinism remained untreated or has been inadequately treated sufficiently long for growth to be restricted, there will usually be some other signs of persistent hypothyroidism, particularly impairment of mental development. With juvenile hypothyroidism (i.e. developing after the first year of life) there may be major effects on growth with little mental impairment.

Nutritional status

Life expectancy is shortened by being substantially overweight or severely underweight. Obesity leads to many complications besides the disability from breathlessness on exertion. Many of the standard tables in common use were prepared from life insurance figures obtained from individuals belonging to social and occupational classes in which the average weights were usually in excess of the ideal. For this reason, it is becoming increasingly common to express nutritional status in terms of the body mass index (BMI) which is derived from the formula Wt/Ht^2, measured in kg/m^2. Subjects may be accessed as being plump when the BMI is between 25–30 and obese if it is in excess of 30. BMI can be calculated from the formula or derived by use of nomogram (p. 356).

The amount of subcutaneous fat can be estimated by measuring the skin fold thickness over the triceps or below the scapula by means of a special pair of calipers. Such a measurement, of course, includes two thickness of skin and subcutaneous fat. A simple clinical estimate can be made by picking up the skin fold between the finger and thumb. Waist-hip ratio may provide a more valuable assessment of visceral adipose fat tissue.

Although the majority of adults in Britain requiring dietetic advice are suffering from the effects of overeating, some are too thin due to undereating or starvation. Undereating results from the anorexia accompanying many organic diseases and psychological disorders such as anorexia nervosa. Chronic alcohol abusers frequently have multiple nutritional deficiencies. In Britain starvation due to poverty is rare, but it is all too prevalent in many parts of the world.

Iron deficiency is common, especially in women, but is usually in part due to blood loss rather than dietary inadequacy. Specific deficiencies of protein and vitamins are rare in Britain and when they occur are usually caused by a visceral disorder. For example vitamin B_{12} is not absorbed in pernicious anaemia due to failure of the production of intrinsic factor by the atrophic stomach. Fat soluble vitamins A, D, E and K are not absorbed normally in obstructive jaundice and multiple deficiencies occur in generalised diseases of the small intestine. Scurvy affecting elderly people living alone is almost the only vitamin deficiency disease of dietetic origin seen in British adults (Plate II). In Asian immigrants vitamin D deficiency is not uncommon and probably results from differences in dietary intake and absorption of the vitamin and decreased formation in the skin.

Abnormalities of fat

In the normal individual fat is stored mainly in the subcutaneous tissues and in the mesentery. In *nutritional obesity*, dietary intake exceeds energy expenditure. Excess fat is widely but not always uniformly distributed. In gross cases, the fat deposits may make palpation of the abdomen uninformative. The face, neck, breasts, buttocks, and thighs will usually also show signs of undue accumulation of fat. As a rule, the amount deposited on limbs is greatest nearer the trunk and tapers towards the wrists and ankles, very little excess fat being deposited on the hands or feet.

In Cushing's syndrome the distribution of fat may be abnormal. This syndrome is due to prolonged elevation of free (i.e. non protein-bound) corticosteroid levels. It can result from the administration of supraphysiological amounts of glucocorticoids such as cortisone or prednisolone, from injections of adrenocorticotrophic hormone, or from excessive endogenous secretion of cortisol. These hormones increase the appetite and may lead to a mixture of simple obesity and the more striking changes due to excessive corticosteroids whereby fat deposition tends to be restricted to the trunk, neck and face, together with an increase of the normal pad of fat over the lower cervical and upper thoracic vertebrae. The limbs remain relatively thin or are actually wasted, the whole impression giving rise to the term 'buffalo obesity'. Osteoporosis causing collapse and wedging of the thoracic and lumbar vertebrae leads to shortening of the spine, increased protuberance of the abdomen, and further exaggeration of the abnormalities described. The face is often florid (p. 46) and round — mooning of the face (Fig. 10.4 p. 307). In contrast the skin is thin due to atrophy of collagen in the dermis, which leads to minor trauma causing bleeding into the skin identical to senile purpura (p. 75); stretching of the skin, especially over the abdomen, thighs and upper arms, may result in purple striae.

Localised deposits of fat which are sometimes tender, may form on the limbs particularly in middle-aged females. Lipomas are commonly found around the trunk and are rather soft, circumscribed, lobulated swellings.

Progressive lipodystrophy is a rare condition in which subcutaneous fat disappears sequentially from the face, neck, arms, chest and trunk. Fat remains or may even be deposited in excess on the lower trunk and thighs, the line of demarcation varying from case to case. Diabetes mellitus is a common accompaniment.

Localised atrophy of subcutaneous fat may occur occasionally in diabetics in areas where insulin is habitually injected. This does not seem to occur when highly purified monocomponent insulin preparations are used.

The significance of a change in weight

A history of a recent change in weight must be regarded critically until it has been explained.

Loss of weight may be due to inadequate intake, malabsorption or a metabolic disturbance. A coincident loss of appetite in a middle-aged person who has previously enjoyed eating should bring the possibility of an underlying malignancy to the doctor's mind. Emaciation may occur in young women suffering from anorexia nervosa; these patients frequently take a great deal of trouble to conceal the fact that their diet is grossly inadequate. Anxiety at any age and depression in later years are common causes of loss of appetite and weight.

Alimentary disease, with malabsorption as a feature may cause loss of weight. Rarely protein loss from the bowel may result in hypoalbuminaemia and oedema and the latter may conceal the change in weight. This may also occur in patients with cardiac cachexia and oedema.

Weight loss accompanied by a history of increased or unchanged appetite suggests the possibility of diabetes mellitus or hyperthyroidism. The former would usually be readily confirmed by examination of the urine for glucose (p. 339), supplemented if necessary by measuring the blood glucose. In patients with hyperthyroidism there are often other symptoms apart from weight loss, measurement of fasting blood glucose and glycosylated haemoglobin. Radiological examination of the chest should be performed if weight loss (p. 67) is unexplained, since pulmonary tuberculosis and primary or metastatic malignancy do not always produce clinical features indicating chest disease.

Because of dietary neglect, chronic alcoholism may be associated with weight loss though in other subjects, the energy value of the alcohol consumed will lead to weight gain.

Gain in weight is frequently encountered in hypothyroidism, in patients treated with corticosteroids or during adolescence, following pregnancy or at the menopause. Endocrine causes of obesity are, relatively rare. Comfort eating during periods of stress, giving up cigarette smoking or moving from an active to a sedentary job are more common explanations. A very rapid increase over a period of days is due to fluid retention, for example in patients with cardiac failure.

Some increase in weight during the luteal phase of the menstrual cycle is normal. In some women, however, this may be excessive and be a contributory factor to premenstrual tension. There is also a circadian pattern with weight being higher in the evening than the morning. This is accentuated in the idiopathic oedema syndrome. Patients with this condition, which is virtually confined to women, have a reduced ability to excrete a water load when standing. This can lead to remarkable fluctuations in their body weight depending on their fluid intake.

The state of hydration

The state of hydration should be assessed in all cases of fluid loss, notably from vomiting, diarrhoea, sweating or polyuria. Unless the possibility of dehydration is given special thought, its existence may be overlooked or its severity underestimated. A detailed history of the nature and quantity of fluid loss is of first importance. If the patient's usual weight is known, much the most satisfactory assessment is obtained by weighing. A dry tongue is apt to be deceptive as it may be due to mouth breathing alone. In an adult, after 4 to 6 litres have been lost, the blood pressure may be low and the skin dry, loose and wrinkled. The finding of a postural drop in blood pressure is a useful physical sign indicating intravascular volume depletion. Loss of elasticity of the skin can be demonstrated by pinching up a fold which then remains as a ridge and subsides abnormally slowly. The eyeballs are soft, due to lowering of the intraocular tension (p. 61). The change of elasticity of the skin with age and the difficulty in manually assessing intraocular pressure make these rather unsatisfactory physical signs. Haematological and biochemical indices may be more helpful than the physical signs. A high haemoglobin concentration or an elevated packed cell volume (p. 345)

provides evidence of the severity of dehydration and serial readings will indicate when treatment has been adequate. Plasma osmolality measurements are even more informative.

Temperature

Body temperature is estimated for clinical purposes by taking readings beneath the tongue or in the rectum. For convenience some use the less accurate sites of axilla, groin or natal cleft. Rectal temperature is usually about 0.5°C higher than the mouth which in turn is 0.5°C higher than the axilla. Rectal readings are more reliable and should be recorded when there is any doubt about the authenticity of recordings from the mouth or axilla.

The normal oral temperature is 37°C. Circadian variations of about 0.5°C occur, the lowest temperature being in the early morning. Fever is usually due to organic disease, though occasionally this is not the case. An otherwise inexplicable transient rise may be due to a recent hot drink or a hot bath. Malingerers sometimes falsify their temperatures by a variety of tricks, including the use of hot-water bottles, in order to feign illness.

The warmth of the skin to the touch usually provides a remarkably good indication of fever, but gives a totally unreliable estimate of normal or low body temperature. The skin of a patient with a normal temperature may feel cold, and an apparently normal skin temperature does not exclude hypothermia. When hypothermia is present, it is commonly overlooked because the ordinary clinical thermometer reads only as low as 35°C and it is not always shaken below this level before a patient's temperature is measured. Clinical thermometers which record lower levels are readily available; temperature as low as 27°C are not uncommon and core body temperatures below 20°C have been recorded in patients who subsequently survived. Hypothermia commonly occurs in elderly patients living alone who have fallen down and are subsequently unable to rise. Other situations in which hypothermia occurs are near drowning and patients who have lain unconscious for a prolonged period of time in low environmental temperatures as a result of drug overdosage, alcohol intoxication or head injury. Medical conditions include hypopituitarism and hypo-thyroidism. Because many of the features of severe hypothyroidism mimic death such subjects may require to be fully resuscitated and rewarmed before assessing viability.

THE HANDS

After the history has been obtained and the opportunity has been taken for making an early appraisal of the patient, the more formal physical assessment usually begins with examination of the hands and pulse.

The hand, directed by the mind, is largely responsible for the dominant position of man in the animal kingdom. It is a highly developed structure and its area of representation on the cerebral cortex is appropriately extensive. While the palmist may claim to read more from the hand than is justified, critical inspection supplemented by palpation can provide much reliable general information. When inspecting the hands, attention should be paid first to general features and then to detailed consideration of individual structures on an anatomical basis. The examination of the function of the hand is described on page 266, and the significance of right or left handedness on page 190.

General features

Grip. The firm determined grip or the soft flabby handshake may reflect the personality of the patient while the inability to relax the grip may be a feature of dystrophia myotonica (p. 57).

Movements. *Gestures* can be most informative while the history is being given (p. 1). There is, for example, the hand pressed flat on top of the head accompanying a complaint of headache and suggesting that this is a psychogenic symptom, 'something weighing on the mind'.

Tremors are studied with the hands at rest and then outstretched; causes include anxiety, hyperthyroidism, alcoholism, parkinsonism and liver, respiratory or renal failure. Characteristic tremors are described on page 217.

Tetany may be recognised by the presence of carpal spasm (p. 338).

Posture. This may be almost diagnostic as ex-emplified by the flexed hand and arm of hemiplegia or the wrist drop of radial nerve palsy. In long standing rheumatoid arthritis there is often ulnar deviation of the hand.

Shape. Trauma is the commonest cause of deformity of the hand. Other examples of unusual shapes include the long thin fingers of arachnodactyly (Fig. 4.1) while a short fourth metacarpal, best seen when making a fist, would strongly support a diagnosis of Turner's syndrome in a girl with primary amenorrhoea. Short metacarpals, especially the fourth and fifth, are found in patients with pseudohypoparathyroidism in which the tissues are resistant to the effects of parathyroid hormone.

Size. Large, broad hands may provide useful clinical corroboration of a diagnosis of acromegaly which has been suspected from the facies (Fig. 4.3). Rings which were previously loose may not now be removed or there may be a history of rings having to be cut off or enlarged. The increase in bulk consists largely of soft tissues; these are also thickened in myxoedema. Oedema may be part of a generalised process or be local from venous or lymphatic obstruction or disuse as with a hemiplegia.

Colour. Pallor of the nails and palmar creases supports the clinical assessment of anaemia. White hands, the skin of which is smooth and soft, are seen in conjunction with similar changes in the face in hypopituitarism. Conclusions regarding pigmentation are similar to those applying to the skin in general (p. 46). The brown staining of the fingers from smoking should be reconciled with the history of cigarette consumption. Coal miners may have small blue tattoo marks in the skin of their hands and in other sites where particles of coal dust have been embedded in the scars of minor injuries. It is worth bearing in mind that professional tattooing within the previous few months may be the source of an acute type B viral hepatitis. The nature of the tattoo may be informative about the personality of the patient (Fig. 4.3). In both miners and professional tattooing the blue colour is due to black particles (carbon or Indian ink) changed in appearance by the scatter of light as it passes through and is reflected back from the skin. This explains why veins normally look blue, while in the elderly, with very thin skin

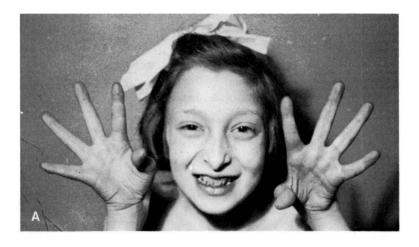

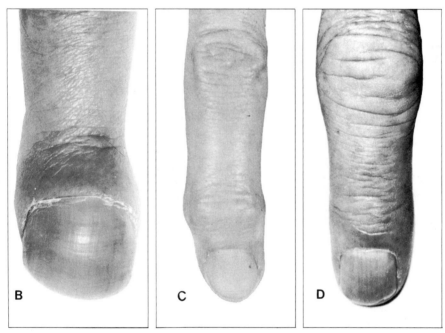

Fig. 4.1 The fingers as a diagnostic aid. (A) Arachnodactyly in Marfan's syndrome. (B) Advanced finger clubbing. (C) Heberden's nodes of osteoarthrosis. (D) Fusiform swelling of proximal interphalangeal joint in rheumatoid arthritis.

from atrophy of collagen, the true red colour of the blood may be seen.

Temperature. In a cold or cool climate the temperature of the patient's hand is a good guide to the blood flow through it. If the hand is warm and cyanosed it can be deduced that arterial oxygen saturation is reduced. In most patients with heart failure the hands tend to be cold and cyanosed due to vasoconstriction in response to a low cardiac output. If they are warm the cause of the heart failure may well be hyperthyroidism or cor pulmonale.

Sweating. The warm moist palms of hyperthyroidism may be contrasted with the cold, clammy hands of the anxious patient. Palmar sweating is also increased in acromegaly.

Detailed Features

Skin. The smooth, hairless hands of a boy should change to the lined and hairy hands of the adult male unless hypogonadism is present. Manual work may produce specific callosities due to pressure at characteristic sites. In contrast, disuse results in a soft, smooth palmar skin like that of an infant, just as occurs on the soles following prolonged recumbency.

The skin may feature a wide variety of specific skin disorders or dermatological manifestation of systemic diseases (p. 77). An example of the former is contact dermatitis due to an external irritant whereas scleroderma may be a sign of progressive systemic sclerosis. The skin has a shiny, glazed appearance and is tightly stretched over the underlying tissues, limiting the movement of the fingers which are held in a semi-flexed position.

Nails. The fact that well manicured nails are things of beauty and a social asset may account for disproportionate distress when an abnormality is present. Injury is by far the most common cause of changes in the nails and may permanently impair their growth. A transverse groove at a similar level on each of the nails dates a systemic disturbance and occasionally indicates a previous illness which has not been mentioned.

Splinter haemorrhages under the nails (Fig. 4.2) are a manifestation of a systemic vasculitis induced by immune complexes which may also cause haemorrhages in the skin and retina and, occasionally, tender nodules in the fingertips (Osler's

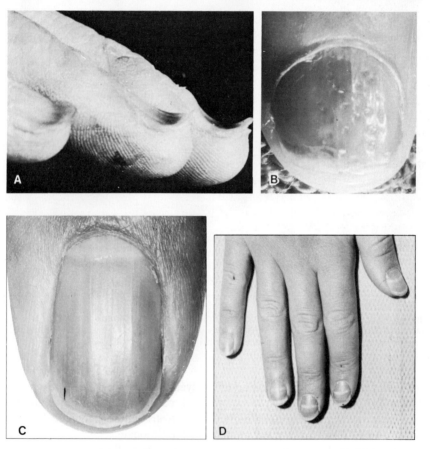

Fig. 4.2 The nails as a diagnostic aid. (A) Advanced koilonychia. (B) Pitting of nail in psoriasis. (C) Splinter haemorrhage and also linear ridges which increase in frequency with age. (D) White bands on nail beds may be a pointer to a systemic disorder such as hypoalbuminaemia.

nodes). Multiple splinter haemorrhages suggest a diagnosis of infective endocarditis.

In long-standing iron deficiency the nails become brittle and then flat and, ultimately, spoon-shaped (koilonychia, Fig. 4.2). The nails may be pitted by psoriasis (Fig. 4.2) which may also discolour and deform them so as to cause confusion with fungal infection. Small isolated white patches (leuconychia) are often seen in the nail plates of normal persons. Whitening of the nail beds (Terry's nails, Fig. 4.2) is much less common but may occur in a systemic disorder such as hypoalbuminaemia. Bitten nails suggest that anxiety neurosis may have to be considered in the final assessment.

Subcutaneous tissues. In Dupuytren's contracture there is thickening and shortening of the palmar fascia resulting in flexion deformities particularly of the fifth and ring fingers. Firm, painless subcutaneous nodules occur in rheumatoid disease but they are much more frequently found over the upper end of the ulna than on the hands. Finger clubbing (Fig. 4.1) is discussed on page 133.

Joints. Arthritis frequently involves the small joints of the hands. Rheumatoid arthritis (Figs 4.1 and 4.3) affects the proximal interphalangeal, metacarpophalangeal and carpal joints and causes pain, stiffness, swelling, restriction of movement and ultimately, often gross deformity. Osteoarthrosis affects mainly the terminal interphalangeal joints and causes little or no disability. At this site the characteristic changes are Heberden's nodes (Fig. 4.1) which are visible and palpable osteophytes projecting from the dorsal surface of the base of the terminal phalanx. If the terminal joints are affected by a diffuse swelling along with apparent rheumatoid changes in other joints, then psoriatic arthropathy should be suspected and skin and nail lesions should be sought.

Muscles. Wasting is common in rheumatoid arthritis. It also occurs in lesions of the lower motor neurone; causes in this category include: syringomyelia, poliomyelitis, lesions of the first thoracic nerve root and motor neurone disease in which fasciculation (p. 217) is very often seen. Specific muscle groups are involved in lesions of the ulnar or median nerves, e.g. in leprosy (Fig

4.3). In the carpal tunnel syndrome there may be selective wasting of the thenar muscles when the median nerve is compressed and this in turn may be a consequence of a generalised condition such as myxoedema, acromegaly, premenstrual fluid retention, pregnancy or rheumatoid arthritis.

Tendons. Tenosynovitis may follow excessive use of a tendon and may result in a 'trigger finger' (p. 268). Tenosynovitis commonly produces a sensation of local crepitus and swelling over the tendon sheath. A common site is the extensor pollicis longus tendon at the wrist where it crosses the radial styloid (De Quervain's tenosynovitis). A tendon may be ruptured from its involvement in hypertrophied synovial membrane on the dorsum of the hand in rheumatoid arthritis.

Bones. Fractures are usually obvious, a notable exception being the scaphoid when the only finding may be tenderness localised in the anatomical snuff-box. Occasionally the bones of the hand, particularly the phalanges, may be involved in granulomatous or other generalised disorders such as sarcoidosis or hyperparathyroidism. Acute dactylitis is characteristic of sickle cell disease in children. Graves' disease, the commonest cause of hyperthyroidism, may be associated with clubbing and periosteal new bone formation usually in the phalanges.

Nerves. Motor changes have already been described. In polyneuropathy there is a characteristic sensory impairment of a glove distribution affecting both hands; the feet are usually also involved. An example, common in the tropics, is the late result of dimorphous or lepromatous leprosy. Secondary infection through abrasions leads to deformities from absorption of the phalanges (Fig. 4.3) or from loss of fingers by ulceration. In tuberculoid leprosy the lesions are likely to be asymmetrical or unilateral.

Blood vessels. Palmar erythema is a mottled, bright red cutaneous vasodilatation often seen mainly over the hypothenar and thenar eminences. Though it is found in normal persons, it is suggestive of liver dysfunction. Arteritis is found in infective endocarditis and in connective tissue disorders; it may cause small necrotic lesions around the base of the nail most commonly in systemic lupus erythematosus. Raynaud's phenomenon is due to arterial spasm and is described on page 93.

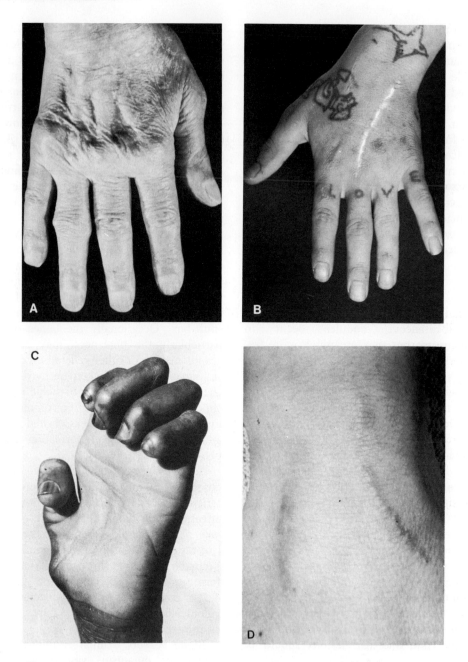

Fig. 4.3   The hands as a diagnostic aid. (A) Rheumatoid arthritis; swelling of one proximal interphalangeal joint of ring finger and of all metacarpophalangeal joints; wasting of small muscles of hand. (B) Aggressive sociopath; scars and pornographic tattoos were also present elsewhere, (C) Leprosy; late median and ulnar nerve lesions causing thenar and hypothenar wasting and claw hand. Sensory impairment has initiated loss of tissue in the terminal phalanges of the index and little fingers due to sepsis and trauma. (D) Linear marks on dorsum of hand following intravenous injection of drugs by an addict.

Occlusive arterial disease due to atheroma is rare in the hands especially when compared to its frequency in the legs. Venous abnormalities are seldom seen but the linear marks following the intravenous injection of drugs of addicts ('main liners') are characteristic (Fig. 4.3).

THE HEAD

For purposes of convenience, the examination of the various components of the head is described in topographical sequence — the cranium, hair, face, eyes, ears, nose and mouth. In practice the examination will probably commence with the structure mainly involved.

The cranium

The examination of the cranium in infancy and childhood can be most informative (Table 10.1, p. 304). This is in striking contrast to the paucity of positive findings in the adult. In the latter, inspection may reveal generalised enlargement in Paget's disease or localised bony bossing overlying a meningioma. The supraorbital ridges often enlarge in acromegaly due to increase in the size of the frontal sinuses. In cranial arteritis the temporal arteries are often visibly and may be palpably enlarged and tender. On auscultation a bruit may occasionally be detected in the presence of an intracranial arteriovenous malformation (p. 239).

The hair

While the examination of the hair of the scalp and face is being described it is convenient to refer to abnormalities of the growth of hair in other sites.

The scalp. In the normal adult male the hair margin of the forehead tends to recede, or at least to become thin at either side; this is described as temporal recession. When present in females it may suggest virilisation. Loss of hair over the frontal region is an almost constant finding in the rare condition myotonic dystrophy. Alopecia totalis is a striking and distressing condition in which all hair may disappear permanently.

The most common local disease of the hair of the scalp is alopecia areata in which the hair falls out in patches; hairs shaped like exclamation marks are found at the periphery of the bald area which is clean and smooth in contrast to fungal infection in which the area is covered with hairs which are broken off close to the skin. Lice and nits of *Pediculus capitis* may also be found (p. 76).

Facial and body hair. Hirsutism is an excessive growth of hair on the face, trunk and limbs in the female. It is a common complaint. The majority of hirsute patients have high levels of salivary testosterone which reflects the free circulating levels of hormone.

In any form of adrenocortical or gonadal dysfunction in the female associated with virilisation, hair appears on the beard or moustache areas and the pubic hair spreads from its normal flat topped distribution up towards the umbilicus, this being described as a male escutcheon. Hair may also appear on the limbs.

Secondary sexual hair on the face in the male, and in the axillae and on the pubis of both sexes, may fail to develop normally in hypogonadism; it may diminish in quantity in old age or be lost in hypopituitarism or as a result of hepatic cirrhosis. In severe hypopituitarism (Fig. 4.4) the loss is ultimately complete, including the hair follicles so that the axillae and pubis return to the smooth appearance seen in childhood (Fig. 4.12).

The early development of pubic hair is related to adrenal androgen production and is called the adrenarche. This occurs in the absence of gonadotrophin secretion. Thus patients with isolated gonadotrophin releasing hormone and hence gonadotrophin deficiency may have early pubic hair but no other signs of pubertal development.

Eyebrows. The amount of hair here varies very widely. Contrary to common belief thinning of the outer third of the eyebrows is so common in normal people as to be of little value in the diagnosis of hypothyroidism.

The face

Some facial appearances are indicative of disease, for example the immobile stare of parkinsonism, the startled appearance of hyperthyroidism, the pale, puffy face of nephritis, the coarse features of myxoedema, the eyes of the patient with Down's syndrome (mongolism) and the risus sardonicus of

ask about:

obstetric history
menstrual pattern
sexuality
previous trauma
fatigue
cold intolerance
thirst
visual problems
headache

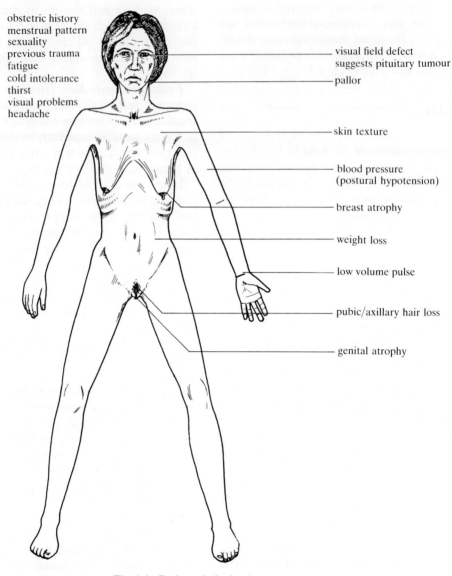

visual field defect
suggests pituitary tumour

pallor

skin texture

blood pressure
(postural hypotension)

breast atrophy

weight loss

low volume pulse

pubic/axillary hair loss

genital atrophy

Fig. 4.4 Panhypopituitarism in a woman.

tetanus (Fig. 10.4 p. 307). In addition, the face, rather like the clothing, may reflect some aspects of the personality and the evidence of time, expense and care devoted to an individual's appearance may be informative. In children, study of the face is particularly rewarding (Figs 10.3 p. 306 and 10.4 p. 307).

In most cases the characteristics which blend to form the facies must each be considered separately. Some examples of the more common and

more significant findings in the eyes, ears, nose and mouth will illustrate the importance of this aspect of the examination.

The eyes

While the history is being taken, the patient's eyes in particular will be under observation. In addition to purely ocular disorders, there are many other diseases which may have manifestations in and around the eyes. These include conditions involving the respiratory system (p. 134), the nervous system (p. 199) and those found in children (Table 10.1 p. 304). The present section deals with features which are not considered in these more specialised fields.

The eyelids. When the patient is alert, and looking directly ahead the eyelids partially cover the upper and lower margins of the iris. In bright light the orbital fissure narrows, while pain, particularly when this involves the eye, may cause spasm of the eyelids (*blepharospasm*). Conditions in which there is a reluctance to face the light (*photophobia*) include any cause of meningeal irritation, such as subarachnoid haemorrhage or meningitis, painful disorders of the eye and migraine.

Retraction of the eyelids, especially the upper, is a common feature of hyperthyroidism (p. 67). The upper lid retraction means that the sclera is visible above the iris while the patient is gazing straight ahead. In hyperthyroidism, when gaze is directed from above downwards, there may be delay in the downward movement of the upper lid; this is a useful sign known as *lid lag*. When sclera is visible below the iris this usually indicates that the globe of the eye has been displaced forwards (*proptosis* or *exophthalmos*).

Swelling of the eyelids occurs readily owing to looseness of the peri-orbital tissues. Swellings due to trauma and inflammatory lesions are sufficiently common to be familiar to the layman. Periorbital oedema may be due to drug hypersensitivity reactions or to contact dermatitis from cosmetics or hair dyes. Systemic causes include glomerulonephritis (Fig. 10.4 p. 307), angiooedema, infection with *Trichinella spiralis* (trichinosis) and in South Americans or travellers from that continent, infection with *Trypanosoma cruzi* (Chagas' disease). Swelling of the eyelids may be conspicuous in patients with right ventricular failure who are sufficiently free from dyspnoea as to be able to lie flat and will be greater on the side on which the patient has been lying. Swelling of the eyelids may occur in thyrotoxicosis as part of the exophthalmos of Graves' disease. It is almost always present in myxoedema.

A meibomian cyst is a painless swelling due to blockage of a tarsal gland on the internal surface of the lid. A persistently *watering eye* suggests that a nasolacrimal duct is blocked; the opening of the upper ends of these ducts can be seen at the medial end of each lid. The lacrimal glands lying in the upper and outer quadrant of the orbits are not normally visible.

Rodent ulcers (p. 78) are most commonly situated on or near the eyelids, though they are frequent elsewhere on the face. Xanthelasma and xanthomatosis are described on page 87.

The eyelashes. A *stye* is due to staphylococcal infection of a hair follicle and *blepharitis* is the term applied to chronic infection of the edges of the lids. *Ectropion* refers to eversion of the lids and *entropion* to inversion; both conditions predispose to conjunctivitis and in the latter the eyelashes tend to damage the cornea.

The conjunctiva. The palpebral conjunctiva of the lower lid may readily be inspected if the lid is gently everted while the patient looks up. The colour gives an approximate assessment of the patient's haemoglobin level but significant anaemia is easily overlooked, particularly in the elderly.

The upper lid may be everted by using the upper margin of the tarsal plate as a hinge. The patient looks down and the lashes and free margin are grasped between the index finger above and the thumb below. By a twisting movement the tarsal plate can be made suddenly to turn back to front (Fig. 4.5) and any foreign body detected and removed.

Conjunctivitis is often accompanied by photophobia, excessive lacrimation and adhesion of the lids by purulent exudate on wakening. Exudate does not accompany the painful, red, subconjunctival injection of scleritis which otherwise closely resembles conjunctivitis. It should be borne in mind that conjunctival injection at the limbus (corneoscleral junction) is also a feature of iritis and glaucoma.

Pingueculae are triangular yellow deposits beneath the conjunctiva between the canthus and the edge of the cornea. They develop with advancing years and are of no clinical significance. *Pterygium* is a patch of progressive fibrosis in the same area which may encroach upon the cornea, particularly in tropical countries.

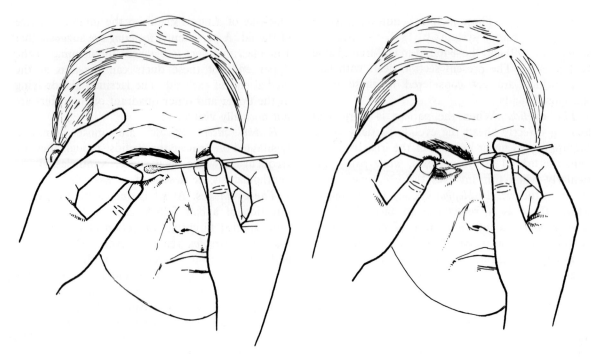

Fig. 4.5 Eversion of the upper lid.

Chemosis is oedema of the conjunctiva and its causes include severe exophthalmos, alcoholism, chronic respiratory failure and obstruction of the superior vena cava; these will be differentiated by other features of the primary condition.

Subconjunctival haemorrhage may obscure the greater part of the sclera and alarm the patient. A bright red colour persists for several days until the blood is absorbed. In the adult it commonly has no obvious cause and may be recurrent. Sometimes it results from coughing, especially whooping cough in children. Occasionally it may be due to basal skull fractures, local trauma or a bleeding disorder.

The sclera. Normal sclera is uniformly white and is the most suitable site for the early detection of jaundice as bilirubin is strongly bound by the plentiful elastic tissue there. It appears blue in osteogenesis imperfecta, a rare hereditary disorder of connective tissue in which the bones are fragile and the sclerae are thin; the blue colour is caused by the choroidal pigment beneath. Recent studies have confirmed Osler's observation that blue sclerae are commonly found in patients with iron deficiency anaemia. In elderly patients scleromalacia often allows the choroidal pigment to be seen as small brown patches on either side of the iris. This condition may also be found in rheumatoid arthritis and may lead to perforation — scleromalacia perforans.

The cornea. Normal cornea is transparent. Haziness of the cornea, accompanied by engorgement of the blood vessels at the limbus, and often an eccentric pupil, are features of acute glaucoma. Even considerable damage to the corneal surface or small embedded foreign bodies may be difficult to recognise without the assistance of fluorescein; with this any breach of the surface will be stained yellow. Opacities of the cornea due to scarring may follow trauma or infection. Corneal damage is more common in patients with exophthalmos or defective tear production. The latter may occur in association with dryness of the mouth (xerostomia) as part of a sicca syndrome or with a connective tissue disease when it is known as Sjögren's syndrome.

Corneal arcus, known also as arcus senilis and arcus lipidus, is a white ring near the outer margin of the cornea; it is commonly present and of no significance in elderly people. In young subjects it may indicate hypercholesterolaemia and be associated with coronary atheroma.

A *Kayser-Fleischer ring* is a yellow or brown deposit of copper at the periphery of the cornea found in Wilson's disease (hepatolenticular degeneration). *Corneal calcification* at the medial and lateral aspects of the cornea-scleral junction is a useful sign suggesting long-standing hypercalcaemia.

The iris. This is inspected while the pupillary reactions are tested. *Iritis* is often a manifestation of systemic disease. Symptoms of *iritis* include pain in the orbit or over the nose or forehead, photophobia and excessive watering of the eye. The vessels of the bulbar conjunctiva at the limbus are dilated and the detailed pattern of the *iris* is blurred. The pupil may be irregular, especially when dilated by a mydriatic, due to adhesions of the iris to the lens (posterior synechiae) which are likely to be permanent.

Intraocular tension. This can be tested digitally but only a very approximate assessment can be made without using a tonometer. The middle, ring and little fingers of both hands of the examiner

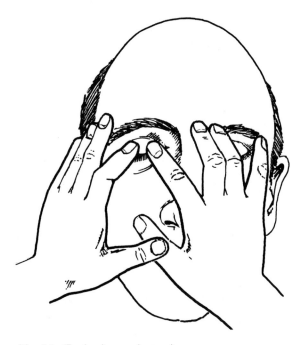

Fig. 4.6   Testing intraocular tension.

should rest on the patient's head in order to steady the hand and the two index fingers are used to test the tension of the globe by eliciting fluctuation (Fig. 4.6). Unless this is done gently, there is some danger of causing retinal detachment, especially if the intraocular tension is high. The importance of detecting the rise in pressure in acute glaucoma is emphasised by the fact that vision is likely to be lost permanently unless treatment is instituted rapidly. The discovery of a low intraocular pressure, though of no importance as regards the eye itself, is useful supportive evidence of dehydration.

Ophthalmoscopic examination. This is described on page 327 to 335.

The ears

The size, shape and form of the auricle vary widely between individuals. Some deformities are of genetic origin; in Down's syndrome the auricles are usually small and the lobule may be rudimentary or absent. The helix of the ear is a recognised site of gouty tophi — white chalky nodules consisting of sodium biurate crystals deposited in the cartilage. Local trauma to the ear may cause haemorrhage which partially organises. This can lead to permanent deformity with the features of 'cauliflower ear'.

Auriscopic examination. The external auditory meatus and the tympanum may be inspected through an auriscope. An improved view of the drum and the meatus will usually be obtained if the auricle is drawn upwards, backwards and slightly laterally in order to straighten the external meatus as much as possible (Fig. 4.7). Wax commonly obscures the view and may be removed by syringing with warm water. A history of middle ear disease or perforation of the drum precludes syringing by the inexperienced. Hard wax may require to be softened by applying a few drops of warm olive oil for two or three nights before removal.

The normal drum appears pearly-grey, with the handle of the malleus visible and lying almost vertically near the centre of the tympanic membrane. A cone of light is reflected from its lower end downwards and forwards to the periphery of the drum (Fig. 4.7).

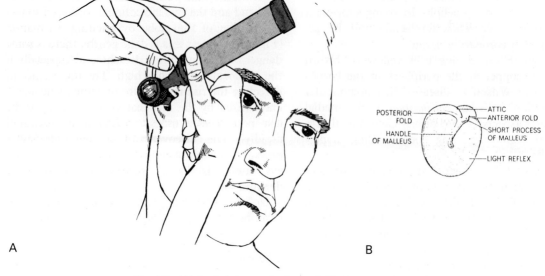

POSTERIOR FOLD
HANDLE OF MALLEUS
ATTIC
ANTERIOR FOLD
SHORT PROCESS OF MALLEUS
LIGHT REFLEX

A   B

Fig. 4.7 (A) Auriscopic examination and (B) the tympanic membrane.

Acute otitis media usually causes earache which may be severe, but in infants it may present as an acute febrile illness without local pain. The common abnormalities on inspection of the drum are acute inflammation and perforation (p. 316). Foreign bodies lodged in the external meatus are not uncommon in children.

The nose and sinuses

The nose may be deformed as a result of an old fracture, or enlarged, red and bulbous (rhinophyma) in the late stages of rosacea. Destruction of the nasal septum by congenital syphilis, local trauma, nasal sniffing of cocaine or Wegener's granulomatosis may produce flattening of the bridge and a 'saddle-nose' appearance. The nose may be narrowed when there is chronic obstruction of the airway in childhood. When associated with mouth breathing this produces the 'adenoidal facies'. Widening of the nose is one of the early features of acromegaly. To test the patency each nostril should be closed in turn by finger pressure and the patient asked to breathe through the other with the mouth closed. The airways should then be examined by direct inspection, preferably with the aid of a nasal speculum. The state of the mucosa and the anterior ends of the inferior turbinates can be visualised; the pearly-grey smooth surface of a polyp or a bleeding point on the nasal septum are two common abnormalities which may be seen. Sniffing of cocaine by addicts may cause ulceration of the nasal mucosa as well as perforation of the septum.

Infection of the frontal air sinuses may cause a headache which characteristically reaches a peak within two or three hours of rising and then spontaneously subsides as the day proceeds. Involvement of the maxillary sinuses may simulate toothache. A purulent nasal or post-nasal discharge is often present and there may be tenderness on pressure over the affected sinus.

The mouth

Routine examination of the mouth, after removal of any dentures, must include inspection of the lips, teeth, gums, tongue, floor of the mouth, mucosa of the cheeks, palate, tonsils and the oropharynx. Any of these structures may be involved by local disease or may show lesions which are part of a systemic disorder. If a mirror is required to examine the nasopharynx and the larynx, then this procedure should be postponed until near the end of the physical examination. The technique of indirect laryngoscopy is described on page 135.

The lips. Exposure to cold commonly causes

dryness followed by desquamation and cracking of the lips. Somewhat resembling this is the much rarer cheilosis of riboflavine deficiency causing red, denuded epithelium at the line of closure of the lips, peeling towards the mucocutaneous junction. A similar appearance may follow the use of lipstick to which the patient is hypersensitive.

Angular stomatitis, consisting of painful inflamed cracks at the corners of the mouth, is often caused by ill-fitting dentures allowing saliva to dribble out of the mouth, followed by infection with *Candida albicans*. Angular stomatitis may also be due to deficiency of iron or riboflavine.

A fissure of the lip in an elderly patient, which fails to heal within two weeks of treatment, should be regarded as a possible epithelioma and requires biopsy.

The teeth. The deciduous teeth are discussed on page 317. Only too often the 32 so-called 'permanent teeth' also have a relatively short life. Inspection of the teeth will give some indication of the patient's attitude to hygiene. The three principal findings are discoloration, caries and missing teeth. Discoloration is usually due to staining from tobacco or from poor hygiene, but devitalised teeth also gradually become grey. Caries may be kept in check for many years by regular dental treatment with fillings. Missing teeth are most commonly the molars; as these are used for grinding rather than biting, their absence is important in connection with alimentary symptoms.

The teeth may be pitted and mottled yellow in fluorosis; notched, separated and peg-shaped upper incisors occur in congenital syphilis (Hutchinson's teeth), and poorly developed (hypoplastic) in juvenile hypoparathyroidism. Eruption of the teeth (Table 13.2 p. 352) may be retarded as part of any disorder responsible for delayed development, especially rickets.

The gums. Gingivitis is very common. At first bleeding is apt to occur, and a narrow line of inflammation can be seen at the free border of the gum, and the interdental papillae are swollen. If the condition progresses, food debris, bacteria and pus tend to accumulate between the teeth and the gum margin (pyorrhoea alveolaris). Halitosis may be apparent and the teeth may become loose. A further hazard is that pus or even a tooth may be aspirated into the bronchial tree and initiate pneumonia. Badly affected gums are associated with frequent transient bacteraemia, the usual organism being *Streptococcus viridans*. This may cause infective endocarditis especially in patients with valvular heart disease. Painful ulceromembranous gingivitis may be due to Vincent's infection (p. 64).

Phenytoin used for the treatment of epilepsy gives rise in some cases to a firm hypertrophy of the gums which may make it desirable to change to some other anticonvulsant. Other abnormalities due to systemic disease are rare, but examples include the soft, spongy haemorrhagic gums of scurvy, the hypertrophied bleeding gums of acute leukaemia and the punctate blue line of chronic lead poisoning.

The tongue. The layman frequently attaches great weight to the appearance of the tongue and may readily develop obsessions about its cleanliness and the significance of any real or imagined changes.

Movement and size of the tongue. The response to the command 'put out your tongue' may provide information about much else besides the movement of the tongue and mandible; for example, a stuporous patient who responds, obviously hears and understands. Even the extent to which a tongue can be protruded may be important; neurological disease, tight frenulum, modesty or a painful condition of the mouth may restrict the movement of the tongue. The symmetry, the size and the shape of the tongue should be noted. Fasciculation (p. 215) should be looked for with the tongue lying at rest within the mouth. It may be seen in motor neurone disease. Wasting of half of the tongue occurs with lesions of the hypoglossal nerve (Fig. 8.22 p. 215) and it is protruded towards the affected side. The tongue is enlarged in Down's syndrome, acromegaly, myxoedema and some cases of amyloidosis. If the organ is asymmetrical, then the possibility of a unilateral lesion must be considered.

The surface of the tongue. This normally varies greatly both in regard to colour and appearance. Shades of pink and red, with a range of grey or even yellow or brown towards the centre, may be acceptable as normal. Variations in colour may be due to foods, particularly coloured sweets, or they may be due to quantitative or qualitative changes in the haemoglobin. Central, cyanosis can best be assessed clinically by inspection of the tongue (p. 132). A clean tongue, often red with prominent papillae, can result from antibiotic treatment.

Small, red, flat elevations can be seen on the surface, especially at the tip and edges; these are the fungiform papillae. The filiform papillae are more numerous at the centre and give rise to the fur. Transient denuded islands (geographical tongue) constitute a symptomless change of no known significance.

Separating the anterior two-thirds from the posterior third of the tongue are the circumvallate papillae (Fig. 8.16 p. 206) set in a wide V with its apex pointing backwards to the foramen caecum. Patients who discover these relatively prominent papillae for themselves are often alarmed by the thought that they might be cancerous. Congenital fissuring of the tongue occurs in varying degrees but has no pathological significance. Iron or vitamin B_{12} deficiency cause a smooth clean looking tongue from diffuse atrophy of the papillae.

Excessive furring, by contrast, is of little significance. It occurs in healthy people and in fever or dehydration. Leukoplakia is characterised by grey opaque areas interspersed with a few red inflamed patches. Occasionally this precancerous condition may be due to syphilis.

The palate. The hard palate comprises the anterior two-thirds, and the soft palate with the uvula lies posteriorly. Deformity such as cleft palate may be noted, and a narrow high arched palate may be found. The latter is of little importance by itself, but may be associated with other congenital abnormalities. The uvula varies much in size and shape; it seldom presents clinical problems except as a source of anxiety to the patient with obsessional disorders focused in the mouth. The examination of movement of the soft palate is described on page 213.

The tonsils. The tonsils are masses of lymphoid tissue which lie beneath the mucous membrane between the pillars of the fauces. In common with lymphoid tissue elsewhere, the tonsils enlarge to reach a maximum between the ages of 8 and 12 years, after which involution takes place. Failure to recognise this normal phase of lymphoid hyperplasia has led to erroneous recommendations for tonsillectomy. Streptococcal tonsillitis must be distinguished from less common causes of sore throats such as infectious mononucleosis, Vincent's infection or diphtheria (p. 65).

Tumours of the tonsils may also occur either in isolation or as part of lymphatic leukaemia or lymphoma.

The pharynx and buccal mucosa. To see the oropharynx adequately it may be necessary to depress the tongue with a spatula and ask the patient to say 'ah' in order to elevate the soft palate. The gag reflex (p. 212) may simultaneously be noted. Small lymphatic nodules can normally be observed on the posterior wall. Mucus or pus consequent on infection in the nose may sometimes be visible trickling down the back of the throat. The nasopharynx can be inspected only with the aid of a suitable mirror and good illumination. After these areas of the mouth and pharynx have been examined, the remainder of the buccal cavity should be checked. A good light or a torch is essential and a spatula is required to separate cheeks and tongue from the teeth and gums. Characteristic abnormalities to be seen here include Koplik's spots (p. 65), aphthous ulcers, and pigmentation.

Pigmentation in the mouth. Melanin deposition in the buccal mucosa is normal in black people and is proportionally less common as the skin becomes lighter, so that usually it is not seen in fair-skinned, fair-haired subjects. Pathological pigmentation in the mouth occurs in Addison's disease. If there are no other suggestive features of this rare condition, the pigmentation is most likely to be congenital in patients with black hair and brown eyes. Other causes which may have to be considered are chronic cachexia, the malabsorption syndrome, haemochromatosis or the rare Peutz – Jeghers syndrome of polyposis of the small intestine with pigmentation around and in the mouth and particularly on the lips and fingers.

The salivary glands. In the course of the examination of the mouth the opening of the parotid duct may be seen on the buccal mucosa as a small papilla opposite the second upper molar tooth. The openings of the ducts of the submandibular salivary glands seldom require identification, but may be found near the midline in the sublingual papilla, adjoining the root of the frenulum of the tongue. Each of these openings is more readily seen if a free flow of saliva is provoked by something tasty. Purulent infections of the salivary glands may be investigated by culturing pus expressed through these orifices.

Causes of enlargement of the parotid gland include mumps, sarcoidosis and tumour. Obstruction of the duct may produce intermittent swelling with pain while eating or may lead to infection of the gland. Obstruction due to salivary calculi is very much more frequent in the submandibular ducts. The submandibular glands may sometimes be affected by mumps in the absence of parotid swelling.

The methods in practice in the diagnosis of some diseases of the mouth

Stomatitis may be a local disorder or an oral manifestation of disease elsewhere.

Ulcerative stomatitis is commonly due to the combination of a spirochaete and a fusiform bacillus which can be seen in a smear taken from one of the ulcers (Vincent's infection). The condition is painful and foul smelling.

Ulcerative stomatitis may also complicate acute leukaemia or agranulocytosis, since these deprive the patient of the normal cellular defence mechanisms against infection. In acute leukaemia the gums often bleed and may be so swollen that the teeth may be largely obscured. Agranulocytosis may present as a sore throat which may progress to an ulcerative stomatitis.

Aphthous stomatitis is characterised by ulcers on the inner sides of the lips, the edges of the tongue, the insides of the cheeks or on the palate. In the earliest stages a small vesicle forms which is quickly destroyed, leaving a shallow ulcer usually surrounded by a red margin. Such ulcers can cause intense discomfort and while they may heal quickly in the course of a day or two, they may progress to form multiple deep indurated ulcers which heal slowly, and may then leave a small scar. The lesions tend to occur in crops; a patient may be free from ulcers for months at a time, only to suffer a relapse. The cause is obscure. They are often seen in patients with ulcerative colitis.

Thrush may occur in the infants of mothers who carry infection with *Candida albicans* in the vagina; it also occurs, particularly in the elderly, in association with febrile or debilitating diseases. It is common in patients being treated with antibiotics, corticosteroids or immunosuppressive drugs. The fungus may be seen as individual or coalescent white deposits adhering to the mucous membrane of any part of the mouth. There is very little evidence of inflammation.

Diphtheria. In this condition a membrane like wash-leather may form particularly on the tonsils and less commonly in the nose or larynx. The affected area bleeds if attempts are made to remove the membrane. The causative organism can be identified on a direct smear and its pathogenicity determined by bacteriological examination. Infectious mononucleosis may also produce a membrane on the tonsils.

Exanthemata (p. 76) often also show lesions of the oral mucosa. In measles small white spots on an erythematosus background are distributed over the mucosa of the cheeks opposite the molar teeth and sometimes throughout the mouth. These Koplik's spots are of particular diagnostic value as they appear before the rash.

Syphilis, in the secondary stage, causes highly infective mucous patches consisting of shallow ulcers with a narrow red margin and a surface covered by a thin white membrane; they resemble snail tracks. The primary ulcer or chancre of syphilis may also occur on the lips, and sometimes in other parts of the mouth.

Carcinoma may be found on the lips, the tongue, the fauces, or the floor of the mouth, usually in the form of an ulcer. Any indolent ulcer requires a biopsy as the only evidence to suggest neoplasia may be the chronicity of the lesion. In the later stages of disease, enlargement of the regional lymph nodes, fixation of the mass, and other signs of malignant disease may appear.

THE NECK

Physical abnormalities in the neck are so common that careful inspection and palpation should be undertaken in any systematic physical examination.

Inspection of the neck will show deformities, abnormal movements, or restriction of movement. Any changes in the skin will be noted, such as scars, unusual pigmentation, rashes, spider telangiectases, abnormal growth of hair, arterial and venous pulsations, or tumours.

Systematic palpation should be carried out, bearing in mind the salivary glands, the lymph nodes and the thyroid gland. From the front the examiner can palpate the back and sides of the neck. The patient should then sit up and the examination continues from behind. Palpation is carried out successively beneath the mandible, over the tonsillar lymph nodes, over the anterior triangles, above the clavicles and especially deep to the sternoclavicular attachments of the sternomastoid muscle where lymph node enlargement may be associated with disease particularly in the chest, and occasionally in the abdomen.

Auscultation over the blood vessels may reveal a murmur arising from carotid or subclavian artery (p. 239).

The thyroid gland

Enlargement of the thyroid gland (*goitre*) is a common occurrence. The presence of a goitre is best observed with the neck slightly extended and identified by its movement when the patient swallows. Palpation is, however, easier from behind with the patient sitting or standing (Fig. 4.8).

Position. The normal thyroid consists of two lateral lobes joined together by a central isthmus which covers the second and third tracheal rings. Hence, the position of a goitre is usually characteristic, but it may extend into the superior mediastinum, or indeed may be entirely retrosternal, and so may not be detected on clinical examination. Rarely, the gland may be located along the line occupied by the thyroglossal duct. When it is situated near the origin on the dorsum of the tongue, the structure is referred to as a lingual goitre. In this situation its nature may be confirmed only by the ability of the swelling to concentrate radioiodine.

Size. The normal thyroid is palpable in about 25% of men and 50% of women. The most frequently used criterion of a goitre (i.e. significant thyroid enlargement) is that the lateral lobes of the

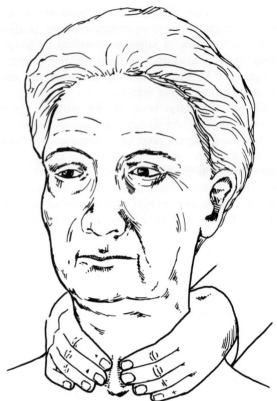

Fig. 4.8 Palpation of the thyroid gland.

thyroid have a volume in excess of that of the terminal phalanges of the thumbs of the patient being examined. The size of a goitre can only be roughly estimated by palpation, but change in the circumference of the neck measured over the point of maximum swelling may be used as an indication of alteration in size. Another method of following changes in thyroid size is to make a frontal plane scan. A ball-point pen is used to outline the goitre and an impression of this is then made on paper moistened with methanol. The paper is then dried and kept as a permanent record in the notes.

Shape. The gland is usually symmetrical in primary hyperthyroidism (Graves' disease) whereas it is irregular in a secondary or nodular toxic goitre. Simple goitres may be relatively symmetrical in their earlier stages, but usually become irregular with time.

Colour changes over a goitre are most unusual, unless it is very big, when distended veins may be responsible for a dusky blue appearance. After exceptionally large doses of radioiodine, thyroiditis occurs and may be associated with slight reddening of the skin, tenderness and perhaps transient dysphagia.

Pain and tenderness may occur in other forms of thyroiditis, particularly the subacute or giant cell variety and may be associated with transient episodes of fever. Dysphagia may also be present.

Mobility. The fact that the thyroid gland is ensheathed by the pretracheal fascia determines its movement on swallowing and distinguishes a goitre from other tumours. However an invasive thyroid carcinoma may lead to fixation of the gland to other surrounding structures and very large goitres may be immobilised because they expand to occupy all the space available in the root of the neck.

Consistency. This may vary from soft to 'stony hard', the latter usually attributable to carcinoma. The texture of the gland may vary from one part to another, just as does the smoothness of its surface. Nodules in the substance of the gland may be large or small, single or multiple.

Enlarged lymph nodes near a goitre will suggest the possibility of carcinoma of the gland particularly if they are firm or hard.

Auscultation. A bruit indicates an abnormally large blood flow. In the untreated state this usually implies hyperthyroidism, but the use of antithyroid drugs may promote an increase in the blood supply sufficient to produce a murmur. It is important not to confuse a thyroid bruit with a murmur arising in the carotid artery or transmitted from the aorta, or a venous hum (p. 111) originating in the internal jugular vein.

Radiological examination of the neck may reveal calcification in the thyroid, narrowing or displacement of the traches, or a retrosternal goitre.

Scanning. A mediastinal swelling is proven to be thyroid if it takes up radioiodine. Radionuclide scanning is also useful in estimating the amount of tissue present, and in detecting 'hot' or 'cold' nodules in the gland. A hot nodule concentrates radioactive iodine more than the surrounding glandular tissue. The overproduction of thyroid hormones by an autonomous nodule will suppress thyroid stimulating hormone (TSH) and hence uptake of the isotope in the rest of the thyroid. A cold nodule will not take up the isotope. A solid cold nodule may require excision to exclude malignancy, whereas a hot nodule is almost always benign. Aspiration cytology may be of considerable value in assessing a cold nodule.

Ultrasonography can usually distinguish between a cystic and a solid tumour (p. 180).

THYROID FUNCTION

The features of thyrotoxicosis include weight loss with increased appetite, heat intolerance, emotional lability, excessive sweating and palpitations. There may be a change in the menstrual cycle and in bowel habit as a consequence of intestinal hurry. In elderly patients however, many of these features may be missing and the condition may be brought to light by the development of atrial fibrillation. Physical signs may include a palpable goitre with bruit, tremor of the outstretched hands (p. 217) and various ocular (p. 59), bone and skin (p. 53) features. Appropriate investigations include measurement of TSH which will be suppressed. Total thyroxine and free thyroxine values are usually raised but may be normal in patients suffering from T3 thyrotoxicosis.

Primary failure of the thyroid gland is associated with an elevated TSH. Circulating thyroid hormones will be reduced. In secondary hypothyroidism, TSH will be low.

Thyroid function tests should also be performed on patients who present with goitre.

THE LYMPHATIC SYSTEM

The lymph nodes should be palpated as a routine in the course of each regional examination. The sites which should be examined include the following: pre- and post-auricular, submandibular, tonsillar, occipital, and posterior and anterior triangles of the neck as described on page 66. The epitrochlear lymph nodes are conveniently felt under the thumb if the patient's right elbow is grasped by the examiner's right hand and vice versa for the left (Fig. 4.9). The procedure is facilitated if, with the other hand, the examiner suspends the patient's arm by the wrist and flexes it at the elbow. The examining hand should then be slid up the inner side of the arm to the axilla,

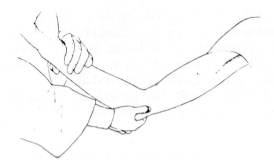

Fig. 4.9   Palpation of the epitrochlear lymph node.

for some lymph nodes lie along the brachial vessels. The right hand should then be used to palpate the vault and medial wall of the left axilla and the left hand for the right axilla (Fig. 4.10). Lymph nodes in the groin and those extending a short distance along with the femoral vessels must also be palpated, though interpretation of the findings in this region is difficult unless enlargement is considerable or change in consistency is unequivocal. While palpating the abdomen it may sometimes be possible to feel gross enlargement of para-aortic or iliac lymph nodes.

Apart from enlargement, there is much diagnostic information to be gained by noting the consistency of the nodes and the presence or absence of tenderness or fixation in accordance with the scheme for the examination of any mass (p. 36). Generalised lymphadenopathy can occur in a variety of viral illnesses, particularly glandular fever. Its finding, if persistent, in male homosexuals, drug addicts, haemophiliacs or others at risk, may suggest the development of the life-threatening acquired immunodeficiency syndrome (AIDS).

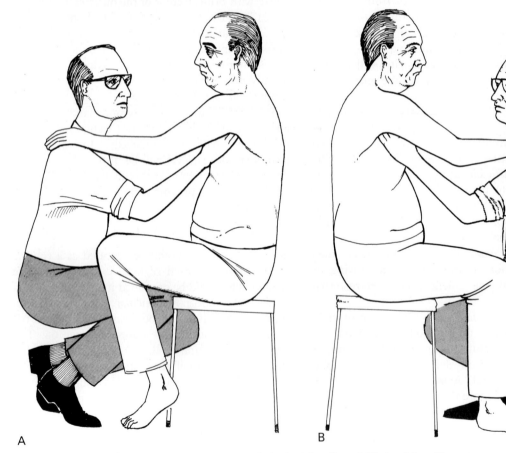

A   B

Fig. 4.10   Palpation of (A) the left axilla and (B) the right axilla.

When there is no obvious local cause for enlarged lymph nodes it is important to examine the reticulo-endothelial system as a whole, including palpation of the liver and spleen. If the outcome points to diffuse involvement, examination of the blood and bone marrow and biopsy of a lymph node may be required. Green needle aspiration or lymph node biopsy is also used in the diagnosis of disseminated neoplasia; biopsy may be helpful in a variety of infections including tuberculosis, bubonic plague, trypanosomiasis and sometimes kala-azar.

THE TRUNK AND LOWER LIMBS

The examination of the trunk and lower limbs is described mainly in the chapters on the nervous and locomotor systems. Fig. 4.12 gives some examples of what can be learned from inspection of the trunk.

The examination of the external genitalia is dealt with in the genito-urinary system and the stages of physical sexual development at puberty are given in the Appendix (Table 13.3 p. 355).

The breasts

General considerations

The female breast is liable to be affected by acute pyogenic abscess, fibrocystic changes and benign and malignant tumours. Since the breast is the most frequent single site of carcinoma in women, a general examination is incomplete unless both breasts have been included. Any mass detected must be regarded as a potentially malignant tumour until this has been excluded.

Breast abscesses are usually preceded by damage to the nipple during the early phase of lactation and seldom cause diagnostic difficulty. With fibrocystic changes, irregular areas of nodularity, usually bilateral, are often combined with tenderness either locally or over a wider area. If changes are localised it may be impossible to exclude carcinoma on clinical examination alone.

Carcinoma characteristically consists of a solitary and often irregular nodule that is firm or hard and usually painless, contrasting sharply in consistency with the surrounding breast tissue. In more ad-

vanced disease there may be evidence of infiltration into the adjacent tissues, fixation to the overlying skin and underlying muscles and enlargement of the regional lymph nodes. Patients with carcinoma of the breast, afraid of cancer, may use denial as a defence mechanism, and occasionally conceal the tumour for many months (Fig. 4.12).

A blood-stained discharge from the nipple may be the only indication of an intraductal tumour which may be so small as to be impalpable. Bilateral inversion of the nipples is a common finding. Unilateral inversion should be an indication to examine the breasts with special care. Retraction or deformity, especially when associated with an eczematous change, developing in a previously normal nipple, is a diagnostic feature of carcinoma. In the male breast carcinoma is rare.

Gynaecomastia (enlargement of the male breast, Fig. 4.12) occurs in about 50% of normal boys at the time of puberty probably because of the relatively high oestradiol levels in comparison to testosterone in the afternoon and evening. Many drugs can cause breast enlargement (e.g. oestrogens used in the treatment of prostatic cancer, spironolactone, cimetidine). It is also found with increased oestrogen production (interstitial cell tumours of the testis, some adrenal tumours, cirrhosis of liver, thyrotoxicosis) or decreased androgen production (hypergonadotrophic hypogonadism, Klinefelter's syndrome, orchitis, hypogonadotrophic hypogonadism). In rare cases there may be tissue resistance to androgens leading to gynaecomastia.

Galactorrhoea suggests that prolactin levels may be elevated. There is usually associated Montgomery tubercle hyperplasia. Spontaneous milk production is uncommon and often galactorrhoea is found only by trying to express milk. The causes of hyperprolactinaemia include physiological processes (pregnancy, postpartum), drugs (dopamine antagonists, dopamine depleting agents), pituitary tumours, hypothalamic and stalk lesions, primary hypothyroidism and renal failure.

Anatomical and physiological considerations

The stages in the development of the female breast are given in Table 13.5 (p. 355). For the purposes of examination and description, the breast may be divided into the nipple, the areola and four quadrants, upper and lower, inner and outer, with the axillary tail projecting from the upper and outer quadrant. The adult nipple consists of erectile tissue covered with pigmented skin which is shared with the areola. The openings of the lactiferous ducts may be seen near the apex of the nipple. The size and shape of the breast in healthy women vary widely in accordance with hereditary factors, sexual maturity, the phase of the menstrual cycle, parity, pregnancy and lactation, and the general state of nutrition. The amount of fat and stroma surrounding the glandular tissue largely determines the size of the breast except during lactation, when the temporary enlargement is almost entirely glandular.

Swelling and some tenderness of the breasts commonly occur in the week before and at the time of menstruation. This engorgement is sometimes attributed to fluid retention associated with fluctuations in the secretion of ovarian oestrogens and progesterone. Palpation may show that the glandular elements of the breasts are more readily detected then than at other times, and they give an impression of radiating strands of firm tissue with a variable degree of granularity. The ease with which the glandular elements of the breast can be felt also varies with the age of the patient, the prominence of the glandular tissue and the quantity of the surrounding fat. There is also a tendency for the strands to be less obvious towards the periphery.

Procedure for examination

Whenever the presence of a carcinoma is suspected, the procedure detailed below should be carried out. If the breast is being examined as part of a general examination, it may be acceptable to use a less complete procedure, palpating the breast as described below, but with the patient in one position only.

An adequate examination of the breasts requires that the patient should be completely undressed to the waist and initially should be seated on a chair. The doctor should sit opposite the patient in a good light and, if male, should be chaperoned. Occasionally special care may be required to avoid

offending the unduly modest patient, but this should never prevent a complete examination.

Before proceeding to palpation, a systematic inspection of both breasts should be undertaken. Any asymmetry should be sought, together with changes in the skin, the nipple and the presence of any local swelling. In order to emphasise any local change, and in particular the presence of a mass or an area of fixation, the patient should be asked to take up each of several positions in turn.

1. The patient's hands are resting on the thighs so that the pectoral muscles are relaxed (Fig. 4.11a).
2. The hands are firmly pressed on to the hips ensuring contraction of the pectoral muscles (Fig. 4.11b) but with the patient sitting symmetrically.
3. The arms are raised above the head, stretching the pectoral muscles as well as the skin overlying and surrounding the breast (Fig. 4.11c).
4. The patient leans well forward so that the breasts are pendulous (Fig. 4.11d).
5. Finally, the breasts are examined while the patient is lying flat on a couch or bed, with the side under review raised by a pillow (Fig. 4.11e).

In each position the breast is inspected, followed by palpation of the four quadrants and the axillary tail in turn. The breasts should be examined with the palm of the hand and the tissue rolled gently against the chest wall. This will have the effect of

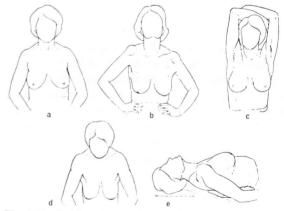

Fig. 4.11 Positions for examination of the breasts. Note in (b) that the patient is not symmetrically positioned and that this is reflected in an apparent difference in the breasts.

accentuating a tumour, while fibrocystic changes become apparent as a more generalised abnormality. If a mass is noted or suspected it should also be felt with the finger-tips so as to elicit the other characteristics of any lump, as described on page 36. One of the features of carcinoma of the breast is 'tethering' of the skin. This may not be obvious at first, but if the breast is elevated gently by the hand, the area of dimpling overlying the tumour may become visible immediately.

A complete examination of the breasts must include palpation of the regional lymph nodes. The examination of the axillae should be undertaken first with the arms relaxed in order to explore the apex of the axilla and then with the hands on the hips in order to tense the axillary fascia and to contract the pectoral muscles. Finally, evidence of any involvement of the supraclavicular lymph nodes should be sought. Findings may be recorded on a simple diagram (Fig. 3.2 p. 37).

The nature of a lump in the breast can often be determined with reasonable certainty by the application of these methods, but it is unusual for a final decision to be reached on clinical grounds alone. Mammography and fine needle aspiration cytology are helpful but for most solid, solitary lesions an excisional biopsy will be required. Mammography has also been introduced to undertake population screening programmes for the early detection of breast cancer.

THE SKIN

Structure and functions

The skin consists of a thin, superficial, avascular, cellular layer (the epidermis) and a deeper, tough fibro-elastic layer (the dermis) which also contains nerves, blood vessels, sweat glands, sebaceous glands and hair follicles. Beneath the skin there is a layer of areolar tissue containing fat. The amount of fat varies widely in different parts of the body and from one individual to another.

The skin protects the deeper parts from trauma, from infection and from extremes of heat and cold. Vitamin D_3 is formed in the skin from 7-dehydrocholesterol in response to ultra-violet light, and harmful effects of this form of radiation are reduced by the melanin pigment also formed in the skin. Mammals are insulated against cold and wet by hair and by the secretions of the sebaceous glands, and heat loss can be minimised by erection of the hairs consequent on contraction of involuntary muscle fibres — the errectores pilorum. A vestige of this reaction is seen in man in the form of 'goose-flesh'. The skin is of vital importance in dissipating heat by vasodilatation and sweating, and it conserves heat by vasoconstriction aided by the insulating effect of the subcutaneous fat. It serves as a channel for the excretion not only of water and electrolytes, but also of normal and abnormal metabolites and drugs.

Disease ensues if any of the main structures of the skin are missing or cease to function. Thus breaches of the surface are liable to lead to systemic infection; ultra-violet light causes sunburn in unpigmented skins; failure of sweating results in death from hyperpyrexia in hot climates; vasodilatation in a cold atmosphere may result in death from hypothermia, a combination which is apt to occur in coma from excess of alcohol; loss of nerve function may result in trophic ulcers; cuts and burns of the skin of the hands accompany the absence of pain and temperature sense in syringomyelia. In addition there is a wide variety of primary disorders of the skin and there are many dermal manifestations of systemic disease.

Examination

When examining the skin, attention must be paid to abnormalities of its structure and function and to any pathological lesions present. The discovery and differentiation of disorders affecting the skin depend largely upon inspection, though palpation sometimes has a useful part to play. Normal practice, especially when the main complaint appears to be a dermatological disorder, should include examination of the whole body surface. This is usually carried out in stages as the various systems are examined.

Colour. Localised or generalised variations in colour are similar to those described for the complexion (p. 46). *Pigmentation* has already been discussed (p. 46). The body may also be somewhat pigmented in the unclean, especially in those instances in which there is infestation with body lice (*Pediculus corporis*). Chronic inflammation, as is often seen in varicose eczema, may give rise to pigmentation. Some localised colour changes are produced by fungal infections such as pityriasis versicolor and numerous other skin diseases. In a patient who has been resident abroad tuberculoid leprosy is a possibility if depigmented anaesthetic patches are found.

The climate in Britain leads to another striking form of pigmentation, *erythema ab igne*, or 'Granny's tartan'. This is commonly seen on the legs of women who sit close to a fire for long periods, and is therefore more often found in the

elderly and in the inactive. The pigmentation is at first red and later brown in colour, and follows the distribution of cutaneous venous plexuses, thus providing the appearance of a coarse net. Even patients with hypopituitarism whose facial pallor is so characteristic, are liable to this form of pigmentation, and indeed these and hypothyroid patients may be specially susceptible because of their intolerance of cold. The discovery of a similar pattern on the skin of the abdomen or elsewhere, due to the local application of heat, suggests chronic pain (Fig. 4.12).

Texture and sebaceous secretion. Normal skin

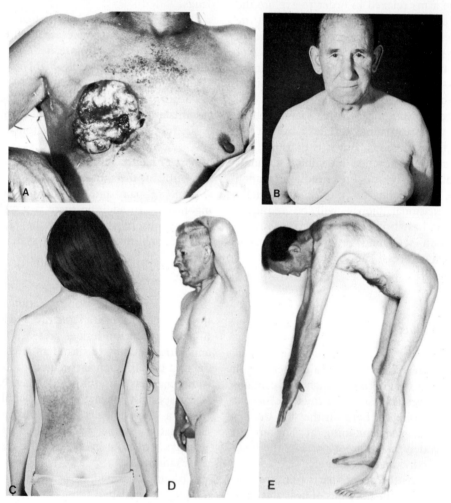

Fig. 4.12 The trunk as a diagnostic aid. (A) Carcinoma of breast, concealed by patient for many months, denial being used as a defence mechanism. (B) Gynaecomastia due to oestrogen therapy for prostatic carcinoma. (C) Erythema ab igne in an unusual site where heat has been applied for chronic pain.(D) Loss of body hair and pallor of the skin in hypopituitarism.
(E) Advanced ankylosing spondylitis with marked loss of flexion of the spine.

has a fine texture and a slightly moist surface. A relatively common disorder is the dry, scaly skin of congenital ichthyoses (fish-skin). In myxoedema the skin also becomes dry and coarse. In contrast is the greasy skin often noted after puberty with its liability to acne vulgaris. Over-active and hypertrophied sebaceous glands become blocked by comedones (blackheads) which consist of plugs of semi-solid secretion capped by horny debris darkening on oxidation. This may develop into an inflamed papule and then a pustule which ultimately bursts. Larger lesions result in permanent scarring. Acne is characteristically distributed over the face, back of the neck, and the front and back of the chest.

Sweating. Diffuse sweating counters the rise of body temperature liable to occur in hot atmospheres, during exercise, in fevers or in hyperthyroidism. Episodes of sweating occur in fainting, in shock, with severe pain, during menopausal flushes, in acute hypoglycaemia or during acute hypertensive episodes caused by a phaeochromocytoma. Sweating on the face, palms, soles and in the axillae is often due to anxiety. Interruption of the sympathetic nerve supply, as in Horner's syndrome (p. 200) or with a more extensive autonomic neuropathy, causes a local loss of sweating.

Sweat contains most of the solutes of blood, but their concentration is much less than in a filtrate of plasma. In cystic fibrosis a characteristic increase can be demonstrated in the concentration of sodium chloride in the sweat (p. 322). In diabetes mellitus the glucose content of sweat is high, and this predisposes to skin infections, particularly with fungi and pyogenic organisms.

A febrile patient, though not sweating visibly, may lose a considerable amount of fluid. Even more serious account must be taken of visible sweating, which may be responsible for the daily loss of several litres of water containing electrolytes in a concentration of about one-third of that in the plasma.

Hyperhidrosis, or excessive and inappropriate sweating, is usually confined to the axillae, the palms, and the soles and its odour may cause considerable embarrassment. Hyperhidrosis predisposes to 'Athlete's foot', a fungal infection which occurs in the interdigital clefts and is characterised by painful cracks in thick, white, sodden skin.

Skin temperature. Differences in temperature between symmetrical regions can be detected with remarkable accuracy by the back of the examiner's fingers, provided that the hand is not cold. Excluding the recent application of heat to the part, a local rise in temperature is due to an increased blood flow. This may be due to inflammation, to Paget's disease of underlying bone, or to tumours with a large blood supply. It may also be due to a recent deep venous thrombosis with a shift of circulation into the skin vessels, or to chronic arterial block which has resulted in the opening up of collateral circulation through the skin.

In contrast to local increases of temperature, local cooling, particularly of a limb or part of a limb, raises the possibility of arterial occlusion (p. 93). In some circumstances, for example with a 'saddle embolus' lodged on the bifurcation of the aorta, both lower limbs might be equally cool.

Nails and hair. Abnormalities of these structures are discussed on pages 54 and 57 respectively.

Lesions of the skin. Specific points in the history may require special attention, for example, the possibility of contact with infectious disease like childhood fevers, scabies, syphilis or leprosy. Contact with animals or occupations involving the handling of animal products introduces the possibility of unusual infections of the skin such as animal ringworm, or erysipeloid, and anthrax. The distribution of the lesions may suggest contact dermatitis, when special enquiry must be made about work, the purchase of new clothing, jewellery, or the application of new cosmetics or hair dyes. Another important factor may be the effects of medicaments which may have been applied with or without medical advice. For example, use of topical steroids may mask or alter many of the common features of various skin diseases including dermatitis and fungal infection. To add to the diagnostic difficulty, many variants of the typical appearance and distribution of the lesions may be seen and further differences may arise from the effects of scratching causing secondary infection.

When assessing the significance of the abnormalities account must not only be taken of their type and distribution but also whether associated lesions are to be found, for example in the mucous membrane of the mouth or nose, the conjunctiva, or the genital area. Enlarged lymph nodes in the drainage area may result from inflammatory or neoplastic conditions of the skin.

Descriptive terms

Most abnormalities can be defined by one or more of the following terms:

Erythema means reddening of the skin, and the term is usually qualified by an adjective such as diffuse, punctate, macular or papular. A *macule* indicates a small circumscribed spot such as a freckle. *Papular* lesions are by definition raised above the surrounding surface of the skin and this can easily be confirmed by running the finger-tips over the affected area. *Vesicular* lesions (blisters) may be superimposed on the changes already mentioned, and consist of collections of fluid in the epidermis or the dermis. Vesicles vary in size, the larger being described as *bullae*. If the fluid within vesicles becomes purulent the lesions are known as *pustules*. *Urticaria* is a raised pale area of skin, varying in width from a few millimetres to several centimetres. It is caused by an increase in interstitial fluid with a high protein content due in turn to increased capillary permeability. The lesions are surrounded by a flare resulting from arteriolar dilatation through an axon reflex. A similar mechanism affecting the subcutaneous tissues gives rise to the less well-defined swelling of *angio-oedema*.

Visible *scaling* or *desquamation* due to abnormal growth of the skin is a feature of many chronic skin lesions. The superficial keratin layer remains nucleated and no longer rubs off imperceptibly. Removal of the epidermis when the lesion is scaly may help to distinguish between psoriasis which leaves a dry surface with bleeding points, and eczema in which a moist, weeping area is exposed.

Linear markings known as *cutaneous striae* may sometimes be seen around the abdomen, shoulders, buttocks and thighs. Those of recent origin are pink, while older striae are white or opalescent. They are found in healthy adolescents after sudden weight gain, in pregnancy and in obesity. In Cushing's syndrome the striae tend to be darker red in colour and more conspicuous than in other conditions.

The observation of *scars* may remind patients of operations which have been forgotten. Puncture marks of hypodermic injections may be noted in diabetics usually in the thighs or anterior abdominal wall. In other circumstances, they should raise suspicions of addiction to drugs such as heroin or cocaine.

Some common dermatological abnormalities and their significance

Examination of the skin seldom fails to reveal some abnormality. Many are of limited significance, for example callosities, moles, freckles, erythema ab igne, warts and acne. Medically trivial skin lesions should be treated with a respect and sympathy which may seem disproportionate to their gravity. The doctor is aware that a few acne pustules on the face of a teenage girl are of no great relevance and that the condition will clear up spontaneously in a few years. From the girl's viewpoint, however, this disfigurement is a social embarrassment which may well influence her behaviour and colour her whole outlook on life.

The student can soon become familiar with common abnormalities by paying attention to the skin in every patient. By so doing, the less usual and sometimes far more important conditions will also be noticed. Some of the more common lesions encountered are discussed separately under the headings of vascular abnormalities, infections, hypersensitivity reactions, cutaneous manifestations of generalised disease, and primary skin disorders, including tumours. Such an outline provides some indication of what can be learned from a careful study of the skin. For a detailed description of individual lesions, the student should consult a textbook of dermatology.

Vascular abnormalities of the skin

Purpura and ecchymosis

Spontaneous bleeding into the skin may be manifest as purpura of various sizes and shapes, or in the subcutaneous tissues it may be visible as ecchymoses (bruises).

Petechiae are the most common manifestations of purpura. They are red or blue lesions of about

1 to 3 mm in diameter visible in the skin deep to the epidermis. Since they consist of extravasated blood they fail to disappear on pressure or on stretching the skin in the affected areas. By contrast, lesions with an intact vasculature can be made to fade and on release of the pressure the colour returns as in spider telangiectasia. Petechiae tend to occur in crops, and unless replaced by fresh lesions, disappear in three or four days. They should be regarded as evidence of abnormal capillary fragility. This can be demonstrated by *Hess's test* in which a sphygmomanometer cuff is applied to the upper arm and maintained between the systolic and diastolic pressure for five minutes. Many purpuric spots appear on the forearm when capillary fragility is increased.

Senile purpura is common in elderly patients and is usually confined to the dorsal surfaces of the forearms and hands. The lesions are dark red and remain so until they fade after many days or even weeks. The skin wrinkles readily and it is so thin that the blood in the veins is seen to be red. The lesions are flat in spite of being up to 2 cm or so in diameter. Small white, often stellate, scars and brown patches may result from previous lesions. The bleeding is produced by shearing strains on the skin which tear the vessels lacking the normal collagenous support. Similar changes occur in patients of any age on long-term treatment with corticosteroids; and in both cases there is a correlation with osteoporosis.

Ecchymoses or bruises usually result from trauma, but their significance may increase in proportion to the triviality of the injury which has produced them. Spontaneous bruising for no demonstrable reason occurs more often in women than in men. Ecchymoses persist longer than petechiae and usually undergo a series of colour changes in the skin from blue to green, yellow and brown as the extravasated blood is broken down. The blood clotting mechanism should be investigated if the liability to bruising from minor injury is acquired.

Significance of purpura and ecchymosis. A liability to bleed into the skin or subcutaneous tissues may be due to one of many defects in the process of blood clotting. Thrombocytopenic purpura may occur either as a result of diminished platelet production or because of increased platelet destruction. Other causes of purpura include a vasculitis as in Henoch's purpura, inadequacy of the capillary intercellular cement substance as in scurvy and toxic damage to the small blood vessels. The last may occur in uraemia, from a wide variety of drugs, or in infections such as meningococcal meningitis. The size and the distribution of the lesions may be very useful guides to the cause of the bleeding. Thus generalised bruises and petechiae, combined perhaps with evidence of bleeding elsewhere in an otherwise healthy patient, are suggestive of thrombocytopenic purpura. Petechiae in a patient who is obviously unwell might suggest leukaemia, infective endocarditis or uraemia. A raised purpuric eruption, usually distributed symmetrically and mainly over the extremities, suggests the Henoch-Schönlein syndrome if associated with abdominal pain or arthralgia. Massive painful bruising of the legs with induration of the muscles, and perifollicular haemorrhage, in an elderly person living alone, are almost pathognomonic of scurvy (Plate II).

Dilatation of blood vessels

Obstruction of the blood flow through main vessels may lead to the development of a *collateral circulation*. Venous collaterals are observed much more frequently than arterial because superficial veins are normally visible and are more obvious when distended. Arterial collateral are seldom detected in conditions other than coarctation of the aorta (p. 94). Dilatation of the small veins (*telangiectasia*) of the face is not necessarily pathological; such an appearance is, however, liable to develop in chronic alcoholics and in those exposed to the rigours of the weather. Small irregular telangiectases also accompany the pigmentation and scarring which follow radiation damage to the skin, and they may be a feature of a number of skin disorders.

Spider telangiectases are characterised by a central arterial dot from which radiate several dilated vessels, all of which are readily obliterated by central pressure. Refilling commences from the central arteriole feeding the vessels. These lesions occur on the face, arms and upper part of the body and are particularly common in patients with hepatic cirrhosis, though they may also be seen in relatively small numbers in pregnancy and hyperthyroidism and occasionally in normal people.

Hereditary haemorrhagic telangiectasia is an uncommon disease in which dilated blood vessels present as dark red spots or larger swellings up to 1 or 2 mm in diameter. They refill readily after being emptied by finger pressure. The lesions occur especially about the face and on the mucous membranes of the mouth and nose, and also at the fingertips. Epistaxis is common and severe iron deficiency anaemia may develop from gastrointestinal blood loss.

Haemangiomas (Campbell de Morgan spots) commonly develop on the chest and abdomen with advancing years. They consist of firm, bright red to purple swellings, about 1 to 2 mm in diameter, usually raised slightly above the surface of the skin. Only with difficulty can they be made to fade on pressure. They have no recognised significance.

A congenital diffuse angioma on the face, colloquially known as a port wine stain, is not uncommon. The disfigurement alone is serious enough for the patient but the lesion may also be associated with a calcifying intracranial angioma causing epilepsy, as well as glaucoma and cataract (Sturge-Weber syndrome).

Infections and infestations of the skin

The *exanthemata* such as scarlet fever, measles, rubella and chickenpox have characteristic skin eruptions. This is also true of *syphilis* in its secondary stage.

Herpes simplex consists of a vesicle or a group of several vesicles on an erythematous base. A dark scab may form as the vesicles dry. The lesions are usually found on the mucocutaneous junction round the mouth but occasionally may occur elsewhere on the skin or mucosae particularly in the genital areas. The condition is due to a viral infection and in susceptible subjects may recur during trivial fevers such as common colds or even as a result of excessive exposure to sunlight. Herpes simplex is also a frequent accompaniment of pneumococcal, meningococcal and malarial infections.

Herpes zoster, ('shingles'), is caused by infection of the posterior root ganglion with the varicella-zoster virus. The ophthalmic division of the trigeminal nerve may be affected and this may lead to corneal ulceration. There may be a prodromal period of several days characterised by pain in the distribution of the appropriate nerve mimicking conditions such as pleurisy, cholecystitis, sciatica, or sinusitis. If the condition is recognised at an early stage and treated with acyclovir the progress of the disease may be altered. Otherwise the skin in the same area develops an irregular erythema upon which groups of vesicles appear. These in turn ulcerate, and in the course of two weeks or more dry up and are replaced by crusted lesions which finally separate. Permanent scarring of the skin is common and may be the only sign in patients with post-herpetic pain, which is sometimes severe and persistent, particularly in the elderly. Occasionally, segmental weakness and muscle wasting accompany or follow the eruption due to involvement of the lower motor neurone. The incidence of herpes zoster is high in patients whose immune mechanisms are impaired by systemic illness or by immunosuppressive drugs.

Bacterial infections of the skin are commonly due to *Staphylococcus aureus* or to *Streptococcus haemolyticus*. The former causes focal lesions such as boils; the latter produces spreading lesions like erysipelas or cellulitis. Both are potent sources of cross infection which may readily become disseminated in surgical wards, children's hospitals, schools and among debilitated persons. Much less common bacterial infections of the skin include diphtheria, tuberculosis, anthrax and erysipeloid.

Infestation of the skin and hair by lice and other insects is not uncommon, and is easily overlooked. Ticks and mites may be acquired from contact with crops or with domestic animals, and their presence should be suspected if bites or itching follow such exposure. Ticks are readily seen. The head is buried in the skin and the body swells as it distends with blood. In *scabies*, a mite (*Sarcoptes scabies*) burrows beneath the epidermis, particularly into the fine skin of the web of the fingers, the wrists, feet and penis, and often leaves a shallow linear track. Itching, especially at night, is a cardinal feature, and scratch marks are common, sometimes becoming secondarily infected. The parasite can be identified under the low power of a microscope if it is picked out of the burrow in the skin with a needle and placed in a drop of 5% potassium hydroxide on a glass slide.

One species of flea, *Pulex irritans*, is fully adapted to man. Infected fleas from rodents are responsible for transmitting plague and endemic typhus fever.

Infestation with *Pediculus capitis* (the head louse) is most readily recognised by the presence of the eggs (nits) on the hair of the host. These superficially resemble flakes of dandruff, but are found to be firmly fixed to the hair. Once eggs are seen the lice can usually be found by using a fine-toothed comb.

Pediculus corporis (the body louse) is found upon the trunk and in the axillae and the ova are laid on the underclothes. *Phthirius pubis* (the crab louse) may be found on the pubis, in the axillae, on the chest wall or on the eyebrows. It is very much smaller than the head or body louse. It may burrow into the epidermis and may easily be overlooked because it remains virtually immobile. Undisturbed, it presents after feeding on blood as a blue spot, and when fasting as a light brown spot about 1 mm in diameter. Infestation with crab lice is transferred only by close contact, and can be classed as a sexually transmitted infection.

Cutaneous hypersensitivity reactions

The antigen may reach the skin by the blood stream or may react with the skin through external contact. Both immediate and delayed types of hypersensitivity occur, as exemplified by urticaria and dermatitis. A specific food such as shellfish may occasionally be incriminated, but nowadays drugs are more usually responsible for immediate hypersensitivity reactions. Enquiry should therefore be made not only about drugs and injections but also about any self-medication. Drugs such as aspirin can easily be overlooked.

An external agent should be suspected from the distribution of a rash; it may be detected by considering the patient's occupation or by obtaining a history of contact with a new garment, cosmetic, soap, watch strap, etc., in accordance with the possibilities raised by the areas involved.

Cutaneous manifestations of generalised disease

A few examples will be given of disease processes in which the importance of the dermatological changes lies in the information they give about disease elsewhere. Skin manifestations often supply part of the evidence of *vitamin deficiency*, as for example follicular hyperkeratosis (vitamin A), cheilosis, angular stomatitis (riboflavin), pellagra (nicotinic acid) and bleeding into the legs in scurvy (vitamin C).

The skin is frequently involved in the *connective tissue disorders*, especially in scleroderma (p. 54), dermatomyositis and systemic lupus erythematosus. In the last an erythematous eruption may be present over the bridge of the nose and adjacent part of the cheeks (butterfly rash, Plate I). *Sarcoidosis* may involve the skin producing papules, nodules or plaques, and is also one of the causes of *erythema nodosum* — a series of red, painful, tender, indurated swellings, varying in size from a few millimetres to several centimetres in diameter (Plate II). They are to be found most constantly over the front of the legs, though they may also extend over the knees and on the thighs, and may even be found on the extensor surface of the arms of forearms. In children and young adults primary tuberculosis or streptococcal infection is responsible more often than sarcoidosis. Erythema nodosum, like *erythema multiforme* (Plate II), may also be precipitated by drugs such as sulphonamides.

Dermatitis artefacta (Plate I) is found in patients with personality disorders. The typical injuries in self-mutilation include superficial lacerations of the wrist and forearms or repetitive minor trauma to the face, neck and other exposed areas of the body.

Xanthomatosis is often associated with hypercholesterolaemia (p. 87).

These examples serve to demonstrate that cutaneous lesions are often present in a wide range of systemic disorders. The skin manifestation may provide the main diagnostic clue. The important lesson is to learn to look at the skin and to question the significance of every abnormality that can be observed.

Primary disorders of the skin

Psoriasis is one of the commonest primary skin disorders. The lesions are usually clearly defined, scaly, erythematous patches with a predilection for the extensor surfaces of the elbows or knees. When the patches are scratched numerous distinctive silvery scales are produced. Involvement of the fingernails (Fig. 4.2) and joints occurs in some cases (p. 55).

Both benign and malignant skin *tumours* may occur. In a *papilloma* all elements of the skin are involved, while other benign tumours may be derived from the individual tissues comprising skin, for example sebaceous cysts, lipomas, neurofibromas and vascular naevi. *Sebaceous cysts* can be distinguished by the fact that they arise in the dermis and therefore move freely with the skin and are attached to it near the central point where a comedo (blackhead) may be present. The swelling, if not too tense, may be indented by pressure. *Neurofibromas* are relatively rare but most frequently arise from small branches of cutaneous nerves causing dermal nodules of varying sizes, some of which may become pedunculated. They are usually associated with scattered patches of brown (café au lait) pigmentation (Plate I). They are important not only because of the disfigurement they cause, but also because they are occasionally associated with tumours of nervous tissue elsewhere, for example, on spinal nerve roots, acoustic neuromas, meningiomas or the tumours of chromaffin tissue forming phaeochromocytomas. *Naevi* are congenital lesions which include *angiomas* (port wine stain) and *melanomas* (moles). The latter may become malignant (Plate I). Any change in a melanoma or any irregularity in its colour, outline or surface may signify malignancy.

Basal cell carcinoma or *rodent ulcer* is a locally malignant tumour which is very frequently seen about the face in elderly persons. These growths start as pearly-white nodules which slowly enlarge until the centre becomes crusted or ulcerated. The *squamous cell carcinoma* or *epithelioma*, in contrast, is a rapidly growing tumour which may spread to adjacent tissues and to the lymph nodes at an early stage. Kaposi's sarcoma is a characteristic skin condition commonly associated with patients infected with HIV. The lesions are violacious in colour and gradually darken with time, becoming elevated firm nodules. They can be widely distributed but occur more commonly in the arms than the legs. These lesions are not usually painful or itchy. *Metastases* to the skin from distant sites such as the lung, the breast, or the kidney usually occur after the primary diagnosis has already been made. Sometimes, however, a carcinoma will first present as a cutaneous metastasis, and if this is suspected biopsy should always be undertaken.

THE METHODS IN PRACTICE: THE DETECTION OF DRUG ABUSE

This example has been chosen because of the prevalence of drug addiction and because it illustrates the need for alertness on the part of the clinician if the condition is to be recognised.

The increasing variety of preparations on which patients become dependent, coupled with the implications that this carries for the doctor who may encounter such patients unexpectedly, makes it important that the few signs which may be present are recognised without delay. Drug addicts are commonly sociopathic and disturbance of behaviour may be apparent particularly when supplies are short or withdrawal is in progress. This is most frequently encountered in alcoholics but corresponding features characteristic of the individual drug may be seen on withdrawal in many other forms of drug abuse, for example when narcotics, cannabis, barbiturates or amphetamines are involved. These may be used in isolation or in various combinations.

The withdrawal syndrome is usually characterised by irritability, restlessness, tremor, sweating, lacrimation, nausea and abdominal pain. An overdose of a powerful narcotic such as heroin may lead to coma with constricted pupils, depressed or periodic respiration, hypotension, and with recovery, vomiting. Evidence may be found of needle punctures, thrombosed veins (Fig. 4.3), ulcers at injection sites, skin sepsis or hepatitis transmitted by infected needles.

The addict will use any subterfuge to obtain drugs such as, for example, feigning illness at a doctor's surgery or at the hospital casualty department. Individuals dependent on drugs are often very knowledgeable about medical and hospital procedures and pass from one doctor or hospital and one town or city to another taking advantage of every opportunity to obtain the drugs they require. Nowadays clinicians should be on the watch for such patients, and be prepared to undertake a careful search for evidence of addiction.

REFERENCES

Bates B 1987 A guide to physical examination and history taking, 4th edition. J B Lippincott Company, Philadelphia.
Burton J L 1990 Essentials of Dermatology 3rd Ed Churchill Livingstone, Edinburgh.
Jamieson M J, McHardy K C, Towler H M A et al 1990 Essential Clinical Signs. Churchill Livingstone, Edinburgh.

Kamal A, Brocklehurst J C 1983 A colour atlas of geriatric medicine. Wolfe Medical Publications, Chicago.
Walker W F 1976 A colour atlas of general surgical diagnosis. Wolfe Medical Publications, Chicago.

5. The cardiovascular system

D. P de Bono

Clinical examination of the cardiovascular system is particulary rewarding in that the symptoms and signs elicited can often be explained in terms of basic physics, anatomy and physiology, and will frequently allow an accurate diagnosis to be made at the bedside. At the same time, recent developments in therapeutics and the increasing scope of cardiac surgery has set new standards for accuracy and completeness of diagnosis and some patients will therefore require further detailed investigation.

THE HISTORY

SYMPTOMS OF HEART DISEASE

Dyspnoea, pain, oedema and palpitations are the principal manifestations of heart disease, and are discussed in detail as their analysis depends on an understanding of their origin and significance. It is the symptoms which provide a measure of functional capacity. However, it is important to appreciate that severe heart disease may be asymptomatic, and come to light only when a complication arises, as, for example, when an arterial embolism occurs.

The general principles which are involved in the assessment of the severity of a symptom have been described in Chapter 1. It is a common practice in the field of cardiology to use the term 'functional grade' to denote the degree of incapacity caused by pain or dyspnoea.

The New York Heart Association Classification of Functional Grade in Heart Disease grades as follows:

Grade I   No limitation of any activities
Grade II   No limitation of ordinary daily activities, but symptoms on vigorous exertion.
Grade III   Everyday activities limited by symptoms, but still ambulant.
Grade IV   All activities very limited — chairbound or bedbound.

Though such a classification may be a useful abbreviation it is no substitute for a succinct record of the patient's description of the symptoms. Questions which often prove helpful include the following: 'What do you now find difficult which you used to be able to do easily?'; 'When you are walking, can you talk at the same time?'; or 'Do you now keep others back?'; or, when there is difficulty in establishing when a symptom occurs (e.g. cardiac pain), it is often useful to say — 'If I wanted to see you with the pain, what could you do to bring it on?'.

Dyspnoea

The analysis of breathlessness is discussed on page 32, but some elaboration is necessary here from the cardiac aspect.

Dyspnoea on effort is usually the first symptom of left heart failure. Exercise leads to increased venous return, and the relatively normal 'right side of the heart' (right atrium and ventricle and the tricuspid and pulmonary valves) transmits this increase through the pulmonary circulation. In the presence of left heart failure the result is pulmonary venous congestion. This stimulates fine nerve endings around the terminal alveoli, and causes a sensation of breathlessness. At the same time, pulmonary interstitial oedema begins to develop. When exercise is stopped, venous return diminishes, congestion subsides and dyspnoea is relieved. Very occasionally severe unaccustomed exercise in the presence of incipient left heart failure leads to progressive pulmonary oedema. The mechanism of dyspnoea and fatigue in chronic cardiac failure is poorly understood, and may include abnormalities of peripheral muscle perfusion.

Paroxysmal nocturnal dyspnoea (p. 35) is a characteristic symptom of left heart failure. It is traditionally attributed to a rise in venous pressure as the patient slips down the pillows but this may be an oversimplification.

Breathlessness demanding the upright position, *orthopnoea*, when due to heart disease, is a symptom of persistent pulmonary oedema and indicates that the heart disease is advanced. In attacks of *acute pulmonary oedema* there is persistent severe breathlessness of sudden onset, accompanied usually by coughing and, generally, considerable alarm. Unless treatment is prompt and effective, the cough, initially repetitive and unproductive, may produce copious watery, frothy and often blood-tinged sputum.

Breathlessness is not a common feature of pure 'right heart failure' (p. 121). However pulmonary hypertension' is often accompanied by severe dyspnoea.

Pain

Angina pectoris. This term was originally used by Heberden in 1772 to describe a characteristic chest pain occurring on exertion and relieved

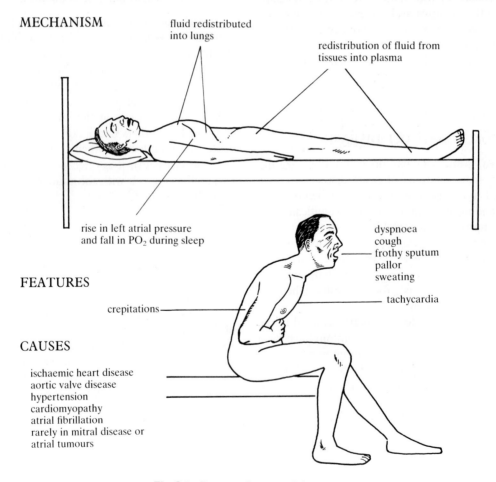

MECHANISM

fluid redistributed into lungs

redistribution of fluid from tissues into plasma

rise in left atrial pressure and fall in PO_2 during sleep

FEATURES

crepitations

dyspnoea
cough
frothy sputum
pallor
sweating

tachycardia

CAUSES

ischaemic heart disease
aortic valve disease
hypertension
cardiomyopathy
atrial fibrillation
rarely in mitral disease or
atrial tumours

Fig. 5.1   Paroxysmal nocturnal dyspnoea.

within 10 minutes by rest which we now know to be the principal symptom of myocardial ischaemia. By extension, the term angina is also used for pain caused by myocardial ischaemia under other circumstances, for example during coronary artery spasm, but 'angina' without further qualification generally means angina of effort (see Fig. 5.2). Typical attacks of angina provoked by less and less exertion, and/or attacks of chest pain like angina occurring at rest with increasing frequency, constitute the syndrome of *crescendo angina* or 'unstable angina' which may precede myocardial infarction. Since angina is frequently the sole symptom, and often unaccompanied by abnormal physical signs, it must be evaluated precisely by analysing the pain along the lines described on page 25 (see table 5.3).

Patients with coronary artery disease and incipient left ventricular failure may get angina on lying flat — *decubitus angina*. Pain which is typical of angina in site and character, but not related to effort nor a symptom of acute myocardial infarction is often attributed to coronary artery spasm. Such pain is sometimes called *variant* or *Printzmetal angina*. Coronary artery spasm is very difficult to confirm by any technique short of coronary angiography, but it may be associated with Raynaud's phenomenon (p. 93) and is much more common in cigarette smokers.

Glyceryl trinitrate hastens the relief of anginal pain, but is also effective in relieving the pain of oesophageal spasm, and its action cannot be regarded as specific.

Other chest pains of cardiovascular origin. *Myocardial infarction* causes a pain which differs from that of angina pectoris mainly in that it is more severe and oppressive and occurs or persists at rest; its type and radiation are similar. The pain or discomfort is often accompanied by a sense of apprehension or of impending death. The patient

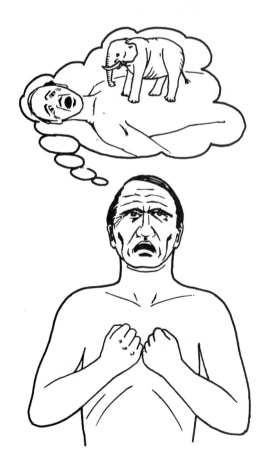

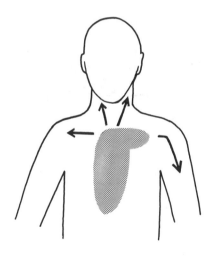

Fig. 5.2 Symptoms of angina.

Site	Sternum (note position of hands)
Character	Tight, band-like constricting, heaviness
Radiation	Arms, wrists, fingers, jaw, back
Duration	Ten minutes
Circumstances	Physical exertion, walking, stairs, emotion, cold, after heavy meals, sexual intercourse
Aggravating factors	Anaemia, obesity, hyperthyroidism
Made better by	Rest, trinitrates, warmth

Table 5.1   Cardiac causes of non-ischaemic chest pain

Cause	Comment
Paroxysmal tachycardia	Usually some underlying ischaemia Patient complains of palpitation Holter monitoring useful
Pericarditis	Retrosternal, shoulder or arm pain Often made worse by inspiration swallowing or lying down. Relieved by sitting forward. Pericardial rub
Pericardial effusion	'Oppressive' pain very similar to ischaemia. Look for signs of tamponade
Dissecting aneurysm	Severe 'tearing' pain, often through to back. May be feeling loss of power in legs
Mitral prolapse	Variety of different pains, some mimicking ischaemia
Pericardial catch	Momentary jab of pain at cardiac apex; never indicates organic disease.

tends to lie still and is generally quiet and pale, often sweats and may have nausea and vomiting. The pain usually reaches a maximum in minutes, or over an hour or so, and then may persist for hours until relieved by analgesics. Occasionally the pain is intermittent or remittent even without treatment. Myocardial infarction is not always painful. In particular, a 'silent' coronary thrombosis may occur in patients with autonomic neuropathy (e.g., diabetes mellitus). Electrocardiographic (ECG) or postmortem evidence of 'silent infarction' may be found in patients who have never had typical symptoms.

Other causes of chest pain of cardiac origin are summarized in Table 5.1. Ischaemic pain may also be confused with the pain of oesophageal reflux (p. 157). Musculo-skeletal pain tends to be a continuous dull ache and is related to movement rather than to exertion. Other causes of chest pain include pleurisy (p. 128) pneumothorax (p. 129) thoracic disc prolapse (p. 256) and transverse myelitis.

Oedema

Oedema is the most characteristic feature of fluid retention in cardiac failure; together with ascites and pleural transudates, it is dealt with on pages 39 to 43.

Other symptoms of heart disease

Palpitation, or awareness of the heart beat, is a common feature of anxiety and can be produced by sympathomimetic drugs such as adrenaline, or isoprenaline; panic attacks are commonly confused with paroxysmal tachycardia. Patients can often say whether the heart beat seems to be regular or irregular, and by tapping with the finger can sometimes indicate the approximate heart rate. Such evidence is of help in diagnosing paroxysmal tachycardias when normal rhythm has returned before the patient is seen. Continuous ambulatory ECG monitoring (p. 31) is of great value in detecting paroxysmal arrhythmias.

Cough, which is repetitive, dry, unproductive and accompanied by tachypnoea, is the herald of pulmonary oedema in some cases. Cough may also be a symptom of aneurysm of the aorta. Compression of the trachea or a main bronchus sometime gives this a trumpeting quality. A dry cough is sometimes a side effect of treatment with angiotensin converting enzymes inhibitors.

Haemoptysis is a feature of pulmonary infarction which is a frequent sequel to pulmonary thromboembolism in bedridden patients. It can also occur in mitral stenosis or pulmonary hypertension.

Syncope is discussed in detail on page 29.

Tiredness is a common symptom in severe heart disease. A feeling of excessive tiredness may precede the onset of acute myocardial infarction. Patients with infective endocarditis may feel prostrated even in the absence of severe cardiac failure. Tiredness is common during the first fortnight of treatment with beta-blockers — it usually improves thereafter but the feeling may persist indefinitely in some patients. However, tiredness is a common feature of many disorders including depression.

The *eyes* may be effected in various forms of cardiovascular disease. Sudden unilateral impairment of vision may result from retinal haemorrhage in severe hypertension, or from emboli to the retina in cases of valvular heart disease.

Often, retinal haemorrhages do not cause noticeable impairment of vision, but are revealed on routine examination with an ophthalmoscope. Unilateral visual disturbances may also result from retinal artery or retinal vein thrombosis (Plate III), or from cranial arteritis. Disturbances of vision effecting both eyes, usually in the form of a homonymous field defect (p. 195) may follow occlusion of a cerebral artery. Patients starting on therapy with a potent diuretic sometimes notice transient visual blurring, possibly related to changes in the hydration of the lens.

Gastrointestinal symptoms. Nausea and vomiting are often features of acute myocardial infarction. They are also the most common presenting symptoms of digoxin intoxication. Sometimes nausea and vomiting accompany worsening cardiac failure, perhaps as a consequence of hepatic or gastric congestion. Diarrhoea may be a manifestation of digoxin toxicity; constipation may result from the dehydration caused by excessive diuretic therapy.

Renal function is dependent on cardiac output, and severe cardiac failure leads to oliguria or even anuria. In less severe cardiac failure the usual diurnal rhythm of urine output may be reversed, with more urine being produced at night than during the day. Acute polyuria sometimes accompanies paroxysmal supraventricular tachycardia

probably secondary to the production of atrial natriuretic factor.

Other aspects of the history

A systematic history must include enquiry into the family history (particularly ischaemic heart disease and stroke), past illnesses, obstetric history, social history, home circumstances and medication. Table 5.2 summarises cardiac components of some important inherited syndromes, Table 5.3 the cardiac components of some multisystem diseases and Table 5.4 drug associations with cardiac disease.

Table 5.3 Cardiac components of multisystem diseases

Disease	Cardiac component
Diabetes mellitus	Atherosclerosis, myocardial infarction, autonomic neuropathy
Alcoholism	Atrial fibrillation, cardiomyopathy, hypertension
Polyarteritis nodosa	Coronary occlusion, cardiomyopathy
Systemic lupus erythematosus	Pericarditis, cardiomyopathy valvular disease
Rheumatoid arthritis or Sarcoidosis	Pericarditis, valvular nodules, cardiomyopathy, conduction disorders

By convention, the term 'cardiomyopathy' should be used only if the cause is unknown, otherwise the condition should be called, for example, 'sarcoid heart muscle disease'. The term cardiomyopathy is used here for brevity, and to emphasise the clinical similarity of the specific heart muscle diseases to idiopathic dilated cardiomyopathy.

Table 5.2 Inherited diseases with important cardiac components

Disease	Cardiac component
Familial hypercholesterolaemia	Precocious coronary disease
Homocystinuria	Coronary disease, thrombosis
Downs' syndrome	AV canal defects, low incidence of atheroma
Turner's syndrome	Coarctation of aorta
Noonan's syndrome	Supravalvar aortic stenosis
Marfan's syndrome	Aortic dissection, mitral reflux
Ehlers Danlos syndrome	Aortic dissection
Friedreich's ataxia	Cardiomyopathy
Dystrophia myotonica	Cardiomyopathy
Neurofibromatosis	Phaeochromocytoma, hypertrophic cardiomyopathy

Table 5.4 Drugs and heart disease

Heart disease	Drugs
Hypertension	Corticosteroids, liquorice derivations, chronic analgesic abuse, non-steroidal anti-inflammatory drugs, oral contraceptives, monoamine oxidase inhibitors, ephedrine alcohol
Fluid retention	Corticosteroids, liquorice, non steroidal anti-inflammatory drugs
Sinus tachycardia	Salbutamol, theophylline derivatives, nifedipine, ephedrine, thyroxine
Tachyarrhythmias	Digoxin, tricyclic antidepressants, theophylline, alcohol, diuretics
Bradyarrhythmias	Beta-blockers, verapamil, digoxin

SYMPTOMS OF PERIPHERAL VASCULAR DISEASE

These can be divided into symptoms of arterial and venous insufficiency, and they will vary according to whether the vascular problem is acute or whether it develops gradually.

Arterial insufficiency

The acute form, as from the embolic occlusion of a large artery, causes pain in the limb, loss of function and altered cutaneous sensation. The limb is often cold to the touch and pale or livid on inspection.

Gradual arterial obstruction, particularly in the lower limb, presents as *intermittent claudication*, an aching pain in the muscles, usually of the thigh or calf, which comes on with exercise and remits with rest. It is often 'aching' or 'squeezing' in nature. Chronic arterial insufficiency in the upper limb is rare, but may follow damage to the brachial artery at cardiac catheterisation. It can cause pain in the forearm and hand during writing. Severe chronic arterial insufficiency may cause *rest pain*. This may be felt deep in the limb or superficially. Often there is altered cutaneous sensation, and there may be a feeling of burning. The patient may seek to relieve discomfort by letting the leg hang over the side of the bed, outside the bedclothes.

Venous insufficiency

The acute form may result from the occlusion by thrombus of a major limb vein such as the femoral or axillary vein. There is usually considerable painful swelling of the limb. The skin may be pale or livid, and the superficial veins are prominent. Sometimes cutaneous blisters form. The limb is usually warm, in marked contrast to features following acute arterial occlusion. It is important to realise that there may be extensive non-occlusive thrombus in, for example, the venous plexuses of the calf with few or no symptoms.

Chronic venous insufficiency usually affects the legs. They may ache at the end of the day or after prolonged standing. Oedema is common. Dilated superficial veins (varicose veins) are common but not invariable. There may be chronic ulceration, usually above or behind the medial malleolus of the ankle, sometimes in front of the tibia.

THE PHYSICAL EXAMINATION

Physical examination of the cardiovascular system has a number of different components. The clinician has to learn how to integrate the different components of the examination so that they answer clinical questions in the most effective way. The examination of the cardiovascular system will be described first under a series of systematic headings:

1. General inspection
2. Examination of the arterial system
3. Examination of the venous system
4. Examination of the heart
5. Examination of the chest and abdomen.

These systematic accounts are followed by a description of an example of a more integrated practical system of examination (p. 119), and later in the chapter by a discussion of the role of clinical examination and the more important cardiac investigations in solving common clinical problems.

1. GENERAL INSPECTION

This should begin even before the examiner starts to take the history, as the patient's appearance, gait, attitude and clothing may all be relevant. A short walk with the patient to the examination room may give valuable information about exercise tolerance. Features such as severe anaemia, Paget's disease, hyper- or hypothyroidism may be apparent at once, or detected only after careful examination.

Hands and face

These areas particularly repay attention in cardiac patients. In practice, their detailed inspection is usually integrated with the examination of the peripheral pulses and the search of oedema, but for convenience the points of special interest are collected here.

The hands. These provide valuable information about the patient's occupation and smoking habits. It is useful, as well as polite, to begin the physical examination by shaking hands with the patient. Warm hands indicate peripheral vasodilatation, cold ones vasoconstriction, and sweaty palms reflect increased sympathetic nervous activity. A blue tinge to the hands may be due to arterial desaturation, but it can also be due to a reduced cardiac output or to stasis of blood in dilated superficial vessels. It should not be regarded as pathological without corroborating evidence. Chronic arterial desaturation, particularly that due to cyanotic congenital heart disease, causes finger clubbing (p. 133) which is also a late sign in infective endocarditis. This last condition may also be associated with splinter haemorrhages (Fig. 4.2 p. 54) under the finger (or toe) nails, or with Osler's nodes (p. 54).

Face. Many varieties of congenital heart disease are associated with abnormalities of the facial skeleton — for example, the high-arched palate of Marfan's syndrome, the hypertelorism (wide-set eyes) sometimes seen in pulmonary stenosis, and the elfin facies (receding jaw, flared nostrils and pointed ears) of supravalvar aortic stenosis. Usually, however, the heart disease draws attention to the facial abnormality rather than vice versa. Some patients with mitral stenosis and a reduced cardiac output have pallid faces with patches of rather dusky erythema over the cheek bones. Although sometimes called the mitral facies, this appearance is not specific as it may be seen in other forms of heart disease and not infrequently in normal subjects.

The *teeth and eyes* should be inspected. Dental disease or its treatment may be responsible for infective endocarditis. Edentulous patients, however, may sometimes develop endocarditis if ill-fitting dentures cause a portal of entry for bacteria. Ophthalmoscopic examination is particularly informative in hypertensive patients (pp. 332).

Xanthomas

These are deposits of lipid in the tendons, skin or soft tissues. They are associated with hyperlipidaemia, and premature coronary artery disease. Tendon xanthomas are felt as thickening of the achilles tendon, or as lumps in the tendons of the extensor digitorum of the hand. They are associated with type II hyperlipidaemia, which is relatively common. Palmar xanthomas occur in the skin creases of the palms and soles are yellowish nodules, often with a rim of erythema. They are characteristic of type III hyperlipidaemia, which is rare. Eruptive xanthomas are similar, but occur over the knees, elbows and buttocks, sometimes in hyperlipidaemia, but also in conditions such as primary biliary cirrhosis.

Xanthelasma is the deposition of lipid in the skin of the eyelids — the upper more commonly than the lower. It may be associated with hyperlipidaemia, but it is sometimes seen in middle aged or elderly people with no evidence of a plasma lipid abnormality.

A *corneal arcus* (p. 60) in a young patient may be an indicator of the presence of hyperlipidaemia.

Cyanosis

This is a bluish or purplish tinge of the skin or mucous membranes which results from the presence of an excessive amount of reduced haemoglobin in the underlying blood vessels. It may be due either to poor perfusion of these vessels (peripheral cyanosis) or to a reduction in the oxygen saturation of arterial blood (central cyanosis). For cyanosis to be observed, there must be a minimum quantity of reduced haemoglobin (about 5 g/dl) in the blood perfusing the skin; cyanosis may thus not be detectable in patients with severe anaemia even if they are gravely hypoxaemic.

Peripheral cyanosis. This is a familiar sight in

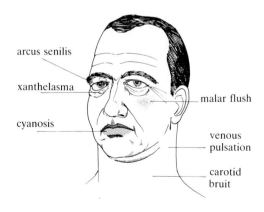

arcus senilis

xanthelasma

cyanosis

malar flush

venous pulsation

carotid bruit

Fig. 5.3 The face and neck in cardiac disease.

cold weather, as a consequence of cold-induced vasoconstriction. It is seen also in patients with a greatly reduced cardiac output, when differential vasoconstriction diverts blood flow from the skin to other organs such as the brain. Peripheral cyanosis is seldom seen in the tongue or buccal mucosa because they are well perfused except in advanced circulatory failure. It can usually be assumed that when cyanosis is present in these sites it is of central (cardiopulmonary) origin. The same assumption can be made when the hands are cyanosed and warm.

Central cyanosis. This can usually be detected when the oxygen saturation of arterial blood falls below 80–85%. It may be due to respiratory (p. 132) or to cardiac causes. The most common 'cardiac' cause is pulmonary oedema, with its associated symptoms of dyspnoea and cough, and the physical sign of crepitations at the lung bases. A less common cardiac cause is an intracardiac or intrapulmonary 'right to left shunt', where venous blood bypasses the lungs and is shunted into the systemic circulation. This is seen in pulmonary arteriovenous fistulae, in Fallot's tetralogy and other rarer forms of congenital heart disease. Patients with a right to left shunt show little or no increase in arterial oxygen saturation when given oxygen to breathe, whereas patients with hypoxaemia from pulmonary oedema or respiratory causes usually show an improvement. Sometimes, hypoxaemia results from pulmonary thromboembolism.

Very occasionally, cyanosis is due to the presence of the *abnormal pigments* sulphaemoglobin or methaemoglobin in the bloodsteam. In these cases, arterial oxygen tension is normal, and the diagnosis can be confirmed by spectroscopic examination of the blood.

2. EXAMINATION OF THE ARTERIAL SYSTEM

Clinicians examine the arterial system partly to assess the patency of the arteries, and partly for information about the function of the heart. The examination of the arterial system is described under the following headings:

a. The pulses

b. Pulse rate and rhythm
c. Pulse volume and character
d. The arterial blood pressure
e. The assessment of peripheral arterial insufficiency
f. The aorta.

a. The pulses

The arterial pulse wave which is felt by the examining fingers is imparted to the column of arterial blood by the contraction of the left ventricle and takes between 0.2 and 0.5 seconds to reach the feet; the blood takes ten times as long to make the same journey. Systolic pressure in excess of 50 mmHg is normally required to detect femoral or brachial artery pulses and corresponding higher values are necessary for more distal pulses to be detected.

The *radial artery* is one of the most accessible of the peripheral arteries. A technique for palpating it is shown in Figure 5.4. Occasionally the radial artery follows an aberrant course traversing the 'anatomical snuff box' and passing over the dorsum of the first metacarpal bone. If both radial pulses are palpated simultaneously a weakness or delay in one of them may give a clue to more proximal arterial disease. The radial and femoral pulses should be checked for synchrony if coarctation of the aorta is suspected (p. 94).

The *ulnar artery* is palpable at the wrist where it crosses the distal end of the radius. Usually both radial and ulnar artery contribute to the blood supply of the hand. This can be demonstrated by asking the patient to make a fist, and then using the thumbs to compress both arteries against the underlying bone. When the fist is released the skin of the palm remains blanched, but colour should return quickly when either artery is released. If there is delay in the return of colour after release of the ulnar artery, then procedures which might damage the radial artery, such as arterial cannulation, should be avoided.

The *brachial artery* is most conveniently felt at the elbow using the examiner's thumb (Fig. 5.4). There is a prejudice against using the thumb for palpating pulses which may be justified when searching for a faint peripheral pulse, but is inappropriate here, where the excellent proprioceptive

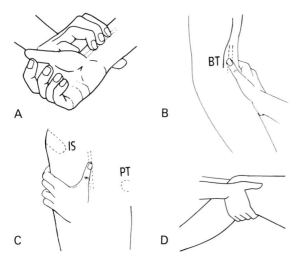

A

B

IS

PT

C

D

Fig. 5.4 Methods for palpating pulses. (A) radial; (B) right brachial medial to biceps tendon (BT); (C) femoral midway between the anterior superior iliac spine (IS) and the pubic tubercle (PT); (D) popliteal. Note that the thumb is shown being used to feel the brachial and femoral pulses. When searching for a very weak pulse, as in the presence of peripheral vascular disease, it is better to use the fingers rather than the thumb, as very faint pulsation in the examiner's thumb may be mistaken for the pulse being sought. The popliteal pulse is felt with the fingertips of either hand, the fingers of both hands being curled into the popliteal fossa.

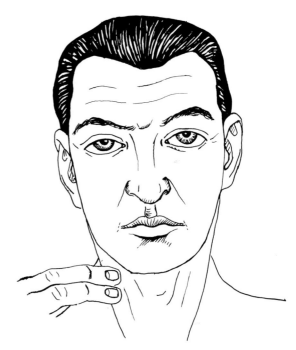

Fig. 5.5 Detecting the carotid artery.

and kinaesthetic sense of the thumb make it ideal for assessing pulse volume and wave form.

The *subclavian artery* is felt from behind by pressing downward with the forefinger above the middle of the clavicle (first part of the artery), or from the front by feeling below the junction of the middle and lateral thirds of the clavicle.

The *carotid artery* is placed adjacent to the trachea, medial to the sterno-mastoid muscle in the lower part of the neck. It is best detected by pressing gently backwards with the fingers or thumb until the pulsation is felt against the front of the cervical vertebra (Fig. 5.5). Pressure on the carotid sinus, which lies at the division of the common carotid into the internal and external carotid arteries, may sometimes induce syncope, and palpation of the carotid artery should be done with the patient lying on a couch.

The *femoral artery* lies halfway between the pubic tubercle and the anterior superior iliac spine at the level of the inguinal ligament (Fig. 5.4).

The *popliteal artery* is felt by pressing with the fingertips in the middle of the popliteal fossa while the patient lies supine with the knee slightly flexed (Fig. 5.4). The artery lies immediately adjacent to the posterior aspect of the knee joint, and is thus one of the deepest structures in the fossa, but with practice it can nearly always be detected unless there is proximal obstruction.

The *posterior tibial artery* is felt behind the medial malleolus, and the *dorsalis pedis artery* is palpable lateral to the extensor hallucis tendon on the dorsum of the foot. Often in the elderly one or both of these vessels will not be palpable. If the dorsalis pedis pulse is not palpable in a young person, there may be an enlarged perforating peroneal artery palpable in front of the lateral malleolus.

b. Pulse rate and rhythm

The rate and rhythm of the pulse reflects the rate and rhythm of the heart, and this is dealt with in detail on p. 105. An irregular cardiac rhythm is associated with a varying pulse volume, since the latter is related to cardiac stroke volume. Sometimes the pulse volume is so small that the pulse is impalpable, and there will be a discrepancy between the heart rate measured by palpation of the pulse and by auscultation. The difference is termed the *pulse deficit*. Although it is not usually difficult to diagnose common abnormalities of rate and rhythm simply by palpation of the pulse, it is always wise to supplement this information by auscultation of the heart, and whenever possible by an ECG.

c. Pulse volume and character

Invaluable information about left ventricular function and left-sided valvular lesions can be gained from a careful assessment of the volume and character of the pulse. The 'closer' to the heart the pulse is palpated the less it is likely to be modified by the properties of the peripheral vessels. The carotid, brachial or femoral pulses are thus more useful for assessing pulse volume and character than the radial pulse.

Pulse volume reflects left ventricular stroke volume; it is increased during or after exercise, in the presence of a fever, or when there is increased 'run off' from the arterial tree through a persistent ductus arteriosus or other arteriovenous fistula. In aortic regurgitation the 'run off' is back into the left ventricle itself during diastole. Conversely, the pulse volume is small in the presence of poor left ventricular function or during tachycardia.

Pulsus alternans is a regular succession of large and small beats and occurs in severe left ventricular failure. It needs to be distinguished from the alternation of pulse volume caused by coupled ventricular ectopic beats, which is much more common.

Pulses paradoxus is a real or apparent decrease in pulse volume during inspiration and increase in expiration. One variety of 'pulsus paradoxus' occurs in severe asthma, where excessive swings in intrathoracic pressure are superimposed on the arterial pressure. In this case systolic and diastolic pressures rise and fall in parallel so there is no consistent change in pulse pressure — but this can be appreciated only with the aid of a continuous intra-arterial recording. In the other variety, or 'true' pulsus paradoxus, there is not only a fall in systolic pressure but a true diminution of pulse volume during inspiration (Fig. 5.6). Although a minor variation in pulse volume in this way occurs

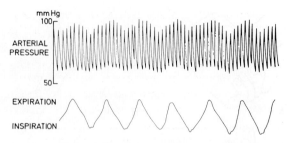

Fig. 5.6 Pulsus paradoxus in a case of pericardial tamponade. Note that systolic pressure and pulse pressure are both reduced during inspiration. (Reproduced with kind permission of Dr L. Fananapazir.)

in normal subjects (so the term 'paradoxus' is a misnomer) its occurrence in such an exaggerated fashion that the changes can be detected by palpation is virtually diagnostic of *cardiac tamponade* — cardiac compression by a tense pericardial effusion. Normally, the physiological changes in intrathoracic pressure during the respiratory cycle are transmitted equally to the four chambers of the heart, so that the swings in left atrial pressure are accompanied by almost identical changes in left ventricular diastolic pressure. In the presence of a tense pericardial effusion, the left ventricle is prevented from responding to the lower intrathoracic pressure during inspiration, its filling is impeded, and stroke volume falls. The right ventricle on the other hand is connected via the right atrium and vena cava to the extrathoracic systemic veins, and its filling can increase at the expense of the left ventricle. The resulting shift in the interventricular septum can sometimes be detected by echocardiography (p. 115). When the increased right ventricular stroke volume is eventually transmitted via the pulmonary veins it tends to accentuate the cyclical variation in left ventricular output.

In patients with a very low cardiac output as a result of cardiac tamponade the radial and brachial arteries may be barely palpable, and pulsus paradoxus is better detected in the carotid or femoral pulses. Sometimes the abnormality is found while the blood pressure is being measured, and this is a good way of confirming an impression of paradoxical pulse gained by palpation.

Delayed pulse. If there is obstruction to blood flow between the heart and the site at which the pulse is felt, pulse volume will be diminished, and the pulse wave itself will be delayed. This can be appreciated clinically only if there is another pulse at a similar distance from the heart which can be used for comparison: for example, the femoral pulses are delayed relative to the radial pulse in coarctation of the aorta, and the left brachial pulse might be delayed relative to the right in the presence of left subclavian stenosis.

The form of the pulse wave. When there is increased 'run off' from the arterial tree the pulse wave may rise normally but then declines abruptly. This is termed a *collapsing pulse*, and the most common association in a resting adult patient is with aortic regurgitation (p.110). In children, a collapsing pulse may be more readily felt in the femoral arteries, and may be an indication of a persistent ductus arteriosus.

A slow rising pulse, best detected in the carotids, is characteristic of aortic stenosis. Turbulence as blood is forced through the narrowed valve is felt as a carotid thrill or shudder. Sometimes the rate of left ventricular ejection is so slowed as a consequence of beta-blocker therapy that a slow-rising pulse is produced, but without a thrill or murmur.

Increasing rigidity of the arteries gives a more rapid upstroke to the pulse; in the elderly, this can obscure the diagnosis of aortic stenosis.

In hypertrophic obstructive cardiomyopathy, left ventricular ejection is initially unimpeded, but is then suddenly 'throttled' by contraction of a muscular ridge in the left ventricular outflow tract. This results in a distinctive 'jerky' quality of the carotid pulses.

Pulsus bisferiens, that is, a pulse with two humps is sometimes felt in patients with aortic stenosis and regurgitation. The earlier explanation was that the first, or 'anacrotic' peak represented the force of left ventricular contraction transmitted through the aortic valve, and the second peak was due to the actual ejection of blood into the aorta. A more recent suggestion is that the 'dip' in the pulse is the result of energy dissipation in the production of a loud systolic murmur.

d. The arterial blood pressure

Ideally, blood pressure should be measured with

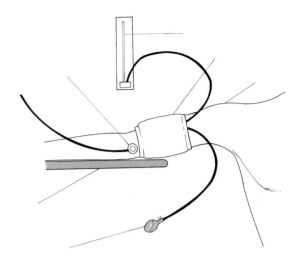

Fig. 5.7 Measuring the blood pressure. (1) no constricting garments. (2) smoothly apply cuff of correct size. (3) palpate brachial pulse before applying stethoscope. (4) support arm at heart level. (5) inflate cuff until radial pulse is impalpable; check systolic pressure by auscultation, deflate at approximately 2 mmHg per second until diastolic pressure is reached.

the patient as relaxed as possible, that is, at the end of the physical examination. However it is often helpful to be aware of an abnormal pressure at an earlier stage, and there is also some risk that if left to the end this very important measurement may be forgotten. One satisfactory method is to measure the blood pressure immediately after palpating the brachial pulse, and then to repeat the measurement at the end of the examination if there is any suspicion of hypertension.

Blood pressure is usually measured by the cuff method (Fig. 5.7). The normal cuff width for adult use is 12 cm — a wider cuff is used for the leg, or for exceptionally fat arms, and a narrower one for children. Too narrow a cuff causes a spuriously high estimate of blood pressure, and this also results if the patients makes a muscular effort in holding up the arm. On the other hand failure to remove tight clothing from the upper arm gives a falsely low estimate. The cuff pressure is allowed to fall slowly until the first Korotkov sounds are heard. This corresponds to the systolic pressure, and the radial pulse becomes palpable shortly afterwards. In this way it is possible to avoid an underestimate of the true systolic pressure resulting from the 'auscultatory gap'

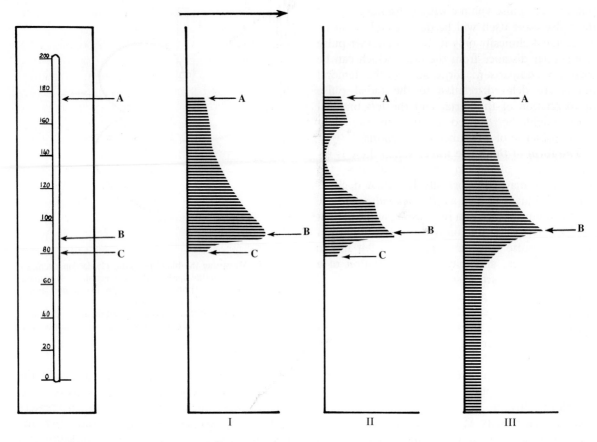

Fig. 5.8 Different patterns of Korotkov sounds. (I) is normal, (II) shows 'silent gap' phenomenon and in (III) muffled sounds persist with no phase 5. At (A) sounds are first heard, (B) sounds become muffled (phase 4) and (C) sounds disappear (phase 5).

phenomenon, where the Korotkov sounds transiently disappear between systole and diastole (Fig. 5.8). As pressure in the cuff continues to fall, the sounds become louder and 'ringing' in nature, then suddenly muffled. This point of muffling is called 'phase IV', and in Britain has previously been used to indicate the diastolic pressure. It does indeed correlate well with diastolic pressure as measured by intra-arterial recordings, but epidemiological studies have shown that there is less variation between observers if diastolic pressure is recorded at the point of complete disappearance of Korotkov sounds, or 'phase V'. For this reason it is now recommended that the phase V value be recorded as the diastolic pressure. In some normal subjects muffled sounds are still

heard as the cuff pressure is reduced to zero, and this is recorded as, for example: 180/90/0. Allowing the pressure in the cuff to fall too rapidly prevents accurate measurement of the diastolic pressure.

There are many possible sources of observer-induced bias in blood pressure recording, and for accurate epidemiological work special apparatus may be needed.

When a difference in the pulse in the two arms is suspected, the blood pressure should be recorded on both sides. When a weak, delayed, femoral pulse is associated with hypertension in the arms (coarctation of the aorta, p. 94) the blood pressure in the legs should also be recorded, using a broad cuff round the thigh with the patient lying prone and the stethoscope applied to the popliteal artery. If the patient is receiving treatment for hypertension or if there is a history to suggest postural hypotension the blood pressure should be taken both supine and erect.

Casual records of blood pressure are less reproducible than repeated records with the patient at rest. Emotional factors may elevate the blood pressure remarkably in some patients, and the systolic pressure may be more than 50 mmHg, and the diastolic more than 30 mmHg higher than in subsequent records when the patient has become accustomed to the procedure. Such falls in pressure on repeated examination are often erroneously attributed to treatment provided for hypertension. Devices which record blood pressure continuously demonstrate the temporary hypertensive effect of doctors approaching the patient's bed. While it has been traditional to discount such 'stress induced' hypertension, epidemiological studies suggest it should not be regarded with complacency.

e. The assessment of peripheral arterial insufficiency

Clinical features. Acute obstruction of the arterial supply to a limb or digit is accompanied by constant severe pain and the distal areas appear pale or white. Later the skin may become livid or discoloured, and finally gangrene or mummification may occur. Conversely, restoration of an arterial blood supply is accompanied by cutaneous blushing (reactive hyperaemia). With a chronically ischaemic limb, there is seldom a striking colour change, but there may be a loss of hair, wasting of subcutaneous tissues, and sometimes ulceration, particularly of areas subject to local pressure.

An ischaemic limb or digit is nearly always cold to the touch. Pressure on the skin produces blanching which is slow to recover when the pressure is removed. Palpation of the peripheral pulses is very important in the diagnosis of peripheral arterial disease — absence of a major pulse in the presence of an adequate central blood pressure is usually good evidence of arterial obstruction. In the feet, absence of the posterior tibial pulse is a more reliable indicator of ischaemia than absence of the dorsalis pedis. In a normal limb, the pulses become easier to feel after exercise; if a pulse is palpable at rest but disappears after exercise there may be proximal arterial obstruction.

Atheroma in a large artery may cause turbulent blood flow, and this can be heard as a murmur (bruit) if a stethoscope is placed over the vessel. It is important to avoid creating a bruit by applying undue pressure on the stethoscope so as to constrict the arterial wall. Care is also needed to distinguish a localised bruit from a systolic murmur transmitted from the aortic valve. Abdominal bruits may be heard in thin healthy subjects but a bruit over the femoral, subclavian or carotid artery, or over the abdominal aorta, is useful evidence of vascular narrowing or irregularity. The converse is not true — there is no bruit over an occluded vessel, and severe stenosis may exist without an audible bruit.

Diagnosis. The pattern of peripheral ischaemia is very helpful in making a diagnosis of its cause. Sudden asymmetric ischaemia with good pulses in the other limbs is usually the result of embolism or occasionally of vascular trauma. Sudden ischaemia of both legs may be due to an embolus lodging at the aortic bifurcation (saddle embolus). Embolism to an arm or a leg, or to a limb and another organ such as eye, brain or kidney suggests a central or cardiac source of emboli. Asymmetric limb ischaemia with chest or abdominal pain may be due to a dissecting aortic aneurysm. Sometimes a systemic vasculitis may mimic multiple embolism, but the ischaemic areas tend to be smaller — individual digits rather than limbs — and there are often characteristic cutaneous lesions. Signs of ischaemia of the skin in the presence of readily palpable pulses may indicate vascular disease affecting arterioles and small arteries rather than larger vessels. Acutely, this may result from cold injury (frostbite) or poisoning with ergotamine. Chronic ischaemia of this kind may complicate diabetes mellitus. Recurrent painful ischaemia of the digits, usually symmetrical and sometimes precipitated by cold or vibration, is called Raynaud's phenomenon, and is due to vascular spasm. Atherosclerosis is the commonest cause of chronic or progressive arterial disease. Although the clinical symptoms may be asymmetric, careful examination will usually reveal evidence of widespread arterial disease in the form of weak or absent pulses and peripheral bruits.

f. The aorta

Coarctation. Narrowing of the aorta may be congenital or acquired, and may affect the thoracic or abdominal part of the vessel. The commonest form is congenital coarctation of the thoracic aorta.

The most important physical signs of aortic coarctation are hypertension in the upper half of the body and delayed femoral pulses relative to the radial pulse (Fig. 5.9). The degree of hypertension ranges from mild to severe, and blood pressure may be higher in the right arm than the left. Blood pressure measured in the right arm is almost always higher than blood pressure in the legs, measured using a wide sphygmomanometer cuff on the thigh, with a stethoscope applied to the

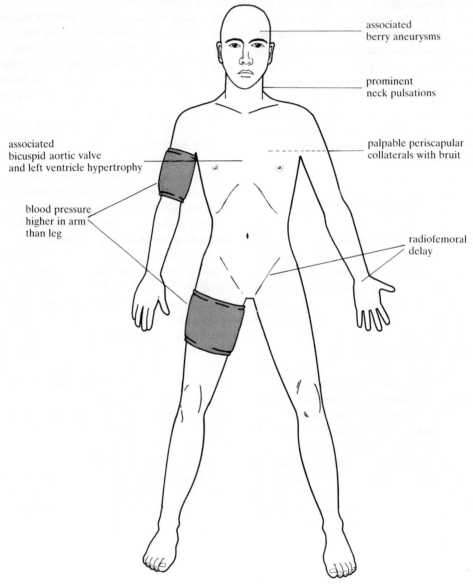

Fig. 5.9   Features of coarctation of the aorta.

popliteal fossa. Congenital coarctation presenting in adolescence or adulthood is usually accompanied by a well developed collateral circulation. There may be exaggerated pulsation in the supraclavicular fossa, and pulsating vessels may be felt over the chest wall and around the scapulae. Blood flow in these vessels may cause a continuous murmur, and it is often possible to hear a systolic murmur to the left of the spine in the third or fourth intercostal space. Congenital coarctation of the aorta is frequently associated with a bicuspid aortic valve (p. 104).

Coarctation of the abdominal aorta is less common; it may be congenital, the result of trauma, or due to an inflammatory, obliterative disease of the aorta and other large arteries called Takayasu's disease. Hypertension and delayed femoral pulses are found as in thoracic coarctation, but there is often an upper abdominal bruit. Collaterals around the neck and shoulders are not usually prominent. Takayasu's disease may affect several arteries and in severe forms all the pulses may be absent or very difficult to feel — the 'pulseless disease'.

Aneurysm. This is an abnormal dilatation or bulge of the aorta. Aneurysms of the thoracic aorta are hard to detect clinically unless they are very large, when they may cause hoarseness by interfering with the recurrent laryngeal nerve, breathlessness or stridor by pressure on the trachea, and pulsation of the sternum of adjacent chest wall. The pulsations of the normal abdominal aorta are often readily palpable in slim subjects. Abdominal aortic aneurysms can usually be felt as pulsatile swellings, the 'expansile' nature of which distinguishes an aneurysm from a solid tumour; the latter is simply transmitting aortic pulsation. In elderly subjects the aorta may elongate and become tortuous, and it may then be difficult to decide whether an aneurysm is present.

Dissecting aneurysms of the aorta are characterised by haemorrhage into the aortic wall, which creates a 'false lumen' separated from the true lumen by a flap of aortic tissue. The dissection may progress proximally or distally along the aorta, and the flap may obstruct major arteries such as the subclavian or carotid vessels. Dissecting aneurysm of the ascending aorta may cause regurgitation at the aortic valve (p. 110). The typical clinical picture is of sudden chest pain often described as tearing or ripping in quality and radiating into the back or between the shoulder blades. The clinical appearances of acute shock with hypotension, pallor, sweating and angor animi are often present. It is important to check for the presence of distal arterial pulses. Depending upon the site and extent of the dissection, there may be variation in the pulse pressures, which may be detected in the arm pulses. Occasionally, neurological symptoms related to the dissection involving the spinal arteries may further complicate the picture. Rupture of an aneurysm may produce sudden death from exsanguination; slow leakage of blood may cause a pleural effusion (usually left-sided) or a retroperitoneal haematoma, sometimes with a palpable abdominal mass and bruising in the flanks.

3. EXAMINATION OF THE VENOUS SYSTEM

As with the arterial system, clinical examination of the venous system gives information about the heart, provided by measurement of the jugular venous pressure and analysis of the jugular venous pulse wave, and information about the patency and function of the peripheral veins.

The jugular venous pressure (JVP)

The central venous pressure (which is the same as right atrial pressure) is an important guide to cardiovascular function, and its elevation is an indication of cardiac failure or fluid overload. A useful estimate of central venous pressure can be made, without resort to instruments, by observing the jugular venous pulse.

The internal jugular veins are collapsible, relatively inelastic tubes in direct continuity with the right atrium. The 'normal' right atrial pressure seldom exceeds 5 mm of mercury, which is equivalent to a column of blood roughly 7 cm high. With a patient lying flat, the jugular veins are distended but not visibly pulsatile (Fig. 5.10). If a patient with a normal right atrial pressure sits upright, the upper part of the vein collapses, but the lower part of the vein remains distended for a vertical height of some 7 cm above the middle of the right atrium. In the upright patient the point

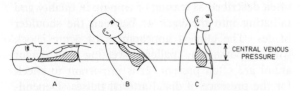

Fig. 5.10 Jugular venous pressure in normal subject. (A) Supine: jugular vein distended, pulsation not visible. (B) Reclining at 45 degrees: point of transition between distended and collapsed vein can usually be seen to pulsate just above the clavicle. (C) Upright: upper part of vein collapsed and transition points obscured by sternum.

of transition between distended and collapsed vein is hidden behind the sternum and clavicles, but allowing the patient to recline at 45 degrees usually makes it visible just above the clavicle, where it can be recognised and distinguished from the carotid pulse by its characteristic features. It is important not to mistake arterial for venous pulsation in the neck. Points of distinction are shown in Table 5.5.

The mean level of jugular venous pressure above right atrial level is a measure of the central venous pressure. Because of the difficulty of 'guessing' the level of the right atrium, it is usual to assume that this lies 5 cms below the level of the manubriosternal angle and this relationship roughly holds true whether the patient is supine or sitting upright. Various causes of elevation in the jugular venous pressure are shown in Table 5.6.

Table 5.5 Ways of distinguishing the jugular venous from the carotid pulse

Jugular venous pulse	Carotid pulse
Varies with posture	No variation with posture
Varies with respiration	No variation with respiration
Two waves per cardiac cycle (in sinus rhythm)	Only one wave per cardiac cycle
Most prominent movement usually inward	Most prominent movement outward
Made more prominent by abdominal pressure	Abdominal pressure has no effect
Often obscured by finger pressure	No effect from finger pressure
Moves ear lobes when venous pressure very high	Does not move ear lobes

Table 5.6 Cause of raised jugular venous pressure

Cause	Comment
Fluid overload	e.g. overtransfusion
Primary or secondary right heart failure	Often with peripheral oedema
Pulmonary embolism	JVP may be very high, but may be missed in supine patient
Chronic pulmonary hypertension	'a' waves often prominent
Pulmonary stenosis	'a' waves often prominent
Pericardial tamponade	Prominent y descent
Constrictive pericarditis	JVP often very high, prominent y descent
Tricuspid stenosis	Slow y descent
Tricuspid reflux	Large 'v' waves
Superior vena caval obstruction	Distended veins without pulsation
Cannon waves	Sharp, often variable, systolic pulsation (p. 97)

The jugular venous pressure normally falls during inspiration as the right atrium and ventricle dilate in response to a lowered intrathoracic pressure. Pressure with the examiner's hand in the right hypochondrium causes a transient rise in jugular venous pressure as the hepatic venous reservoir is compressed — *the hepatojugular reflux*. In patients with constrictive pericarditis the jugular pressure may rise during inspiration (Kussmaul's sign) because the congested liver is compressed by the descending diaphragm and the right atrium and ventricle are prevented from distending by the rigid pericardium. This sign is also seen occasionally in severe right ventricular failure.

A low jugular venous pressure may result as a consequence of any condition causing a reduction in pre-load for example haemorrhage or dehydration. An unexpectedly low venous pressure in patients with other signs of cardiac disease is commonly due to diuretic therapy.

Although the external jugular veins are often distended when venous pressure is high, they are an unreliable guide since there is often a valve-like constriction where the external joins the internal jugular. A grossly elevated jugular venous pressure may sometimes be missed because the distended veins do not pulsate: pulsation may become apparent if the patient is placed in a more upright position, or it may be observed that the arm veins remains distended until the patient's hand is raised well above the head.

The jugular venous pulse

Confusion is apt to arise in descriptions of the wave form of the jugular pulse, because jugular pulsation is often difficult to detect in subjects with normal hearts, and patients with readily-discernable jugular pulsation very commonly have some cardiac abnormality. Figure 5.11 shows a pressure tracing recorded from the internal jugular vein in a patient with a normal cardiac function. The *a* wave coincides with atrial systole, and the early part of the *x* descent following it is due to atrial relaxation. Continuation of the *x* descent is due to retraction of the tricuspid valve during early right ventricular systole. Continuing venous return while the tricuspid valve is closed causes right atrial pressure to rise again, and it reaches a second peak, called a *v* wave at the end of ventricular systole. Ventricular relaxation and tricuspid valve opening then cause a second fall in atrial pressure (the *y* descent) as the pent-up venous blood floods into the ventricle. The *c* wave, an extra wave transmitted from the carotid artery, is sometimes seen between *a* and *v* waves.

Exaggerated *a* waves in the jugular pulse are a hallmark of right atrial hypertrophy. This may be due to tricuspid stenosis, or more commonly to right ventricular hypertrophy with an associated increase in ventricular 'stiffness'. They are readily recognised by being presystolic, especially when timed against the carotid pulse. The prominence of the *x* descent is usually related to the size of the *a* wave. In cases of atrioventricular dissociation, for example complete heart block, atrial and ventricular systole sometimes coincide. Atrial contraction against a closed tricuspid valve then causes a strikingly large venous pulsation, called a cannon wave. Regular cannon waves may occur in patients with a ventricular pacemaker but intact retrograde conduction from ventricle to atrium, and are easily mistaken for a sign of tricuspid regurgitation.

Tricuspid regurgitation, whether resulting from damage to the tricuspid valve or simply from dilatation of its annulus secondary to right ventricular failure, is characterised by exaggerated systolic venous pulsation (Fig. 5.12). Traditionally these waves are called *v* waves, which is unfortunate as their mechanism and timing are different from the physiological *v* waves described above. However to coin a new name for them would only add to confusion. The *v* waves of tricuspid regurgitation occur in mid-systole, are often accompanied by palpable venous pulsation, and in severe cases a tricuspid regurgitant murmur and a pulsatile liver can also be detected.

When the JVP is elevated, the *y* descent after

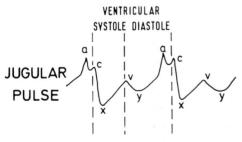

Fig. 5.11 Form of the venous pulse wave tracing from internal jugular vein. a = atrial systole; c = transmitted pulsation of carotid artery at onset of ventricular systole; v = peak pressure in right atrium immediately prior to opening of tricuspid valve; a − x = x descent, due to atrial relaxation; v − y = y descent at commencement of ventricular filling.

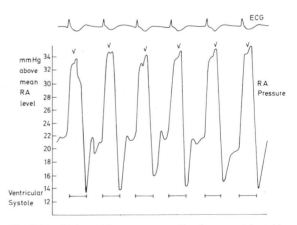

Fig. 5.12 Right atrial pressure recording in severe tricuspid regurgitation. Systolic pulse waves of large amplitude are present, and unlike the physiological *v* waves (Fig. 5.11) they start in early systole. Atrial fibrillation is present, so *a* waves are absent.

tricuspid valve opening is usually the most prominent feature of the venous pulse, provided tricuspid regurgitation is absent. In the presence of right ventricular failure ventricular stiffness is increased and this tends to produce some 'damping' of the y descent. In constrictive pericarditis however initial ventricular filling is unimpeded, only to be brought to a sudden halt as the limits set by the pericardium are reached. The resulting combination of a raised venous pressure and a precipitous early phase of the y descent is often striking. Tricuspid stenosis on the other hand gives a slow y and x descent, together with large a waves.

The patency and function of peripheral veins

The principal abnormalities of the peripheral venous system are thrombophlebitis, deep vein thrombosis and varicose veins.

The characteristics of superficial venous thrombosis and a deep venous thrombosis affecting a lower limb are given below.

Thrombosis of the axillary or subclavian vein occurs relatively infrequently. It will cause pain or swelling in the arm with a distension of veins around the shoulder. If the superior vena cava is involved, swelling and venous congestion affect the neck and face.

Superficial venous thrombosis (thrombophlebitis):

Causes: Intravenous infusions
Insect bites
Trauma
Spontaneous
Rarely, a manifestation of malignant disease (and then often recurrent: thrombophlebitis migrans)
Site: Superficial veins of arms, legs and trunk
Features: Pain, redness, oedema, lymphadenopathy. Vein can be felt as a hard tender cord
Differential Diagnosis: Infection
Outcome: Spontaneous resolution

Deep vein thrombosis of the lower limb:

Causes: Stasis — from prolonged immobility e.g long distance flights

Post-operative
High dose oestrogens
Intra-abdominal infection
Intra-abdominal tumours
Site: Deep veins of calf, thigh, pelvis, axillary or subclavian vein
Features: Often clinically silent. May be aching and swelling in leg, with prominence of superficial veins. May be tenderness over femoral vein.
Differential diagnosis: Partial rupture of gastrocnemius muscle, rupture of semimembranosus bursa of knee joint (Baker's cyst).
Confirmation of diagnosis: Venogram, impedance plethysmography, Doppler scan
Outcome: Risk of pulmonary embolism from thrombus which extends above the calf. Risk of permanent damage to venous valves of leg veins ('post-phlebitic syndrome').

Varicose veins. These are distended superficial veins of the legs. Predisposing factors include incompetence of the venous valves in the long and short saphenous veins, and especially in the perforating veins which connect the deep and superficial venous systems of the leg. Varicose veins will only be seen with the patient in the erect posture. Competence of the valves in the long saphenous vein can be tested by first 'emptying' the veins by elevating the leg, then compressing the saphenofemoral junction with a finger or light tourniquet and asking the patient to stand up. If the varicosities are due solely to saphenofemoral incompetence they will not fill until the finger is removed. Commonly, there will be some filling of the varices via perforating veins even while the long saphenous vein is occluded. The precise sites of the perforating veins can often be established using multiple points of compression.

4. EXAMINATION OF THE HEART

The methods used are inspection, palpation, percussion (occasionally) and auscultation.

Inspection

Inspection of the chest with particular relevance to the heart includes the detection of deformity and both normal and abnormal pulsation.

Emphysema and severe kyphosis or scoliosis

may be recognised by inspection alone; either of these conditions can lead to heart failure. A minor degree of sternal depression or pectus excavatum (p. 137) is common and harmless, but is sometimes associated with a soft systolic murmur and minor ECG abnormalities. Skeletal abnormalities such as pectus excavatum or kyphoscoliosis may also be part of Marfan's syndrome, in which abnormalities of the heart and aorta are common. In those forms of congenital heart disease in which gross pulmonary artery hypertension is a feature during the growing period, e.g. in some large ventricular septal defects, there may be prominence of the left chest over the hypertrophied right ventricle, and a bilateral Harrison's sulcus (p. 137) may be seen. The tense pulmonary arteries reduce lung compliance, the pull of the diaphragm is increased and the chest wall may be indrawn at its attachment to the ribs just as in those who suffer from severe asthma during the growing period.

The forceful apical thrust of left ventricular hypertrophy, the left parasternal impulse of right ventricular hypertrophy, and the pulsation of an enlarged pulmonary artery in the second left intercostal space may all be detected on inspection. In patients with a dilated and hypokinetic left ventricle as a consequence of myocardial infarction or cardiomyopathy an extensive but diffuse area of apical pulsation can often be seen more easily than felt. In hypertrophic cardiomyopathy the apical impulse often has a characteristic 'double beat' quality which again may be more easily seen than felt. An aneurysm of the aorta may produce a pulsation in the second right intercostal space or of the upper sternum. When the heart is much enlarged the chest wall may be seen to move with each heart beat.

Epigastric pulsation transmitted from the abdominal aorta is a normal finding, particularly in thin people. Abnormal pulsation in this region may be due to enlargement of the right ventricle, abdominal aneurysm, pancreatic cyst or to pulsation of the liver as a result of tricuspid regurgitation.

Palpation

Discriminating palpation of the chest is one of the most valuable methods in the examination of the heart, and can often enable prediction of some of the findings on auscultation. The right hand is first placed on the left chest wall with the middle finger lying in about the fifth intercostal space in the anterior axillary line. The position of the apex beat is then defined, if possible, and the quality of the apical impulse noted. Abnormal vibrations (see thrills below) are also sought. The hand is then placed to the left of the sternum and then on the manubrium and any pulsations and thrills again noted.

Apex beat. The position of the apex beat is best defined as the furthest point downwards and outwards on the chest wall where the finger is lifted by the cardiac impulse. The patient should be semi-recumbent, because the heart moves to a variable extent on standing or turning to one side. The normal apex beat is within the mid-clavicular line in the fifth interspace. The second costal cartilage is at the level of the manubriosternal angle whence the interspaces can readily be identified. When displaced, the site of the apex beat should be localised in terms of intercostal space and with reference to mid-clavicular, anterior axillary and mid-axillary lines. Many students are puzzled by the fact that the finger is lifted during systole, when the ventricle is contracting. This due to the complex rotatory movement of the heart with systole, one effect of which is a forward movement of the apex. Sometimes the apex beat cannot be felt. The common causes of this are obesity or emphysema, and in the latter case the heart sounds may be faint or inaudible. A pericardial effusion may also make the heart beat impalpable. The apex beat may be displaced, or even impalpable, because of disease of the lung or pleura when the trachea may be deviated (p. 136) and abnormalities found on examination of the chest. Very rarely as a congenital abnormality the heart lies on the right side (*dextrocardia*), but this should be revealed if due attention is paid to the site of maximum intensity of the heart sounds.

The apex beat may also be displaced because of cardiac enlargement. The apex impulse is abnormally forceful in left ventricular hypertrophy, and the terms heaving, thrusting or sustained are commonly used to describe it. In mitral stenosis, on the other hand, the abnormally increased shock of closure of the mitral valve may be palpable in which case the sensation is like that of an unusually hard knock on the other side of a closed door and the impulse is described as 'tapping'.

The best evidence of right ventricular hypertrophy is a diffuse impulse to the left of the sternum. However in emphysema there may be considerable right ventricular hypertrophy which cannot be detected in life, because the over-inflated lung intervenes between the heart and the chest wall.

Thrills. Murmurs (p. 107) may be so loud as to be palpable as thrills, examples being the apical diastolic thrill of mitral stenosis and the basal systolic thrill of aortic stenosis (often accompanied by a suprasternal thrill and carotid 'shudder' p. 108). Thrills are best appreciated when the patient leans forward with the breath held in expiration, with the exception of the thrill of mitral stenosis which is most easily felt when the patient turns on to the left side. The back of a purring cat traditionally and accurately provides the nearest palpable equivalent to the diastolic thrill of mitral stenosis; systolic thrills are more nearly imitated by a bluebottle trapped in the hand. The upper left parasternal systolic thrill of pulmonary stenosis, and the lower left parasternal systolic thrill of a ventricular septal defect, are the the most common examples among the congenital causes. A diastolic thrill over the sternum is very uncommon, occurring only with gross aortic regurgitation. A suspected thrill is denied by the subsequent finding that there is either no murmur or only a very quiet one. The sudden development of a thrill is an important manifestation of acute valve failure, for example in infective endocarditis, or when there is mechanical failure of an artificial heart valve.

Other palpable abnormalities. When the semilunar valve close under an abnormally high pressure there may be a palpable shock at the upper end of the sternum. When this is due to closure of the pulmonary valves, it is often most readily appreciated to the left of the sternum. An aneurysm of the arch of the aorta may produce a pulsation which is generally maximal in the second right intercostal space, but which may also lift the sternum. Likewise, a dilated pulmonary artery may give a palpable pulse to the left of the sternum at about the second left intercostal space. Occasionally pericardial friction (p. 112) is palpable.

Percussion

There is usually an area of dullness to percussion to the left of the sternum where the heart lies against the chest. This area is reduced or absent in cases of emphysema. There may be abnormal dullness to percussion to the right of the sternum when a large pericardial effusion is present. Massive enlargement of the left atrium occurs occasionally in rheumatic disease of the mitral valve, usually with gross mitral regurgitation and the resultant dullness posteriorly has been mistaken for a pleural effusion. A large aneurysm of the aorta may produce an area of abnormal dullness to the right of the upper sternum. Percussion is usually employed only when these conditions are suspected. A radiograph of the chest provides more reliable evidence.

Auscultation

Expertise comes with time and practice. In the first few months the student will be doing well if the first and second heart sounds can be identified, and murmurs accurately classified as systolic or diastolic. It is best in describing auscultatory findings to be modest but accurate rather than detailed but wrong.

Correct *timing* is essential, and it is good practice to feel the patient's carotid pulse with the thumb of one hand whilst the other hand holds the stethoscope to the precordium. The author starts auscultation at the cardiac apex, but others prefer to begin in the pulmonary area; students need to establish their own routine. Whatever the order, it is essential to listen at the apex, to the left and right of both upper and lower parts of the sternum, and beneath the clavicles. It is best to make a rapid survey of all these sites using the diaphragm of the stethoscope, and then to return for a longer period to those sites where an abnormality was heard, or to the best sites (see below) for detecting specific lesions suggested by the history and other parts of the examination. The bell of the stethoscope, with the chestpiece pressed

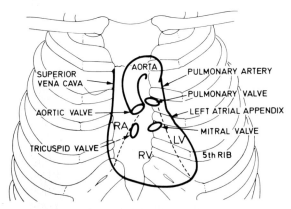

Fig. 5.13 The surface markings of the valves in relationship to the radiological outline of the heart. The directions in which sounds and murmurs are preferentially conducted from the valves are described on pages 107 to 111.

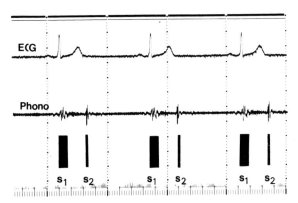

Fig. 5.14 Auscultatory notation. The relationship between a phonocardiogram (the graphic recording of the heart sounds) and the conventional 'shorthand' auscultatory notation.

lightly against the skin, is best for conducting low pitched sounds such as mid-diastolic murmurs or the third heart sound. The diaphragm, pressed firmly against the skin, selectively filters out low pitched sounds, and thereby emphasises high pitched ones such as the second heart sound or early diastolic murmurs.

Pulmonary valve closure and pulmonary ejection murmurs are usually best heard in the second or third intercostal spaces to the left of the sternum, and aortic ejection murmurs in a corresponding site to the right of the sternum. These sites are sometimes called the *pulmonary and aortic areas* respectively, but it must be appreciated that they are several centimetres away from the surface projection of the valves themselves (Fig. 5.13). At these sites, it is advisable to use the diaphragm of the stethoscope. At the apex, it is necessary to listen with both the diaphragm and the bell. It is essential to auscultate with the patient rolled on to the left side if mitral stenosis is to be excluded. Conversely, the second heart sound and early diastolic murmurs are best heard if the patient sits up and leans forward.

Auscultatory notation

Traditionally, the first and second heart sounds are said to sound like 'lub-dup'. This type of description, though evocative, is clumsy and lacking in precision when applied to more complex auscul-

tatory findings. Phonocardiography, a technique for visually displaying heart sounds either on paper or on an oscilloscope screen, has provided the basis for a more flexible graphical notation for auscultation. Figure 5.14 shows a phonocardiogram recorded from a normal heart. The first and second heart sounds appear as vertical 'blips' on either side of a baseline. The height of the blip depends on the loudness of the sound, and the width on its duration. The conventional shorthand auscultatory notation is simply a sketch of what might be seen on phonocardiography, using vertical lines or oblong blocks to represent the heart sounds, and shading to represent murmurs. Ventricular systole is represented by the space between the first and second heart sounds. Ventricular diastole can be subdivided into early diastole which ends with the opening of the mitral and tricuspid valves, mid-diastole which physiologically represents passive ventricular filling, and late diastole (or presystole) which corresponds with atrial systole and is graphically represented by the space before the first heart sound. The significance of these sub-divisions will become clearer when the timing of individual murmurs and other sounds is discussed presently.

The heart sounds

Conventionally, there are first, second, third and fourth heart sounds. The first and second sounds (S_1 and S_2 in shorthand) are virtually always audible. The third and fourth (S_3 and S_4) become prominent only under special circumstances. Other sounds audible during the cardiac cycle but distinguished from murmurs by their short duration are sometimes grouped together as 'added sounds', although their causes are very diverse. They include the opening snap of mitral stenosis, ejection clicks arising in the aorta or pulmonary artery, mid-systolic clicks associated with mitral valve prolapse, and the sounds associated with mechanical prosthetic heart valves. The student will find that if attention is concentrated initially on the first and second heart sounds, identification of other heart sounds will come later.

The first heart sound. This is principally the sound of mitral valve closure. Tricuspid valve closure is usually very quiet, but may be loud if right ventricular pressure is elevated.

The first heart sound is recognised as:

1. The 'lub' in 'lub-dup'
2. The sound which immediately precedes the main apical impulse
3. The sound which immediately precedes the carotid pulse wave.

It is well heard with both the bell and the diaphragm of the stethoscope, and is usually loudest at the apex, or between the apex and the lower left sternal border.

The loudness of the first heart sound varies with the position of the mitral valve cusps at the onset of systole. If the cusps are wide apart they are 'slammed' together to produce a loud S_1, but if they are close together at the onset of systole then S_1 tends to be quiet. The first sound thus tends to be prominent in patients with an increased cardiac output, and may be almost inaudible in severe cardiac failure. Beat to beat variation in intensity of S_1 occurs in atrial fibrillation, and also in atrioventricular dissociation, where the relation between atrial and ventricular systole is constantly changing. A loud S_1 is also characteristic of mitral stenosis, but the mechanism is different; here the abnormal valve acts as a rather stiff diaphragm which is suddenly tensed by the chordae tendineae as the ventricle contracts. The resulting shock wave is not only heard as a loud S_1 but may also be felt on palpation of the precordium.

The second heart sound. This is due to the closure of aortic and pulmonary valves at the end of ventricular systole.

The second heart sound is recognised as:

1. The 'dup' in 'lub-dup'
2. The sound which follows the apical impulse
3. The sound which immediately follows the carotid pulse wave.

It is usually best heard at the upper left sternal edge using the diaphragm of the stethoscope. During quiet expiration the components of S_2 which are due to aortic valve closure (sometimes called A_2) and to pulmonary valve closure (P_2) are virtually inseparable. During inspiration P_2 tends to be delayed because of increased venous return, while A_2 occurs a little sooner because left ventricular filling is slightly reduced. The second heart sound may then become *split* — the earlier component is due to aortic and the latter to pulmonary valve closure (Fig. 5.15). This normal or

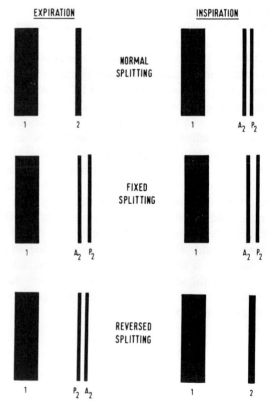

Fig. 5.15 Splitting of the second heart sound. Shown in diagrammatic representations of phonocardiograms.

physiological splitting of the second heart sound is easy to detect in children or young adults, but becomes much more difficult to hear in older patients. Like sinus arrhythmia, physiological splitting of the seond heart sound disappears in the presence of heart failure.

Delayed closure of the pulmonary valve tends to occur when the right ventricle is dilated, when there is obstruction to right ventricular emptying as in pulmonary stenosis, or when there is delay in the electrical activation of the right ventricle as indicated by the appearance of right bundle branch block on the ECG. All these can lead to exaggerated splitting of the second heart sound, but the width of the split still tends to increase with inspiration and decrease with expiration.

In atrial septal defect the increase in right ventricular stroke volume as a consequence of a left to right shunt at atrial level causes wide splitting of the second heart sound, but because right and left atria are in free communication right and left ventricular stroke volumes vary in the same way during the respiratory cycle. The result is *fixed splitting* of the second heart sound which is pathognomic of atrial septal defect.

Chronic pulmonary hypertension does not in itself cause exaggerated splitting of the second sound, because, although the right ventricle is ejecting blood against a higher pressure, the actual ejection time of the hypertrophied ventricle is not appreciably prolonged. Both systemic and pulmonary hypertension may cause the second sound to be excessively loud, but the effect is more striking with pulmonary hypertension because the pulmonary valve lies closer to the chest wall. With severe pulmonary hypertension the shock of pulmonary valve closure may be palpable.

If left ventricular ejection is abnormally delayed, P_2 may occur before A_2, and the second sound splits in expiration and comes together in inspiration. This *reversed splitting* of the second sound is often striking in hypertrophic obstructive cardiomyopathy (p. 109). It may also occur in left bundle branch block and in aortic stenosis, but here it can be difficult to detect because rigidity of the valve may make A_2 very quiet.

The third heart sound (S_3). This sound coincides with the onset of the rapid period of ventricular diastolic filling. It is analogous to the

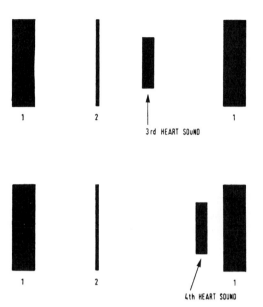

Fig. 5.16 Third and fourth heart sounds. The third sound coincides with the onset of ventricular filling, and the fourth sound with the ventricular filling which results from atrial contraction. The third and fourth sounds are heard at the cardiac apex when they arise in the left ventricle, and to the left of the lower sternum when their origin is in the right ventricle. (Diagrammatic representations of phonocardiograms.)

sound produced when a slack sail suddenly fills with wind. Usually S_3 is low-pitched and best heard at the apex with the stethoscope bell; it is sometimes palpable. Occasionally S_3 is loud and the casual auscultator mistakes it for S_2 (Fig. 5.16). This may occur particularly in mitral regurgitation where the murmur may partly obscure S_2.

A third sound is 'physiological' in healthy young adults and particularly in athletes, with their slow resting pulse rate and large stroke volume. In older patients, and especially when it is associated with tachycardia and other signs of cardiac failure, its presence indicates impaired ventricular function, and specifically, a raised end-diastolic pressure. The combination of tachycardia and a loud S_3 gives a characteristic cadence to the heart sounds described as a *gallop rhythm*, or more prosaically, a *triple rhythm*. A third sound can originate from either ventricle, and the one responsible is usually deduced from the circumstances rather than the quality of the sound.

Table 5.7 Normal and added sounds related to events and timing of the cardiac cycle

Sound	Event	Timing
First sound	Closure of AV valves	
Ejection sound	Opening of semilunar valves	SYSTOLE
Second sound	Closure of semilunar valves	
Opening snap	Opening of abnormal AV valves (e.g. in mitral stenosis)	
Third sound	Ventricular filling begins	DIASTOLE
Fourth sound	Ventricular filling increases with atrial contraction	

The fourth heart sound (S_4). This sound accompanies, and is due to, atrial systole. It can be heard only in the presence of sinus rhythm. Although phonocardiography can detect a quiet S_4 in many normal subjects, it tends to become particularly prominent when a hypertrophied left atrium pumps blood through an unobstructed mitral valve into a stiff left ventricle; these conditions are most often fulfilled in ischaemic heart disease or systemic hypertension. It is usually a rather low-pitched sound best heard at the apex with the bell of the stethoscope. Tachycardia with a fourth heart sound may also produce a triple or gallop rhythm. In patients with a sufficiently slow heart rate it is sometimes possible to make out fourth, first, second and third heart sounds, but as the heart rate increases third and fourth sounds tend to merge.

The opening snap. This is a high-pitched sound which occurs in patients with mitral stenosis when the stenosed valve moves forward towards the left ventricle at the beginning of diastole. It is best heard with the diaphragm of the stethoscope, and is sometimes more obvious at the left sternal edge than at the apex. Occasionally it is mistaken for a widely split second sound. A loud opening snap implies that the valve, though stenosed, is still mobile. As the valve stiffens and calcifies the

opening snap may become quieter or disappear. The interval between the second heart sound and the opening snap gets shorter with increasing left atrial pressure, and thus with more severe mitral stenosis.

Ejection clicks. These are high-pitched sounds which closely follow the first heart sound. They originate from either the aortic valve and aorta or pulmonary valve and pulmonary artery. Aortic ejection clicks tend to be best heard in the 'aortic area' at the upper right sternal edge, and pulmonary ejection clicks in the 'pulmonary area' to the left of the upper sternum. Aortic ejection clicks are most commonly associated with congenitally bicuspid aortic valves or congenital aortic stenosis, and are probably due principally to the opening of the abnormal cusps. Ejection of blood into a dilated ascending aorta may also play a part. Similarly, pulmonary ejection clicks are most commonly due to valvular pulmonary stenosis, but can also be heard in patients with idiopathic dilatation of the pulmonary artery, or with pulmonary artery dilatation caused by pulmonary hypertension.

Mid-systolic clicks. Mitral valve prolapse (p. 109) is the commonest cause of these added sounds. A small pneumothorax may also produce a regular systolic click (p. 147).

Prosthetic valve sounds. Replacement heart valves may be grafts of suitably treated animal (usually porcine) tissue, or may be artificial mechanical valves such as the Starr-Edwards ball valve or the Bjork-Shiley disc valve. 'Biological' heart valves produce similar heart sounds to the natural valves they replace. Mechanical valves usually produce two sounds or clicks for each cardiac cycle: a quiet opening click and a louder closing sound. With a mitral prosthesis the loud closing sound accompanies (and largely constitutes) the first heart sound, and the opening click follows the second sound in a similar position to the opening snap of mitral stenosis. Conversely, with an aortic prosthesis the opening sound follows S_1 in a similar position to an ejection click, while the louder closing sound accompanies S_2. Careful recording of prosthetic sounds is important in reviewing patients after heart valve replacement, because disappearance or muffling of a previously-documented opening sound is an early indication of thrombosis on the valve.

The relationship of the normal and added sounds to the events and timing of the cardiac cycle is summarised in Table 5.7 (p. 104).

The rate and rhythm of the heart

The heart rate. *Tachycardia* is a heart rate faster than 100 per minute, and *bradycardia* is a rate slower than 50 per minute, but the appropriateness of the tachycardia or bradycardia is more significant than its absolute value. Sinus tachycardia is to be expected during exercise or in a febrile patient. It accompanies anxiety, shock and most forms of cardiac failure, and it is a normal finding in infants or young children. Sinus bradycardia is common during sleep, and often occurs at rest in healthy and athletic young people. On the other hand it may be a feature of the 'sick sinus syndrome', of hypothyroidism or hypothermia, or of raised intracranial pressure. Ectopic beats (extrasystoles), when they alternate with normal beats and produce no palpable pulse, may cause an illusion of bradycardia, but auscultation will reveal them.

In complete heart block the heart rate is usually less than 50 per minute, and may fall as low as 20. In *paroxysmal supraventricular tachycardia* the pulse rate is usually between 140 and 180 per minute, and may be more rapid in children. Carotid sinus massage (p.112) may terminate the attack, or, by increasing the atrio-ventricular block, produce a transient but abrupt fall in pulse rate. *Atrial flutter* is a variant of atrial tachycardia with a rapid atrial rate of about 300 per minute. The ventricles usually respond to alternate atrial beats (2 : 1 atrio-ventricular block) giving a regular pulse of 150 per minute, but carotid sinus pressure may cause a sudden reduction to 100 per minute (3 : 1 block) or slower. Atrial fibrillation is considered under heart rhythm (p. 106).

Ventricular tachycardia may produce a rate so rapid that the pulse is impalpable and the patient may lose consciousness. At slower rates it may be difficult to distinguish from atrial tachycardia without the help of the ECG. Carotid sinus pressure does not affect the rate in ventricular tachycardia, but this is not a reliable point of distinction as some cases of atrial tachycardia also fail to respond.

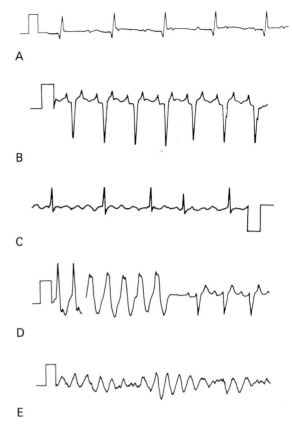

Fig. 5.17 Some examples of cardiac arrhythmias. (A) Complete heart block in a patient with an anterior myocardial infarction (lead V1 — note the Q wave). (B) Atrial tachycardia with a 2:1 block (lead V1). (C) Atrial fibrillation with controlled ventricular response (lead V1). (D) Ventricular tachycardia rising from a left ventricular focus confirmed by concordant positivity from V1–V6. The arrhythmia was abolished following an IV bolus of lignocaine (lead V1). (E) Ventricular fibrillation — note the chaotic pattern (lead 11).

Heart rhythm. The commonest irregularity is *sinus arrhythmia* — this is an acceleration of the heart rate during inspiration and a slowing at the beginning of expiration. It is particularly prominent in adolescents or athletic young adults, or in circumstances of increased vagal tone. It is not found in patients with cardiac failure, with autonomic neuropathy (e.g. in diabetes) or with a large atrial septal defect.

Ectopic beats are recognised by their prematurity; they occur earlier than the next expected regular beat. The more premature the ectopic beat, the smaller the pulse volume, and very premature beats may not be detected at the wrist. Ectopic beats are followed by a compensatory pause, and because of this the succeeding pulse may be of greater than normal volume; it is this beat, rather than the extrasystole, which is often noticed by the patient. In theory, atrial and ventricular extrasystoles can be distinguished by the length of the compensatory pause, but the ECG does so more reliably. In some patients extrasystoles disappear on exercise as the heart rate increases, but in others, and especially in patients with ischaemic heart disease, they may be induced by exertion.

Intermittent heart block causing 'dropped beats' may also cause an irregular pulse, although much less often than extrasystoles. Atrio-ventricular conduction may fail sporadically and unpredictably, or there may be a regular numerical relationship between atrial and ventricular beats (Wenckebach block). In the latter, it is as though succeeding atrial beats found it increasingly difficult to 'get through' to the ventricle, until one beat fails to do so and a pause results which allows the conducting system to recover (Fig. 5.18). The resulting pulse cadence is accurately described, in Wenckebach's own expression, as a 'regular intermission of the pulse'.

Atrial fibrillation causes an 'irregularly irregular' pulse. Both the interval between, and the volume of, consecutive pulses vary from beat to beat. Aus-

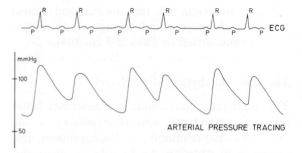

Fig. 5.18 The Wenckebach phenomenon. ECG and pulse trace showing 3:2 atrioventricular block; every third P wave on the ECG is not followed by a QRS complex, and a pulse beat is 'dropped'.

cultation confirms the irregularity of heart rhythm, and the intensity of the heart sounds is also variable. In general, the first heart sound tends to be louder after a long diastole and softer after a short one, but the converse may be true at slow heart rates. The atrial rate is always very rapid and strictly speaking it is incorrect to refer to a controlled ventricular rate as 'slow atrial fibrillation'. The irregularity of rhythm is reflected in beat to beat variation of blood pressure — the systolic and diastolic pressures have to be expressed as an approximate average over several beats. When the ventricular rate is fast, as is often the case at the onset of atrial fibrillation, some of the pulse beats are too weak to be palpable, and there is a pulse

Table 5.8 Causes of atrial fibrillation

Cause	Clues	Tests
Valvular disease (especially mitral)	Auscultation	CXR, echocardiography
Alcohol	History, parotid or liver enlargement	Liver function, echocardiography
Thyrotoxicosis	History, tremor, goitre, eye signs. Classic features often absent in the elderly	Thyroid function
Ischaemia or hypertensive heart disease	History, blood pressure	ECG, echocardiography exclusion
Sick sinus syndrome	History	Ambulatory ECG monitoring
Carcinoma bronchus	Smoking history	CXR
Atrial septal defect	Auscultation	CXR, echocardiography

deficit between the apical rate and the rate counted at the wrist. As the ventricular rate slows, either spontaneously or in response to digoxin, the pulse deficit tends to become less. A fourth heart sound, which is associated with atrial systole, is never heard in atrial fibrillation. No *a* waves are seen in the jugular venous pulse, but *v* waves and tricuspid regurgitant waves may be present. Sometimes the heart rhythm is so close to being regular that its true nature is appreciated only from the ECG. Patients with atrial fibrillation sometimes complain of palpitations but often the arrhythmia is discovered only on examining the patient with cardiac failure or arterial embolism, or during a routine medical examination. Some important causes of atrial fibrillation are shown in Table 5.8.

Murmurs

Attention must be paid to the intensity, quality and timing of a murmur. Murmurs arise from turbulent blood flow and they tend to be propagated in the same direction as the flow. Obviously, the louder a murmur is, the further it will be propagated, irrespective of its site origin. In the analysis of a murmur its timing and quality are the most important distinguishing features, and the latter has to be learned from experience, although recordings may be of help. In regard to timing, murmurs are classified, in the first instance, as systolic, diastolic or continuous. The timing of a murmur can be assessed by reference to the first and second heart sounds or by checking it against the carotid pulse.

The intensity of a murmur is often described in terms of grades, as follows:

Grade 1. Just audible in a quiet room, with the patient's breath held and using a good stethoscope
Grade 2. Quiet
Grade 3. Moderately loud
Grade 4. Loud, and accompanied by a thrill
Grade 5. Very loud
Grade 6. Audible without a stethoscope and with the head away from the chest.

Such a murmur may sometimes be heard with the stethoscope chest-piece on top of the patient's head, on the sacrum or at the wrists and even by the patient's spouse.

Murmurs of Grade 4 and louder are accompanied by a palpable thrill. It is unusual for competent observers to record more than one grade difference after listening to the same murmur. The record should state, for example, Grade 5/6 murmur, i.e. fifth out of six grades, so that the number of grades used is made clear.

Systolic murmurs.

These are divided into (1) ejection systolic murmurs, (2) pansystolic murmurs (sometimes called holosystolic in the United States) and (3) late systolic murmurs.

1. Ejection systolic murmurs. These result from turbulent blood flow through distorted or stenotic semilunar valves, or occasionally from turbulence caused by increased bloodflow through normal semilunar valves. The murmur increases to a crescendo about the middle of systole, then diminishes and ceases just before the second heart sound. The murmur may be preceded by an ejection click (p. 104). The crescendo-decrescendo nature of the murmur gives a 'diamond shaped' pattern on the phonocardiograph (Fig. 5.20) and this is also used in the 'shorthand notation' for the murmur (Fig. 5.19). It is wrong however to speak of 'diamond shaped murmurs'.

Examples of ejection systolic murmurs. The murmur of *aortic stenosis* (Figs. 5.19 and 5.20) was called a 'bruit de scie' (i.e. a saw-like murmur) by Laënnec, the founder of the stethoscopic art. The acoustic quality and the acceleration and deceleration of the saw provide a precise analogy. It is usually loudest in the second right intercostal space or suprasternal notch, and radiates to the

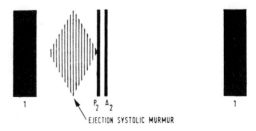

Fig. 5.19   Ejection systolic murmur (aortic stenosis). The aortic element of the second heart sound is delayed and a split second heart sound results.

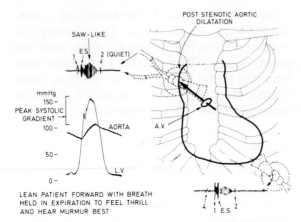

Fig. 5.20 Aortic stenosis. There is a systolic pressure gradient across the stenotic aortic valve (AV). The resultant high velocity jet (arrow) impinges on the wall of the aorta and the diaphragm placed near to this on the chest detects the murmur best: alternatively the bell may be placed in the suprasternal notch. The phonocardiograms show the ejection systolic murmur preceded by an ejection sound (ES). A fourth heart sound may be heard at the apex.

neck. With calcific aortic stenosis it sometimes has a mewing quality like the cry of a seagull. If the aortic stenosis is severe, and left ventricular function well preserved, there is usually an accompanying thrill, and in the carotid arteries the turbulence is felt as a carotid shudder. With the onset of cardiac failure the murmur may become surprisingly soft. The murmur is generally better heard at the apex than it is over the right ventricle, and occasionally may be louder at the apex than it is at the base. An ejection click (p. 104) strongly favours valvular stenosis; in every other respect the murmur of the much rarer subvalvular stenosis is clinically similar. In elderly patients with valvular stenosis an ejection click is seldom present—either because the cusps are calcified and immobile, or because the stenosis is due to calcific accretions at the base of the cups rather than to cusp rigidity or fusion.

Pulmonary stenosis. This murmur is of similar quality to that of aortic stenosis, and at the same level, but loudest in the second left intercostal space. The murmur radiates towards the left shoulder. The loudness of the murmur is a better guide to the severity of pulmonary stenosis than of aortic stenosis.

Atrial septal defect. The increased pulmonary blood flow of an atrial septal defect also may produce a pulmonary ejection systolic murmur but this is not usually of more than grade 3/6 intensity. The flow of blood through the defect itself does not produce a murmur. The second sound may be split throughout the respiratory cycle in both pulmonary stenosis and atrial septal defects, due to delay in onset, or a prolongation, of right ventricular ejection, but fixed splitting is a characteristic of atrial septal defect (p. 103). A mid-diastolic murmur in the tricuspid area indicates turbulent flow at tricuspid valve and strongly favours an atrial septal defect; it is the only diastolic murmur which sounds like a systolic murmur. It never rumbles like that of mitral stenosis.

2. Pansystolic murmurs. These are so called because they extend throughout systole, and they are the result of escape of blood from a ventricle into an area of low pressure, as with a leaking atrioventricular valve, or a small ventricular septal defect. The murmur has little mid-systolic accentuation, and, unlike the ejection murmur, starts simultaneously with the first heart sound and may spill over into early diastole, for the pressure gradient responsible for the abnormal flow persists after closure of the semilunar valves (Fig. 5.21). The distinction between an ejection type systolic murmur and a pansystolic murmur can usually be made with the stethoscope, but occasionally may be impossible even with a phonocardiogram.

Examples of pansystolic murmurs. Mitral regurgitation of significance usually produces an apical pansystolic murmur, radiating to the axilla and often heard over the lower left chest at the back. It may be as loud as grade 5/6. The increased forward flow through the valve in diastole often produces a low-pitched short mid-diastolic

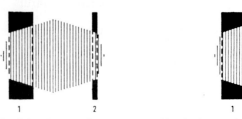

Fig. 5.21 Pansystolic murmur as with mitral regurgitation.

murmur of abrupt onset, or a third heart sound. When some mitral stenosis coexists atrioventricular flow is throttled, the murmur is less abrupt in onset and a third heart sound is not present.

Tricuspid regurgitation usually produces a pansystolic murmur audible over the right ventricle to the left of the sternum in the fourth intercostal space. A much enlarged right ventricle may extend to the left anterior axillary line, and under these circumstances the murmur is often mistaken for that of mitral regurgitation. The explanation already given for the diastolic murmur or third sound of mitral regurgitation applies to a similar murmur or sound at the left sternal edge in the fourth interspace accompanying tricuspid regurgitation. A tricuspid regurgitant murmur is usually accompanied by a systolic jugular venous pulse wave and often by systolic expansion of the liver. These findings may occur in heart failure from rheumatic or ischaemic heart disease, or with chronic cor pulmonale.

Ventricular septal defect. A pansystolic murmur to the left of the sternum is the characteristic murmur of a jet of blood through this defect. It has a typical rough quality, like the tearing of fabric, and is usually accompanied by a thrill. When the defect is small this is the only physical sign. When it is larger the shunt is responsible also for an apical mid-diastolic murmur because of increased flow through the mitral valve.

3. Late systolic murmurs. These are systolic murmurs which do not start immediately after the first heart sound, but begin later in systole.

Hypertrophic obstructive cardiomyopathy is sometimes associated with a ejection systolic murmur, but in other patients the obstruction to left ventricular ejection develops only in mid-systole, and the result is a mid or late systolic murmur. The timing of the murmur, as well as its intensity, may vary with left ventricular volume, and can be affected by posture or the Valsalva manoeuvre (p. 113). In addition, there may be a loud S_4 and reversed splitting of S_2.

Mitral valve prolapse is another cause of a late systolic murmur. In this condition elongation or rupture of the chordae tendineae tethering the mitral valve to the left ventricular papillary muscles allows a portion of one of the mitral valve

leaflets to prolapse into the left atrium during systole. The prolapse itself may be accompanied by a mid-systolic click (p. 104) and the mitral regurgitation which may result gives rise to a murmur. Sometimes the mid-systolic click (or clicks) is not associated with a murmur, and in other patients prolapse occurs at the onset of systole and the resulting pansystolic murmur is indistinguishable from that due to other causes of mitral regurgitation. Both the click and the murmur of mitral prolapse may vary strikingly with posture and phase of respiration; in some cases they can be heard only when the patient stands up. Echocardiography (p. 116) is very useful in confirming the diagnosis.

Diastolic murmurs

The three main types of diastolic murmur are (1) those of leaking semi-lunar valves, which are loudest in early diastole when the pressure gradient is highest, and which are decrescendo; these are termed *early diastolic murmurs;* (2) the murmurs of turbulent blood flow at the atrioventricular valves, which start slightly later in diastole and are therefore sometimes called *mid-diastolic* or *delayed diastolic murmurs;* and (3)

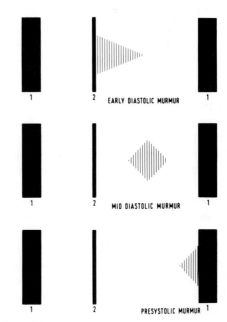

Fig. 5.22 Diastolic murmurs.

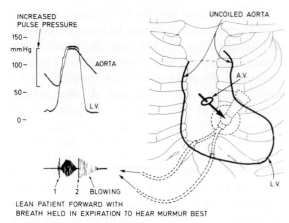

Fig. 5.23 Aortic regurgitation. The pulse pressure is usually increased; the jet from the aortic valve (AV) impinges on the interventricular septum (arrow) during diastole, producing a high pitched murmur which is best heard with the diaphragm. The phonocardiogram also shows the systolic murmur which is common because of the increased flow through the aortic valve in systole.

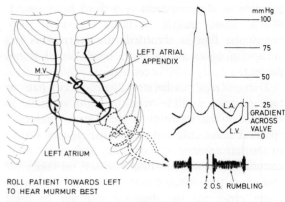

Fig. 5.24 Mitral stenosis. There is a pressure gradient across the mitral valve; in this example it continues throughout diastole. This causes a sharp movement of the tethered anterior cusp of the mitral valve at the time when flow commences and the opening snap (OS) results. The jet through the stenotic valve (arrow) strikes the endocardium at the cardiac apex. The murmur which results is best heard with the bell lightly applied there.

murmurs due to turbulence at one of the AV valves resulting from atrial contraction, so-called *presystolic*, or *atrial systolic* murmurs (Fig. 5.22).

Examples of diastolic murmurs. *Aortic regurgitation* produces a blowing early diastolic murmur of all grades of intensity (Fig. 5.23). When very soft it resembles a breath sound, and can then be detected only when breathing is arrested in expiration, and with the patient leaning forward. In aortic regurgitation of rheumatic origin the murmur is usually loudest to the left of the sternum in the fourth intercostal space; in syphilitic aortic regurgitation the murmur is often louder to the right of the sternum. Even the quietest aortic diastolic murmur cannot be ignored, and finding it may be of great clinical importance when infective endocarditis is suspected. In practice the murmur is often overlooked, either because the examiner is not attuned to hear the high-pitched noise or because auscultation is not performed in the proper manner and over a wide enough area.

Pulmonary regurgitation produces a murmur which is similar in quality and site to that of aortic regurgitation. A loud second heart sound to the left of the sternum or other features associated with pulmonary arterial hypertension favour pulmonary regurgitation as the cause of the murmur. Pulmonary regurgitation is much less common than aortic regurgitation. The murmur of pulmonary regurgitation is often called the *Graham Steell* murmur after the cardiologist who first described it; he called it the murmur of high pressure in the pulmonary artery long before it was possible to measure this pressure in man. It occurs with pulmonary arterial hypertension, e.g. in some cases of mitral stenosis or pulmonary arterial thromboembolism.

Mitral stenosis betrays itself to the stethoscope even when in all other respects the patient is normal (Fig. 5.24). The jet through the stenosed mitral valve impinges on the endocardium of the left ventricle at the apex, and the resulting turbulence shows itself as a murmur best heard at the site of the apical impulse. The auscultatory findings in mitral stenosis have been described as FFOUT-TA-TA-ROU, where FFOUT represents the loud first sound (though LUP might be better), the first TA the second heart sound, the second one the opening snap, and the ROU the low-pitched rumbling mitral diastolic murmur which is reminiscent of the rumble of rocks in a mountain river in flood. The murmur is best heard, in most cases, when the patient is turned half on to the left side, thus bringing the apex a little nearer to the chest wall, and by increasing the turbulence of mitral valve blood flow by slight exertion. When the reduction of the mitral valve orifice is only slight, the characteristic rumbling murmur is heard only during the increased blood velocity of atrial systole — the so-called presystolic murmur. Presystolic accentuation does not occur if there is atrial fibrillation. The murmur of mitral stenosis causes a low-pitched vibration of the chest wall which can often be damped out by pressure with the bell of the stethoscope. It is not generally appreciated that two people can listen to the same area, in the same patient, with the same bell stethoscope, and yet disagree because one person presses the bell harder against the skin than the other. A short rumbling apical mid-diastolic murmur is sometimes heard in patients with gross aortic regurgitation but without mitral stenosis, and is called after *Austin Flint*, who first described it. It is due to the aortic regurgitant jet interfering with the normal opening of the antero-medial cusp of the mitral valve. The label is usually reserved for patients who have aortic regurgitation which is not due to rheumatic heart disease, for in the latter case co-existent mitral stenosis would be the more likely cause of the murmur.

Tricuspid stenosis produces a murmur which is similar in timing to that of mitral stenosis, loudest to the left of the lower sternum, and in quality is higher pitched and harsher, and hence more like a systolic murmur. Its intensity usually increases during inspiration.

Continuous murmurs

Arteriovenous murmurs.   The characteristic murmur of an arteriovenous fistula is continuous throughout systole and diastole. A persistent ductus arteriosus, though not strictly an arteriovenous fistula as it joins the aorta to the pulmonary artery, provides a good example of this murmur, and in this case it is maximal in the second left intercostal space and generally accompanied by a thrill (Fig. 5.25).

Venous hum. A continuing roaring noise is often audible above either clavicle when the head and shoulders are higher than the heart (i.e. when the patient is sitting, standing or reclining against pillows). It is audible in most children when sitting. It is due to blood flow through the jugular

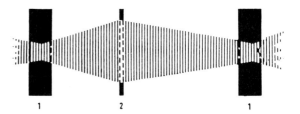

Fig. 5.25   Continuous murmur of persistent ductus arteriosus.

veins, and is abolished by pressure with the hand against the side of the patient's neck above the stethoscope, or by the patient assuming a horizontal or head-down position. It alters in intensity with changes in position of the head, and when loud may be heard surprisingly far away, e.g. to each side of the lower sternum. Its importance rests on the fact that it is extremely common, and often gives rise to a mistaken belief that there is a persistent ductus arteriosus. However, a venous hum lacks the late systolic accentuation characteristic of the murmur of a persistent ductus (Fig. 5.25).

Flow murmurs

These are murmurs produced by increased blood flow through normal valves. Soft ejection systolic murmurs are common after vigorous exercise, in the presence of anaemia, or during pregnancy, and characteristically disappear when the cause of an increased cardiac output is removed. Echocardiographic demonstration of valvular normality adds to the confidence with which they can be diagnosed. Diastolic flow murmurs are much less common, but are sometimes heard in children with torrential mitral or tricuspid valve bloodflow resulting from an intracardiac shunt.

Exocardiac 'noises'

Since murmurs are by definition sounds produced by turbulent bloodflow within the heart, it is best to use some other term for sounds recurring with each heartbeat but originating outside the heart. Pericardial rubs and the 'clicking' of a small pneumothorax (p. 147) are examples. Pneumomediastinum, which follows oesophageal rupture, or may complicate pneumothorax, may give rise to a spectacular exocardiac noise which sounds like a loud systolic murmur and is called a mediastinal crunch. Otherwise, exocardiac noises are seldom mistaken for murmurs.

Pericardial friction

The characteristic physical sign of acute pericarditis is a systolic and diastolic *pericardial rub* which is generally maximal to the left of the lower sternum, sounds like friction between rough surfaces and seems near to the stethoscope. It is accentuated when the patient leans forward, and by pressure with the stethoscope. Pleura overlies some of the heart and a pleural rub at this site may be indistinguishable from pericardial friction (p. 148). Some causes of a pericardial friction rub are shown in Table 5.9. The features of pericardial tamponade — with its acute development — and chronic pericardial constriction are summarised below.

Table 5.9 Causes of a pericardial friction rub

Causes	Other diagnostic features
Acute viral pericarditis	Usually benign. Serial antibody titres
Pyogenic pericarditis	Usually severe systemic symptoms. Effusion common. Blood cultures
Tuberculous pericarditis	Effusion common. Often few other features when acute. May lead to chronic constrictive pericarditis
Acute myocardial infarction	History, ECG
Dressler's syndrome	2–6 weeks following myocardial infarction. High ESR
Acute rheumatic fever	Other features of rheumatic fever (see text)
Systemic lupus erythematosus	Rash, renal impairment, serology
Rheumatoid arthritis	Effusion common, joints, serology
Uraemia	Plasma urea

All types of pericarditis can cause a pericardial effusion, though this is more common with some than others. When an effusion forms a pericardial rub may become inaudible.

Pericardial tamponade
Clinical Features:

    Raised Jugular Venous Pressure
    Hypotension
    Parodoxical pulse
    Oliguria

Causes: Trauma, e.g. stabbing
    Acute pericarditis (see Table 5.9)
    Metastases from malignant tumours
    Myxoedema

Diagnosis: Echocardiography

Chronic pericardial constriction
Clinical Features:

    Raised Jugular Venous pressure
    Hepatomegaly
    Ascites
    Peripheral oedema
    JVP rises with inspiration
    (Kussmaul's sign)
    Rarely, systolic indrawing of
    left lower ribs posteriorly
    (Broadbent's sign)

Causes: Tuberculosis
    Following viral infection
    'Idiopathic'

Diagnosis: Calcification on radiograph
    (especially lateral film)
    Cardiac catherisation
    Echocardiography

Cardiac and vasomotor reflexes

The normal function of the heart and vascular system is co-ordinated by a series of reflexes. Attempts to elicit these reflexes in patients with suspected disease may throw light on cardiovascular function on the one hand, and on that of the autonomic nervous system on the other.

The carotid sinus reflexes. Bradycardia is produced by pressure on the carotid sinus and in some patients this may also cause vasodilatation. *Carotid sinus massage* is a useful manoeuvre for transiently increasing vagus nerve activity. It is helpful in the diagnosis and treatment of tachycardias and sometimes in the assessment of blackouts and 'funny turns' (p. 29). It depends on stimulating the blood pressure receptors in the carotid sinus, which lies at the bifurcation of the common carotid into internal and external carotid arteries. Sometimes this bifurcation lies quite low in the neck; more commonly it is just beneath the angle of the jaw. Carotid sinus massage should be performed gently and only on one side at a time. The patient should lie supine as there is a risk of syncope in those with a sensitive reflex.

Tachycardia and vasoconstriction are mediated via carotid sinus and aortic arch baroreceptors to compensate for circumstances such as a change in posture which might otherwise result in hypotension. There is normally an increase in pulse rate when a person stands up, but this is not seen in patients, e.g. diabetics, with autonomic neuropathy. The response is also reduced by beta-blockade. If the vasoconstrictor response is deficient, postural hypotension may occur; the commonest cause is medication with antihypertensive drugs, but sometimes postural hypotension may be due not to a deficient reflex, but to hypovolaemia.

The Valsalva manoeuvre. This is a forced attempt at expiration when the mouth is shut and the nose held closed. The Valsalva manoeuvre is worth trying in patients with paroxysmal supraventricular tachycardia in an attempt to arrest the arrhythmia. It should be performed in a supine position and seems to be more effective in younger patients with this condition.

The Valsalva manoeuvre can also be used, in the absence of cardiac failure, to ascribe a murmur to the left or right side of the heart. Murmurs originating on either side tend to become quieter during the attempted expiration because venous return is reduced, but murmurs arising on the right side become louder immediately straining ceases, while those arising on the left regain their intensity about six beats later. An exception is the systolic murmur of hypertrophic obstructive cardiomyopathy (p. 109) which gets louder during the straining because reduced ventricular filling tends to increase the degree of obstruction.

5. EXAMINATION OF THE CHEST AND ABDOMEN

The detailed examination of the chest and abdomen are described elsewhere (p. 136 and p. 167) and only those points especially relevant to the cardiovascular system will be emphasised here.

The pattern of breathing is frequently altered in patients with cardiac problems. Pulmonary congestion or oedema decrease lung compliance, and tend to lead to rapid shallow breathing with a short inspiratory phase and rapid expiration. Patients with chronic obstructive lung disease tend in contrast to have a prolonged expiratory phase. It should be noted that patients with pulmonary disease may have secondary cardiac problems (cor pulmonale). Patients with severe cardiac failure and a low cardiac output may have periodic (Cheyne-Stokes) respiration.

The shape of the chest is sometimes relevant. Children with reduced lung compliance secondary to a large left to right shunt tend to develop indrawing of the lower ribs, sometimes associated with a bulge over the precordium. These changes may persist to adult life despite surgical or spontaneous correction of the shunt. A congenital funnel chest (p. 137) is sometimes associated with a systolic murmur and ECG abnormalities. Thoracic scoliosis may be a manifestation of Marfan's syndrome and its associated cardiovascular anomalies.

Pleural effusions may occur as part of the general process of fluid retention accompanying cardiac failure. They may be unilateral or bilateral, and their position may vary with the posture in which the patient has been lying.

Crepitations at the lung bases are important evidence of early pulmonary oedema if they persist after the patient has been asked to take a deep breath or to cough. As pulmonary oedema becomes more severe the crepitations become more extensive, and eventually they can be heard all over the chest.

In the abdomen, hepatic enlargement may be due to venous congestion resulting from cardiac failure — if so, the jugular venous pressure will also be elevated. Expansile pulsation of the liver may occur in severe tricuspid regurgitation. Abdominal palpation also reveal an aortic aneurysm. In patients with hypertension it is important to palpate for enlarged kidneys and to listen for renal artery or aortic bruits.

THE INTEGRATION OF THE PHYSICAL EXAMINATION

Every clinican needs to develop an efficient and thorough 'drill' for carrying out a physical examination which will ensure that nothing important is omitted, yet allows flexibility for emphasis on points suggested by the history. One technique which has been found satisfactory is as follows:

Start with a general inspection as described on p. 86. The first physical contact with the patient may be by means of a handshake, which is not only polite but gives information about skin temperature and anxiety, and allows the hands to be examined. Feel the radial pulse, and obtain a preliminary impression of heart rate and rhythm. The brachial and carotid pulses are palpated next. The blood pressure measurement may be made now or deferred until the patient is more relaxed. Next examine the neck to assess jugular pulsation; this should start with the patient reclining and the thorax at an angle of 45° to the horizontal, but if the jugular pressure is high the patient may need to sit up for it to be assessed properly. The precordium is then palpated, and the heart auscultated. If mitral stenosis is a possibility and a mid-diastolic murmur has not been heard it may become more apparent when the patient rolls onto the left side, and if the examination is repeated after exercise. Pericardial friction rub and early diastolic murmurs are best heard with the patient sitting up and leaning slightly forward with the breath held in full expiration. The sitting position now provides the opportunity to check for sacral oedema and to auscultate the back of the chest with particular attention to the lung bases.

The abdomen is examined after the chest; ideally the patient should be asked to lie flat, but orthopnoea may not allow this. An enlarged liver resulting from cardiac failure is often tender. The examination is completed by palpating the femoral and leg pulses and testing for oedema in the lower limbs. In appropriate cases it may be important to examine the optic fundi (hypertension), to test the urine for protein (hypertension; oedema), and to look for varicose veins with the patient erect.

FURTHER INVESTIGATION

The standard aids to the diagnosis of disorders of the cardiovascular system are radiography, electrocardiography and echocardiography. These can be supplemented with phonocardiography, ultrasonography, cardiac catheterisation, angiography and radionuclide studies.

Radiography

A standard film of the chest, namely a postero-anterior exposure with at least six feet in distance between the X-ray tube and the film, provides valuable information, in particular about the size of the cardiac shadow, the main pulmonary artery, aorta and it also provides information about the peripheral pulmonary vascularity, especially useful in paediatrics and, for example, in Eisenmenger's syndrome. Enlargement of the left atrial appendage appears as a bulge on the left border of the heart and is a usual feature of mitral stenosis; the left atrium may often be seen as a dense almost circular opacity within the cardiac outline. The shadow of an enlarged right atrium encroaches upon the right lung field. The relative contribution of each of the two ventricles to cardiomegaly is often impossible to determine in a posterior-anterior film and is unreliable even when lateral films are used. Both electrocardiography and clinical examination are usually better tools for this purpose.

A standard radiograph is valuable in indicating that a pericardial effusion has developed, particularly if a recent film is available for comparison. However, the pericardium is a relatively inelastic sac and acute pericardial effusions may occur with little increase in the size of the cardiac shadow on a chest X-ray. Pulmonary oedema, hydrothoraces and pulmonary infarction may be more certainly established by radiography than by clinical examination; radionuclides are used in the investigation of suspected pulmonary embolism (p. 150). Pulmonary arterial hypertension, and both increased and reduced pulmonary blood flow may also produce characteristic changes in the vascular shadows.

Image-intensifier screening is more efficient

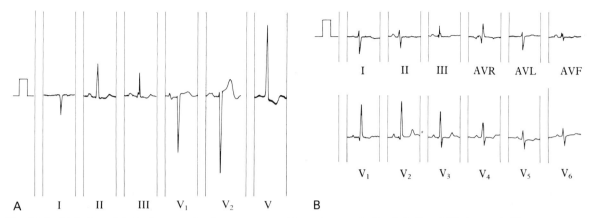

Fig. 5.26 (A) Left ventricular hypertrophy from a woman with aortic stenosis. Leads I, II and III show only T wave inversion. Note the enormous voltages, broadened QRS complex and T wave inversion and V_2 and V_5 (B) Right ventricular hypertrophy from a woman with pulmonary hypertension. Note the dominant R wave in lead V_1 and V_2 and predominant S wave lead I and V_6.

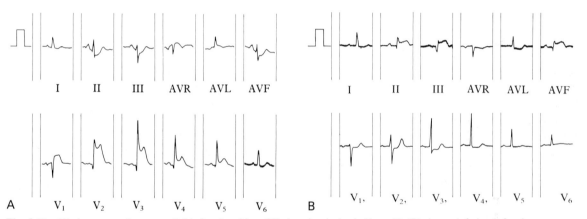

Fig. 5.27 (A) Acute anterior mycardial infarction. Note ST elevation in leads V_1 to V_4 (B) Acute inferior infarction. Note ST elevation in leads in II, III and AVF.

than the plain radiograph in detecting valvular calcification, but the same information can also be obtained by echocardiography. Screening may also detect calcification in the coronary arteries, and is particularly useful in studying the movement of artificial heart valves, especially when these include a radio-opaque marker in the ball or disc.

Electrocardiography

The electrocardiograph amplifies and records electrical activity originating from the heart and detected via electrodes applied to the skin. Standard combinations of electrode positions are called leads, and it is conventional to record 12 leads which 'look at' the electrical activity of the heart from different directions (Fig. 5.28).

The ECG is invaluable for elucidating arrhythmias (see Fig. 5.17 p. 105) for detecting hypertrophy of each of the cardiac chambers (see Fig. 5.26) and above all for providing evidence of acute injury to heart muscle from ischaemia (including myocardial infarction) (see Fig. 5.27) or metabolic disturbances. It is possible to perform 24 hour ambulatory monitoring of patients to look for paroxysmal cardiac arrhythmias.

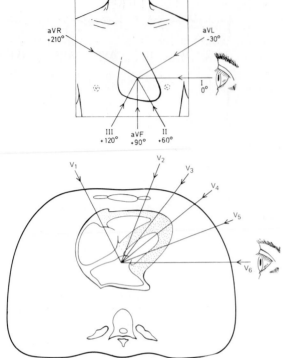

Fig. 5.28 Electrocardiography. Diagram to show the directions from which the 12 standard leads 'look at' the heart. The transverse section is viewed from below like a CT scan and 'looks at' rotation of the heart — clockwise and counterclockwise.

Echocardiography

This technique uses ultrasound to study the disposition and movement of valves and other structures within the heart and also the pericardium. It depends on the reflection of ultrasound waves at interfaces between liquid (e.g. blood) and more solid tissues. In 'M mode' echocardiography the ultrasound is focused into a narrow beam, and the output is a graph against time of the movement relative to the chest wall of those structures through which the beam passes (Fig. 5.29). By tilting the beam, the operator can study the movement of the anterior and posterior walls of the left ventricle, the mitral valve cusps, or the aorta and left atrium. Characteristic patterns of movement are produced in, for example, mitral stenosis, and pericardial effusions are easily recognised. Accurate measurements can be made of cardiac size.

In two-dimensional (2D) real time echocardiography, the ultrasound beam is swung rapidly

back and forth over an arc or sector; this is done mechanically or, in some machines, electronically. The resulting information is synthesised into a two-dimensional map or picture of the position of reflecting structures in a sector-shaped 'slice' through the heart (Fig. 5.30). The structures shown in the 'slice' will of course depend on the position of the ultrasound crystal and the direction of oscillation of the beam. Because the beam oscillates very rapidly, the ultrasound picture accurately reproduces the movements of the structures in the living heart. This type of echocardiography is particularly good at detecting intracardiac masses, such as thrombi or tumours, endocarditic vegetations and the function of prosthetic valves. It is also very useful in sorting out complex structural abnormalities in congenital heart disease.

Transoesophageal echocardiography is performed using a small echo probe which can be passed

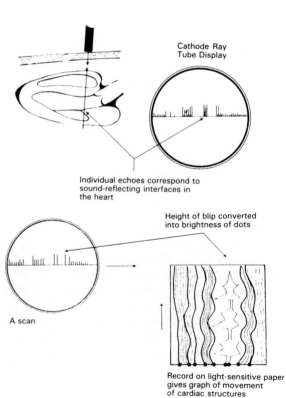

Cathode Ray Tube Display

Individual echoes correspond to sound-reflecting interfaces in the heart

A scan

Height of blip converted into brightness of dots

Record on light-sensitive paper gives graph of movement of cardiac structures

Fig. 5.29 Principles of M-mode echocardiography. The reflected echoes of ultrasound are converted into blips of light on a cathode-ray tube. The blips can be used to plot a 'graph against time' of the position of cardiac structures on a moving strip of paper.

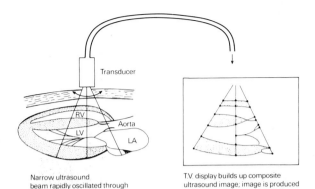

Fig. 5.30 Principles of two-dimensional (2D) real time echocardiography. A moving, two-dimensional image of the echoes detected from a 'slice' of heart can be built up by swinging the ultrasound beam rapidly back and forth.

down the oesophagus. Because the oesophagus lies close to both the descending aorta and left atrium with no intervening lung tissue, excellent echocardiographic images can be obtained. The technique is particularly valuable in diagnosing dissecting aortic aneurysm, left atrial thrombus, endocarditic vegetations on the mitral or aortic valves, and (with the aid of Doppler) mitral regurgitation.

The advent of echocardiography has made it possible for information, previously accessible only by cardiac catheterization and angiocardiography, to be made available without an invasive procedure, and if necessary, without moving the patient from bed.

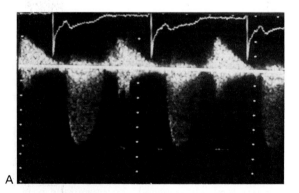

Fig. 5.31 Continuous wave Doppler ultrasound recording from a patient with severe aortic stenosis. The ultrasound beam is aligned with blood leaving through the aortic valve (it also picks up some blood flow through the mitral valve). The maximum velocity across the aortic valve is five and a half metres per second indicating an aortic gradient radiant of over 100 mm of mercury.

Phonocardiography

This records heart sounds and murmurs and may help to elucidate difficult problems of auscultation. Examples of phonocardiograms are given in Fig. 5.14 (normal), Fig. 5.20 (aortic stenosis), Fig. 5.23 (aortic regurgitation), and Fig. 5.24 (mitral stenosis).

Doppler cardiography

The frequency of ultrasound reflected from erythrocytes moving towards or away from a probe undergoes a shift which varies with the relative velocity of movement of the cells. The frequency shift can be detected, analysed and displayed either as a graph of frequency shift against time (Fig. 5.31) or as a colour overlay to a 2D echocardiographic image. 'Pulsed' Doppler samples velocities in a particular location chosen with reference to echocardiographic landmarks. Continuous wave Doppler assesses frequency shifts along a pencil-like track through the heart. When blood passes from a high pressure chamber to a low pressure chamber across a restriction such as

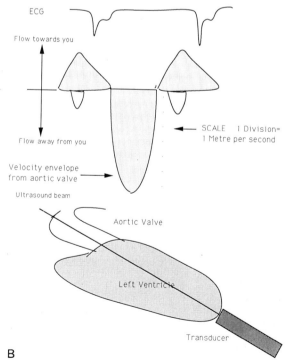

Table 5.10   Types of radionuclide scan in cardiology

Type	Isotope	Use
Gated blood pool scan (labelled red cells)	Technetium	Left ventricular volume and ejection fraction, less reliably right ventricular volume and ejection fraction.
Perfusion scan	Thallium	Thallium taken up by viable myocardium. Used in conjunction with exercise to detect viable but ischaemic myocardium
Perfusion scan	Technetium-labelled pyrophosphate	Taken up by damaged muscle. Used to detect ischaemic damage
Platelet scan	Indium-labelled platelets	Detects thrombi and endocarditic vegetations

a stenosed aortic valve, the maximum velocity (Vmax) of the jet of blood is approximately related to the pressure drop (P1–P2) by the equation:

$$(P1–P2) = 4 \,(Vmax)^2$$

Vmax will be underestimated unless the Doppler probe is carefully aligned with the jet of blood. The combination of 2D echocardiography and Doppler is called duplex ultrasound scanning. It is particularly useful in assessing valvular heart disease and congenital heart disease. It can also be used to measure pulmonary artery pressure if there is any tricuspid regurgitation, since the velocity of the regurgitant jet will give an estimate of peak right ventricular pressure.

Radionuclide studies

The availability of radioactive isotopes of short half-life emitting gamma rays, together with sophisticated equipment (the gamma camera) for detecting this radiation has made it possible to use radionuclides for studying cardiac function. Two basic types of technique are available (see Table 5.10).

*1. **Blood-pool scanning.*** The radionuclide is injected into the bloodstream and mixes with the circulating blood. The gamma camera detects the amount of radionuclide in the heart at different phases of the cardiac cycle, and also the size and 'shape' of the cardiac chambers. By linking the gamma camera to the ECG it is possible to collect information over several cardiac cycles. Blood-pool

scanning gives an accurate and reproducible measure of left ventricular function, and is also used for detecting left ventricular aneurysms. The main disadvantage is the high cost of the equipment.

*2. **Myocardial scanning.*** Although this uses the same gamma camera, both the isotopes and the concepts involved differ from those in blood-pool scanning. The object is usually to distinguish between ischaemic and non-ischaemic myocardium (using radioactive thallium) or between normal and damaged myocardium (using radioactive pyrophosphate). Much care and attention to detail is needed if reliable results are to be obtained.

Catheterisation and angiography

In contrast to the investigations described above, these are invasive techniques, which require the insertion of tubes or catheters into the patient's arteries or veins. This may be done percutaneously or after a surgical 'cut-down'. A catheter inserted into a vein can be advanced into the right atrium, and then manipulated into the right ventricle and pulmonary artery. In the presence of an atrial septal defect or patent foramen ovale, venous catheters can also enter the left atrium and left ventricle. If the atrial septum is intact, access to the left ventricle is usually by retrograde passage of a catheter across the aortic valve. Left atrial pressure can be measured directly by puncturing the interatrial septum with a special long, curved needle via a catheter passed up the femoral vein to the right atrium. For many purposes, however, a satisfactory approximation to left artial pressure can be recorded by 'wedging' an end-hole venous catheter in a branch of the pulmonary artery. Cardiac catheters are usually manipulated under radiographic control using an image-intensifier, but if a venous catheter is provided at its distal end with a small balloon which can be inflated when the catheter is in the right atrium then the bloodstream itself will guide the catheter through the right ventricle and into the pulmonary artery. The balloon also makes it easy to 'wedge' the catheters so as to estimate left atrial pressure. These Swan-Ganz catheters are being used increasingly in intensive and coronary care units, where they can be inserted without the need to transfer the patient to a radiology department.

Pressure measurements obtained through cardiac catheters can be used to assess the severity of valvular stenoses, and measurement of ventricular end-diastolic pressures gives an indication of ventricular compliance and indirectly of ventricular function (see Fig. 5.32). Measurement of oxygen saturation in samples withdrawn via the catheters at different sites in the heart allow the detection of intracardiac left to right or right to left shunts, and also allows calculation of pul-

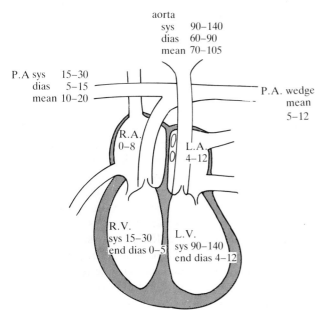

Fig. 5.32 Normal resting pressures in mm mercury in the chambers of the heart.

monary and systemic blood flow. Cardiac output can also be measured by dye-dilution or thermo-dilution techniques. Catheters also allow the injection of radio-opaque contrast medium into individual chambers of the heart, the aorta or pulmonary artery, or, using specially shaped catheters, into either coronary artery. Coronary angiography can be combined, in selected patients, with angioplasty whereby suitable stenotic lesions in proximal vessels are dilated without recourse to surgery.

Angiography of peripheral arteries is usually a prelude to possible vascular surgery or angioplasty. Radio-opaque contrast can be injected into the artery through a needle or catheter, or computer imaging techniques used to obtain a clear image after a venous injection of the radio-opaque dye (digital subtraction angiography). Venous angiography (venography) is useful in detecting venous thrombosis.

THE METHODS IN PRACTICE

So far, we have tended to consider points of history-taking or physical signs either in isolation or in the context of an orderly clinical examination. In practice, it is often clear from an early stage that the diagnosis will lie in a particular direction, and it is helpful to concentrate on certain specific points in the examination and subsequent investigation. Four common diagnostic problems have been selected to exemplify this approach, and also to demonstrate the integration which is often required between the physical examination and further investigation. The examples chosen are cardiac failure, systolic and diastolic murmurs and hypertension.

Cardiac failure

Cardiac failure is not a diagnosis, or at least, not a complete one. It is necessary to specify whether the failure affects the left or right 'side' of the heart, or both together and as far as possible to identify the underlying pathological process. Left heart failure characteristically presents with breathlessness and pulmonary oedema is an early manifestation. Pure left heart failure is seldom associated with much peripheral oedema, because pulmonary oedema develops so rapidly and causes symptoms before peripheral oedema has time to accumulate. Very commonly, however, left and right heart failure occur together, either because reflex pulmonary vasoconstriction in response to a raised pulmonary venous pressure causes secondary right heart failure, or because a process such as myocardial disease affects both the right and left ventricles simultaneously. In this situation pulmonary oedema, or at least pulmonary congestion may co-exist with a raised jugular venous pressure and peripheral oedema. In contrast, peripheral oedema is often a prominent feature, together with a raised jugular venous pressure and hepatomegaly, of pure right heart failure. This is not because the mechanism of oedema is different in right and left heart failure but because the relative absence of breathlessness often allows the insidious accumulation of considerable amounts of peripheral oedema before the patient complains.

Mechanisms of cardiac failure

Cardiac failure may be due to (1) volume overload, (2) inflow obstruction, (3) myocardial disease and (4) outflow obstruction. These can involve either the left or right side of the heart.

1. Volume overload. The simplest example of this is when a patient with a healthy heart is over-transfused with blood or plasma. As the venous pressure rises, cardiac output increases (a manifestation of Starling's law), and this is reflected in increased venous return. Until the excess fluid is excreted, the patient will have a raised venous pressure, a bounding pulse, tachycardia and an active or hyperkinetic apical cardiac impulse. If transfusion is continued, pulmonary oedema develops. The patient then begins to cough, becomes breathless and confused, and will rapidly die unless urgent measures are taken.

A less dramatic presentation occurs when there is an excessively low peripheral vascular resistance over a prolonged period. This may result from surgical or congenital arteriovenous fistulae, from anaemia, from extensive Paget's disease of bone, or from various skin diseases causing cutaneous vasodilation. It may also be due to vasodilating drugs. The kidneys interpret the low blood pressure as evidence of volume depletion and retain salt and water. Blood volume is expanded, the jugular venous pressure rises, and there may be peripheral oedema. Occasionally the patient becomes breathless because of pulmonary congestion. There is tachycardia, the pulse volume is large, and there is a wide interval between systolic and diastolic blood pressure. The left and right ventricles respond by dilating, and the cardiac apex becomes displaced laterally and is hyperkinetic. Systolic flow murmurs are common. Sometimes, a continuous murmur can be heard over the site of an arteriovenous fistula.

The volume overload in atrial septal defect is confined to the right atrium and ventricle, in persistent ductus arteriosus to the left ventricle and atrium, while in aortic regurgitation the 'run-off' from the arterial tree is back into left ventricle itself. Mitral regurgitation is also characterised by the need for an increased left ventricular stroke volume to compensate for the leaking mitral valve, but here the clinical picture is modified by the increase in left atrial pressure caused by the leak.

2. Inflow obstruction. The inflow of blood to the ventricles may be obstructed at the tricuspid or mitral valve. The resulting turbulence of the bloodflow causes characteristic murmurs (tricuspid stenosis p. 111, mitral stenosis p. 110). The chamber upstream of the obstruction (the left atrium in the case of mitral stenosis) is subjected to increased pressure and tends to enlarge. Left or right atrial enlargement may eventually lead to atrial fibrillation. Any rise in left atrial pressure is of course transmitted to the pulmonary veins, and pulmonary oedema may result; alternatively reflex pulmonary vasoconstriction causes secondary right heart failure.

A different form of inflow obstruction occurs when ventricular filling is limited either by excessive stiffness of the ventricle or by an external constraint, such as pericardial fluid in pericardial tamponade or a rigid pericardium in constrictive pericarditis. In the last two conditions signs such as pulsus paradoxus and Kussmaul's sign help to make the diagnosis, but when the restricting factor is 'built-in' to the ventricle, as in restrictive cardiomyopathy or endocardial fibrosis the diagnosis may be difficult.

3. Myocardial disease. This is by far the commonest cause of left heart failure, which in this instance can truly be called left ventricular failure. Impaired myocardial function may be secondary to coronary artery disease, may result from specific disease of the myocardium such as viral myocarditis, or may be caused by one of the many myocardial disorders of uncertain aetiology encompassed by the term cardiomyopathy. It may also follow long-standing ventricular outflow obstruction (see below), probably as a consequence of diffuse myocardial ischaemia. Many of these processes can affect the right ventricle as well as the left.

There are few specific physical signs to indicate myocardial disease, and its diagnosis is often made by a process of exclusion. The heart sounds tend to be quiet when the cardiac output is low, and a gallop rhythm may result from the presence of a third heart sound. When the left ventricle is dilated and contracts weakly a diffuse apical impulse is often felt over a wide area. A history of angina or myocardial infarction may suggest the aetiology of the myocardial damage.

4. Outflow obstruction. The afterload against which the ventricles have to work may be increased either because outflow of blood from the ventricles is 'throttled' as in pulmonary or aortic valve stenosis, or because the resistance in the pulmonary or systemic circulation is high, as in pulmonary or systemic hypertension. In either case the ventricle involved responds by undergoing hypertrophy, which may affect the character of the apical impulse. The hypertrophied myocardium demands an increased blood supply, and, if the coronary circulation is unable to provide this, the patient may suffer angina on exertion. The hypertrophied ventricle is less compliant, so left atrial pressure tends to rise, and left atrial hypertrophy causes an audible fourth heart sound. Characteristically, patients with ventricular outflow obstruction tolerate the condition with few symptoms for a prolonged period, but when symptoms appear deterioration is rapid. With left-sided obstruction, pulmonary oedema is the usual result, and this frequently presents as paroxysmal nocturnal dyspnoea.

Increased pulmonary vascular resistance resulting from chronic lung disease is by far the commonest cause of chronic right heart failure in Northern industrial countries, and the combi-

nation is given the name of *cor pulmonale*. Two different mechanisms seem to be involved — pulmonary vasoconstriction resulting from hypoxia, and destruction of the vessels in the lung parenchyma in chronic emphysema. Right heart failure often develops for the first time during an infection of the respiratory tract. There is peripheral oedema, hepatomegaly and a raised jugular venous pressure. Arterial oxygen desaturation is common, but many patients have a depressed respiratory drive and may not complain of dyspnoea. Carbon dioxide retention is almost invariable and tends to cause peripheral vasodilatation; the warm hands and bounding pulse which result seem at first sight incompatible with cardiac failure.

Investigation. Chest radiography frequently shows enlargement of the heart in patients with cardiac failure; this may be generalised, or affect a single chamber. In general, ventricles tend to dilate in response to a volume load, or as a consequence of muscle damage, and hypertrophy in response to a pressure load. Hypertrophy may not be apparent radiologically until a late stage. In acute ventricular damage, for example following a myocardial infarction, the pericardium restrains the heart from dilating and the heart size may be normal on the initial radiograph. Chest radiography may also show pulmonary oedema or upper lobe venous diversion in left-sided heart failure.

The ECG may reveal myocardial infarction, or indicate dilatation or hypertrophy of a specific cardiac chamber.

Echocardiography provides a direct measurement of atrial and ventricular size and contractility. Good ventricular contractility is a feature of volume overload or valvular incompetence; poor contraction results from myocardial disease, either primary or resulting from prolonged volume overload or outflow obstruction. Inflow obstruction may also produce a characteristic alteration in the pattern of ventricular filling.

Doppler cardiography can indicate the severity of valve stenosis or incompetence, and measure cardiac output.

Radionuclide ventriculography measures ventricular function, and can also assess intracardiac shunts.

Cardiac catheterisation is a specialised technique

for investigating cardiac failure, but in many cases a definitive diagnosis can be made from clinical examination and non-invasive investigation alone.

Systolic murmurs

The significance of a systolic murmur depends very much on its context. Thus a soft systolic murmur in a healthy active adolescent may be of trivial importance but should not be ignored as it may be caused by a valvular anomaly which could predispose to infective endocarditis; for example bicuspid aortic valve.

The site, radiation and character of a murmur give clues about its origin (p. 107). This information must be integrated with the findings on examination of the pulse, JVP and palpation of the precordium. Atrial fibrillation is more common with mitral valve disease than other causes of murmurs. Frequent ventricular extrasystoles sometimes occur in patients with mitral valve prolapse. The arterial pulse waveform is altered in aortic stenosis, giving a characteristic 'slow-rising' pulse best appreciated on feeling the carotid artery, whereas in hypertrophic cardiomyopathy the pulse is 'jerky', starting normally then suddenly cut off. Palpating the precordium may reveal the 'sustained' apical impulse of left ventricular hypertrophy in aortic stenosis or hypertrophic cardiomyopathy, or a displaced apical impulse indicating cardiac enlargement. The jugular venous pressure is likely to be raised if there is cardiac failure. Look for the systolic venous waves of tricuspid regurgitation; if this is severe there may be systolic pulsation of the liver.

The extent to which the loudness of the murmur reflects the haemodynamic severity of the underlying lesion depends on the cause of the murmur. Provided the patient has a normal cardiac output, there is a correlation between the intensity of the murmurs of aortic or pulmonary stenosis and the severity of the stenosis, but if the cardiac output is reduced the murmurs will become quieter. The relationship between loudness and severity for aortic stenosis becomes less good with increasing age. The pansystolic murmur of mitral regurgitation also tends to become louder with increasing mitral incompetence, but sometimes very severe regurgitation occurs with a quiet murmur, and

conversely mitral prolapse may give a very loud murmur in the presence of trivial regurgitation.

A small congenital ventricular septal defect may produce a very loud murmur yet be of little haemodynamic consequence. On the other hand a large ventricular septal defect with pulmonary hypertension (Eisenmenger's syndrome) may not cause a murmur because right and left ventricular pressures are equal. An acute ventricular septal defect occurring as a complication of myocardial infarction will produce a murmur whose intensity tends to reflect the size of the left to right shunt.

Innocent systolic murmurs. In an otherwise healthy and asymptomatic patient a soft systolic murmur (grade 2/6 or less) loudest at the left sternal edge, with normal first and second heart sounds, no JVP elevation, a normal arterial pulse contour and no clinical cardiac enlargement is extremely unlikely to indicate a haemodynamically significant cardiac lesion.

Investigation. A chest radiograph provides information about the size and shape of the heart and about the pulmonary circulation. An ECG gives evidence of any atrial or ventricular enlargement or hypertrophy. The role of echocardiography is discussed on page 115. Cardiac catheterisation is considered only if the non-invasive investigations have not provided a complete diagnosis.

Diastolic murmurs

The most common diastolic murmurs are the mid-diastolic and presystolic murmurs of mitral stenosis and the early diastolic murmur of aortic regurgitation. An Austin Flint murmur (p. 111) may also be heard. Pulmonary regurgitation and tricuspid stenosis are relatively rare. It is important to confirm the diastolic nature of a murmur by timing it against the carotid pulse.

As with systolic murmurs, examination of the pulsewave and palpation of the precordium are very useful. The characteristic pulse of severe aortic regurgitation is 'collapsing'. The apex beat tends to be displaced, and there is an 'active' feel to the precordium as a consequence of the large stroke volume. In mitral stenosis the loud first heart sound can often be felt as well as heard, and the apex beat has a 'tapping' character. In

Table 5.11 Causes of secondary hypertension

Cause	Clues	Tests
Aortic coarctation	Radiofemoral delay, bruits	Angiography
Cushing's syndrome	Facial and bodily appearance, striae, fluid retention	Plasma and urinary cortisol, dexamethasone suppression, CT scan, (adrenals, pituitary, ectopic sources of ACTH)
Conn's syndrome	Polyuria, muscle weakness	Electrolytes, renin, aldosterone, abdominal scan
Phaeochromocytoma	History, disproportionately severe ocular changes	Urine metanephrins, abdominal CT scan
Polycystic kidneys	Abdominal masses	Ultrasound, urography
Renal disease	History, proteinuria bruits	Creatinine clearance urography, angiography
Congenital adrenal hyperplasia	Primary amenorrhoea with virilisation (11β-hydroxylase deficiency). Without virilisation (17α-hydroxylase deficiency)	Hormone assays

tricuspid stenosis the most striking features are the raised jugular venous pressure and characteristic venous pulse contour.

Investigation. This is as for systolic murmurs. Patients with aortic regurgitation should have serological tests for syphilis (p. 241). Occasionally a connective tissue disease (e.g. Marfan's syndrome, p. 48) may cause aortic regurgitation and investigation must be directed accordingly.

Systemic hypertension

This common condition has no specific symptoms; it is recognised either on routine examination, or because of its complications, which include cardiac failure, renal failure and stroke. The clinical examination of a hypertensive patient has two main aims — to seek a specific cause for the hypertension, and to evaluate the extent of the damage done as the result of it.

A specific cause for hypertension is likely to be elicited only in a minority of patients, but is more commonly found in younger subjects. In the history, attention should be paid to a story of paroxysmal headaches, vomiting, sweating, weight loss and other features of excessive sympathomimetic activity, as this may indicate the presence of a phaeochromocytoma. Rarely, such a tumour is so large as to be palpable in the abdomen. A history of recurrent urinary tract infections, or persistent enuresis in an adolescent, may give warning of renal disease. Specific enquiry should be made about alcohol intake and chronic analgesic abuse, which may cause analgesic nephropathy. During the history and physical examination it is important to pay particular attention to excluding a secondary cause. (Table 5.11).

The effects of hypertension on the heart are manifest initially as left ventricular hypertrophy, with a characteristic quality of the apex beat, and a fourth heart sound reflecting secondary atrial hypertrophy. Later, ventricular dilatation and cardiac failure may ensue. The optic fundi show characteristic changes with hypertension. This comprises thickening of the arterial walls, 'nipping' at arteriovenous junctions, flame haemorrhages and exudates both soft and hard (Plate IV). In accelerated hypertension, papilloedema (p. 331) may develop. Such changes may be a clue to intermittent hypertension even if the blood pressure is normal when the patient is seen.

Investigation. This includes urine analysis for protein, microscopy for blood cells and casts, and estimation of plasma urea and creatinine to assess renal function. Plasma potassium concentration may be reduced in primary or secondary hyper-aldosteronism. Plasma glucose and cholesterol measurements help to assess the risk of ischaemic heart disease. The ECG and chest radiograph are useful 'baseline' investigations in determining prognosis and allow subsequent changes to be more easily recognised. Renography and other renal investigations are indicated when history, examination or other investigations point to a possibility of renal disease. Selected patients may need a renal arteriogram to investigate the possibility of renal artery stenosis. Patients with severe or paroxysmal hypertension should have a 24-hour urine collection for catecholamine metabolites as a screening test for phaeochromocytoma.

FURTHER READING

Leatham A 1987 Jubilee editorial: auscultation and phonocardiography — a personal view of the past 40 years. British Heart Journal 57: 397–403

Lembo N J, Dell'Italia L J, Crawford M H, O'Rourke R A 1988 Bedside diagnosis of systolic murmurs. New England Journal of Medicine 318: 1572–1578

Mittal S R 1985 Jugular venous pressure — a reappraisal. International Journal of Cardiology 8: 109–112

6. The respiratory system

G. K. Crompton

Many of the methods of physical examination still in clinical usage differ remarkably little from those described by Laënnec in his *Treatise on the Diseases of the Chest*, published in 1819. Inspection, palpation, percussion and auscultation are still used to detect abnormalities in the bronchi, lungs and pleura and by analysis of the various physical signs to determine the gross pathology of the lesions. Advances in physiology, pathology, immunology, microbiology, radiology, endoscopy and thoracic surgery have, however, permitted not only the diagnosis of respiratory disease with more precision but also a reappraisal of the value of clinical investigation in its various forms. Nowadays, for example, more weight is placed on careful history-taking than on the elicitation of elegant, but possibly misleading, physical signs. Indeed in many disorders the disease process may reach an advanced stage before any abnormal signs can be detected and unless symptoms are promptly investigated, serious delays in diagnosis and treatment may result.

THE HISTORY

The approach to history-taking in patients thought to have respiratory disease differs according to the nature of the illness, the main distinction being that between an acute or subacute illness and a chronic respiratory disorder. The methods used to obtain a coherent account of the patient's symptoms are, however, the same in the two types of case. Firstly, a narrative history is taken, as outlined in Chapter 1. Specific enquiry is then made about any of the principal respiratory symptoms not mentioned in the narrative history. At this stage the clinician should consider all the conditions which might conceivably be responsible for the patient's symptoms. This will seldom be a formidable list, perhaps three or four items in an average case. The doctor should then ask a series of supplementary questions designed to provide evidence for and against each possible diagnosis. In the course of this interrogation the patient may have to be asked to confirm or expand some of the information previously given. This method of integrating and rationalising the history has an important place in the diagnosis of respiratory disease because it facilitates the recognition of certain characteristic symptom-patterns, such as those presented by chronic bronchitis and bronchial asthma, in which physical signs and even specialised investigations may be of limited diagnostic value.

In an *acute respiratory illness* it is important to enquire carefully about the onset of the illness, which may provide a valuable clue to its nature. In pneumococcal pneumonia, for example, systemic disturbance (rigor, pyrexia, malaise) seldom precedes the first respiratory symptom (often pleural pain) by more than a few hours, while in viral pneumonia the patient may be generally unwell for several days before there are any symptoms or signs to suggest pulmonary involvement. Acute dyspnoea is a presenting symptom of particular importance since it often demands urgent treatment, and an error in diagnosis between, say, tension pneumothorax, an acute attack of bronchial asthma and left heart failure may have catastrophic consequences. There, too, a carefully taken history, from a relative if the patient is too breathless to give a coherent account of the illness, may enable such a mistake to be avoided. The nature and effect of treatment prescribed before the patient is seen should also be carefully noted.

In *chronic respiratory disorders* history-taking is a complex and time-consuming procedure. Care must be taken to record not only major incidents in the course of the illness but also to describe and assess the interval or background symptoms. In the case of acute episodes, such as exacerbations of chronic bronchitis, an enquiry should be made into the events which preceded them and the effects which they appeared to have on the course of the disease. Most chronic respiratory disorders pursue a fairly predictable course, and if a patient exhibits symptoms out of line with the established pattern of the illness, the development of another disease should be suspected. The course of disease may also be adversely influenced by treatment of coexisting disorders, for example, a beta-adrenoreceptor blocking drug for hypertension or angina in a patient with chronic asthma. The influence of environmental factors, such as weather and time of year, changes of temperature and exposure to smoke and dust, should be recorded. Such information, in addition to its diagnostic value, may be relevant to prevention and treatment.

SYMPTOMS OF RESPIRATORY DISEASE

The six principal symptoms of respiratory disease are cough, sputum, haemoptysis, chest pain, breathlessness and wheeze. Most of these symptoms may occur in the absence of primary respiratory disease. Certain types of central chest pain, for example, may be of cardiac, pericardial or oesophageal origin, breathlessness may be due to pulmonary oedema secondary to left ventricular failure, and haemoptysis may be the presenting symptom in mitral stenosis or disorders of the blood clotting mechanism. Nevertheless, lateral chest pain and the other five principal symptoms are usually indicative of respiratory disease, and will be discussed in that context.

Cough

This is the most frequent symptom of respiratory disease. It may be caused by stimuli arising in the mucosa of any part of the respiratory tract from the pharynx to the smaller bronchi. Stimuli arising in the parietal pleura may, on rare occasions, also produce cough, for example during the aspiration of a pleural effusion. The frequency, severity and character of cough are dependent on several factors including (a) the situation and nature of the lesion responsible for the cough, (b) the presence or absence of sputum and (c) coexisting abnormalities such as vocal cord paralysis, impairment of ventilatory function and pleural pain.

Types of Cough. 1. Cough produced by stimuli arising in the *pharyngeal mucosa* occurs in pharyngitis or may be caused by secretions trickling down the posterior pharyngeal wall from the nasal sinuses. It is typically a persistent cough, but may be paroxysmal.

2. Cough arising in the *larynx* has a harsh, barking quality and may be painful, especially in acute laryngitis. If a vocal cord is paralysed, a cough, whatever its site of origin, will lose its normal explosive force and will cease to be as effective in clearing the respiratory tract of secretion. Whooping-cough is characterised by prolonged severe paroxysms culminating in a long, stridulous, inspiratory whoop produced by laryngeal spasm.

3. Cough arising in the *trachea* is usually caused by tracheitis, in which it is harsh, dry and painful at first, becoming loose, productive and painless later. Cough caused by a malignant tumour partially obstructing the trachea is associated with stridor (p. 130), persistent and at times severe and suffocating. Such patients may become deeply cyanosed and even unconscious during paroxysms of coughing.

4. Cough of several different types may be produced by stimulation of nerve endings in the *bronchial mucosa*.

Cough in *acute bronchitis* is often preceded or accompanied by transient wheeze and a feeling of diffuse tightness in the chest. In the early stages it sounds dry; later it becomes loose and productive usually of purulent sputum.

Cough in *chronic bronchitis* tends to occur in prolonged paroxysms, which usually culminate in the production of sputum. Bouts of coughing often produce breathlessness, frequently accompanied by wheezing, and may be very distressing. When the sputum is very tenacious, however, or if there is serious impairment of ventilatory function, the patient, exhausted by the effort of couging, may abandon the attempt to clear the bronchi of secretions and the coughing comes to an indecisive stop. Cough in chronic bronchitis has other typical features. It is particularly troublesome when the patient retires to bed at night and, even more so, on getting up in the morning, because of sudden changes in posture and in the temperature and humidity of the inspired air. Sleep is seldom disturbed by coughing, but most patients with chronic bronchitis waken in the morning with cough, wheeze and a sensation of tightness in the chest. These symptoms do not improve until sputum is brought up by violent bouts of coughing which may continue for long periods. Cough in chronic bronchitis is also stimulated by bronchial irritants such as smoke, fumes or dust, and by the sudden increase in the depth of ventilation which occurs with exertion and laughter. Some patients may experience cough syncope (p. 30) during bouts of prolonged and violent coughing.

Prolonged paroxysms of coughing may also occur in patients with *chronic asthma*. The cough, which invariably aggravates wheeze and breathlessness often wakens the patient in the middle of the night. Associated breathlessness and wheeze may be wrongly attributed to left ventricular failure (p. 119).

In *bronchial carcinoma* cough may be an early and persistent symptom. At first it is a frequent short dry cough, but later may become more severe and distressing.

Cough in *bronchiectasis*, uncomplicated by chronic bronchitis or asthma, is characteristically loose and readily productive of sputum. It may be brought on by changes in posture, e.g. by stooping if the bronchiectasis affects the lower lobes. Patients with severe unilateral bronchiectasis prefer to sleep on the affected side in order to prevent cough being stimulated by the dislodgement of sputum. Cough in *pneumonia* is dry and irritant at first, later becoming loose and productive. When pleural pain is present, cough is typically short and partially suppressed. Cough in *acute pulmonary oedema* secondary to left heart failure is generally short, persistent and exhausting. A similar type of cough may occur in *allergic* and *fibrosing alveolitis*.

Sputum

When a patient has sputum, information should be obtained as to amount, character, viscosity and taste or odour.

Amount. This can seldom be accurately estimated by the patient although statements that it is very large (e.g. a teacupful per day) or very small (one or two spits per day) are usually reliable. If it is important to obtain precise information about the amount of sputum, the patient should be given a container and a 24-hour collection measured. Some patients deny cough while admitting to the presence of sputum, saying that they bring it up merely by clearing the throat. A specific enquiry about sputum should, therefore, be made in every case. Most children and some women swallow their sputum, even when it is being produced in large amounts. The sound of the cough, if it is loose or moist, will, however, indicate that sputum is present.

Character. This is seldom described accurately by the patient and, wherever possible, a specimen should be inspected by the doctor. Apart from haemoptysis, there are four types of sputum — serous, mucoid, purulent and mucopurulent (Table 6.1). The term 'dirty spit' used by many patients is misleading as it may refer either to purulent sputum or to mucoid sputum containing soot particles. Mucoid sputum may be copious and frothy in some cases of chronic bronchitis and

Table 6.1 Sputum

Type	Appearance	Cause
Serous	Clear, watery, frothy. May be pink	Acute pulmonary oedema. Bronchioalveolar-cell carcinoma (rare)
Mucoid	Clear, grey, white. May be frothy or black (soot)	Chronic bronchitis. Chronic asthma
Mucopurulent or purulent	Yellow, green, brown	All types of bronchopulmonary bacterial infection. (Eosinophils can cause sputum to appear purulent)
Rusty	Rusty, golden yellow	Pneumococcal pneumonia

asthma. Hysterical patients may spit out large amounts of saliva which they claim to be sputum.

Viscosity. Mucoid sputum is often more viscous than purulent sputum and for that reason is often more difficult to cough up. Sputum is particularly viscous in the early stages of pneumococcal pneumonia and in severe asthma. Serous sputum is watery with a low viscosity.

Taste or odour. When this is described as 'nasty' the patient may merely be referring to the normal taste of purulent sputum. Only when terms such as offensive, nauseating or putrid are used can it be assumed that the sputum is fetid (as in bronchiectasis or lung abscess with anaerobic bacterial infection). The observer's own sense of smell should be used to assess odour.

Haemoptysis

Coughing up blood from the lower respiratory tract occurs in many disorders (Table 6.2). When no cause can be found the oropharynx should be examined for a source of bleeding. The blood is bright red at first but may later become dark red. It is often frothy and may be mixed with sputum. Although most patients realise whether blood has been coughed up or vomited, haemoptysis is occasionally confused with haematemesis.

Whenever a history of haemoptysis is obtained, questions must be asked about its type, degree, frequency and duration. In some cases the events preceding it may be of importance in diagnosis, e.g. deep venous thrombosis in a lower limb or a respiratory infection.

Frequency and duration of haemoptysis. Frank haemoptysis may be massive and fatal, but usually the blood becomes progressively darker for 24 to 48 hours or even longer after the bleeding ceases. When, however, small amounts of fresh blood are coughed up frequently, either as frank haemoptysis or blood-stained sputum, for example daily for a week, this strongly suggests a diagnosis of bronchial carcinoma. Regular blood-streaking of mucoid sputum, sometimes only in the mornings, should always raise the suspicion of bronchial carcinoma. Recurrent episodes of haemoptysis over many years, usually associated with purulent sputum, are a feature of bronchiectasis.

Chest pain

Three types of chest pain are directly due to respiratory disease:

1. *Upper retrosternal pain* of the type experienced in acute tracheitis (p. 130).

2. *Retrosternal pain associated with lesions of the mediastinum,* e.g. tumours, acute mediastinitis and mediastinal emphysema. This type of pain, which is an uncommon but important symptom, has a constrictive or oppressive character similar to that of cardiac pain and may radiate into the arms or neck, but is seldom severe and is not related to exertion.

3. *Pleural pain,* caused by stretching of an inflamed parietal pleura, can occur in all forms of pleurisy. Identical pain is produced by fractures of ribs. Pleural pain is recognised by its sharp, stab-

Table 6.2 Causes of haemoptysis

Common	Uncommon	Others
• <u>Pulmonary infarction</u> <u>Bronchial carcinoma</u>	Mitral stenosis	Foreign body inhalation
• <u>Tuberculosis</u>	Aspergilloma	Chest trauma
• Bronchiectasis	Bronchial adenoma	Iatrogenic: bronchoscopy
Lung abscess	Tracheal tumours	transbronchial biopsy
⋆ Acute bronchitis	Metastatic pulmonary malignant disease	transthoracic lung biopsy
⋆ Chronic bronchitis	Laryngeal tumours	
	Connective tissue diseases	
	Idiopathic pulmonary haemosiderosis	
	Goodpasture's syndrome	
	Blood dyscrasias and anticoagulation	
	Hypertension	

————— Most important causes
•　　　Most common causes of frank/massive haemoptysis
⋆　　　Diagnosis assumed only after exclusion of other causes

bing character and by its relationship to breathing and coughing. It may be present only at the end of a deep inspiration or during a cough; with more severe degrees, even shallow breathing may produce intense pain. The pain is aggravated by exertion (which causes an increase in the depth of breathing) and occasionally by movements of the thoracic spine. Pleural pain often, but not invariably, subsides when an effusion develops.

In spontaneous pneumothorax pleural pain may be present, particularly if the amount of air in the pleural space is small. More often, however, after a brief initial episode of severe unilateral pain the patient complains mainly of tightness across the front of the chest, which may later become localised to the affected side. Rarely, there may be central retrosternal pain resembling that of myocardial infarction, with radiation into the neck and upper limbs. This type of pain may be due to mediastinal emphysema, with which spontaneous pneumothorax is occasionally associated.

Other intrathoracic diseases may produce central chest pain, e.g., lesions of the heart and great vessels (p. 82) or of the oesophagus (p. 157). Piercing unilateral chest pain may be due to involvement of a spinal nerve root by a vertebral lesion or by herpes zoster (p. 76). Pain caused by invasion of the chest wall by malignant pulmonary tumour or by a metastatic deposit in a rib is constant, severe, aching and usually unrelated to breathing, while that produced by simple rib fractures or Coxsackie B infection (Bornholm disease) resemble pleural pain. Chest pain in the absence of organic disease may be a manifestation of anxiety.

The characteristics of any form of chest pain should be fully analysed as described on page 25.

Breathlessness (Dyspnoea)

This has been analysed on pages 32 to 36. A clinical assessment of pulmonary function is an essential component of the history of every patient with respiratory disease.

Apnoea

Apnoea or cessation of breathing can occur during life in a number of circumstances:

1. Breath may be voluntarily held for short periods.

2. Periods of apnoea alternate with over-ventilation in Cheyne-Stoke breathing (p. 138).

3. Apnoea during sleep is of two main types:

a. Obstructive sleep apnoea occurs when the upper airway is intermittently obstructed during sleep and is more often seen in obese short-necked adults who snore loudly.

b. Central sleep apnoea. Breathing may occasionally cease for up to ten seconds in healthy people. Pathological central sleep apnoea can occur with prolonged and frequent periods during which there is no activity of the respiratory muscles. The cause and clinical significance of central sleep apnoea are poorly understood.

Wheeze

When a patient complains of wheeze it is important to discover what is meant by the term. Some patients use it merely to describe noisy and laboured breathing while others apply it to the rattling of secretions in the upper air passages. Wheeze should, however, be applied only to the musical sounds produced by the passage of air through narrowed bronchi. It is invariably louder during expiration and is often confined to that phase of the respiratory cycle. It is more conspicuous during deep breathing and sometimes may become audible only when the depth of respiration is increased. Many patients become so accustomed to wheeze that they cease to be aware of its presence until a relative or friend draws attention to it. Patients with stridor (p. 130) may describe it as wheeze. Care must be taken to distinguish between these two sounds because stridor is usually caused by partial obstruction of a major airway by a tumour or an inhaled foreign body, and thus demands urgent investigation and treatment.

SYMPTOMS OF DISEASE OF THE UPPER RESPIRATORY TRACT

Nose and nasopharynx

The most frequent symptoms of disease in the nose and nasopharynx are obstruction of the nasal airway, often described by patients as 'catarrh', and nasal discharge. Not uncommonly, these two symptoms co-exist.

It is necessary to enquire whether the *nasal obstruction* consistently affects the right or left nasal airway (or both), or whether it changes from one side to the other, according to the position of the head. Persistent obstruction is usually due to adenoidal enlargement, a deflected septum or to polypi, whereas intermittent obstruction is more often caused by mucosal oedema and excessive secretions. Bilateral nasal obstruction may lead to chronic mouth breathing, which, in children particularly, is often the reason for seeking medical advice.

The amount, nature and colour of any *nasal discharge* should normally be recorded in lay terms, e.g. profuse and watery, scanty, tenacious or green, unless a specimen is inspected by the doctor, and then technical terms, such as serous, mucoid or purulent, can be used.

Factors which precipitate recurrent nasal obstruction and discharge, e.g. the inhalation of dust or grass pollens, should be identified whenever possible. An enquiry should also be made about excessive *sneezing*, a common feature of allergic rhinitis, and *headache* which may accompany acute infection of the nasal sinuses.

Epistaxis may give rise to apparent haemoptysis if blood in the posterior nares is inhaled and then coughed up.

Larynx

The two chief symptoms of laryngeal disease are hoarseness and stridor, but lesions of the larynx may also produce cough and pain.

Hoarseness may vary in degree from a slight harshness of the voice to complete loss (aphonia). The voice may have a croaking quality in hypothyroidism (p. 47). Enquiries should be made about the duration of hoarseness and about events which may have preceded its onset, such as a head cold, abuse of the voice, chronic cough or an operation on the neck or throat. It should be noted whether it is improving, worsening or remaining static.

Cough of a short, dry, barking character almost invariably accompanies hoarseness caused by an or-

ganic lesion within the larynx. The bovine cough of laryngeal paralysis is described on page 213.

Laryngeal stridor is a high-pitched crowing sound occurring during inspiration. It may be produced by a foreign body lodged between the cords or by laryngeal spasm, exudate or oedema related to acute viral or bacterial infection. The sound is aggravated by coughing.

Laryngeal pain of mild degree occurs transiently in acute laryngitis; constant severe pain is a feature of advanced tuberculous laryngitis and laryngeal carcinoma.

All patients with stridor and those in whom a marked degree of hoarseness persists for more than a fortnight should have a laryngoscopy (p. 135).

Trachea.

Diseases of the trachea may produce pain, cough, stridor and dyspnoea.

Tracheal pain is referred to behind the sternal manubrium. In the early stages of acute tracheitis it may be severe and become momentarily intense on coughing but subsides as soon as the cough becomes productive.

Tracheal stridor is usually due to obstruction of the tracheal lumen by a malignant tumour and is always accompanied by breathlessness. It is lower in pitch than laryngeal stridor, is heard best during inspiration and is accentuated by coughing. Stridor may also be present when a tumour partially obstructs one or both main bronchi. If stridor is suspected the patient should be asked to cough and then breathe deeply in and out with the mouth widely open. Listening carefully close to the patient's mouth during the first few breaths after coughing can often confirm the presence of stridor at an early stage.

History of previous illness

When the present illness appears to be involving the respiratory system, information of considerable value in diagnosis, prognosis, and treatment may be obtained from the past medical history. The following conditions are of particular importance:

Tuberculosis. Primary tuberculous infection in childhood may be responsible for lobar or segmental bronchiectasis in later life. Post-primary tuberculosis, if inadequately treated, may relapse. Extensive bilateral tuberculosis, even when no longer active, produces severe pulmonary fibrosis which may ultimately cause respiratory and heart failure. Bronchiectasis at the site of an inactive tuberculous lesion, or an aspergilloma in a 'healed' tuberculous cavity, may give rise to haemoptysis. If a history of tuberculosis is given, full details of the nature and duration of treatment should be obtained, if necessary from the hospital or chest clinic which the patient attended.

Enquiry should be made into the history of BCG vaccination which is offered to most tuberculin-negative British children at the age of 13 and in some countries is given to all new-born infants. Successful vaccination affords considerable protection against tuberculosis.

Pneumonia and pleurisy. Some chronic respiratory disorders, e.g. pulmonary fibrosis and bronchiectasis, date from an attack of pneumonia, sometimes described by patients as pleurisy or congestion. A long history of recurrent pneumonia, particularly if it occurs in the same site each time, is suggestive of bronchiectasis, or, if the history is short (e.g. less than a year), of bronchial carcinoma. Rarely, recurrent pneumonia may be a feature of myelomatosis or hypogammaglobulinaemia and it is common in children with cystic fibrosis. It may be a complication of bulbar or pseudo-bulbar palsy (p. 215) or of aspiration from the oesophagus as in achalasia of the cardia.

Other respiratory illnesses. Severe attacks of measles or whooping cough in childhood may cause bronchiectasis. With the reduced incidence of these infections, bronchiectasis in children is now rare, but is still encountered in adults either as a sequel to such illnesses in childhood or as a complication of allergic broncho-pulmonary aspergillosis which itself is a rare complication of bronchial asthma.

Chest injuries and operations. It is necessary to enquire into the circumstances and nature of any chest injury or operation and to consider whether it might be related to the patient's current illness. For example, surgical or accidental trauma may produce deformities of the chest wall. A traumatic haemothorax, particularly if complicated by infection, may result in gross pleural thickening. A foreign body lodged in the lung may cause recurrent haemoptysis or be responsible for the development of a chronic pulmonary abscess or bronchiectasis.

Other surgical procedures. Any major operation may be complicated by pulmonary embolism and infarction. The inhalation of septic material during dental extractions or tonsillectomy under general anaesthesia may result in the development of a pulmonary abscess. Any abdominal or thoracic operation, particularly an operation on the upper abdomen, may give rise to collapse of the lung; subsequent bacterial infection causes pneumonia and bronchiectasis may develop if resolution is incomplete.

Acute abdominal conditions. A perforated peptic ulcer or acute cholecystitis, may mimic pulmonary disease, and subphrenic abscess, amoebic liver abscess, pancreatitis or ovarian malignancy may produce a pleural effusion.

Allergic disorders. Patients who are believed to have an allergic disorder, such as bronchial asthma or allergic rhinitis, should be asked about previous manifestations of allergy, e.g. eczema, urticaria, and angio-oedema. A detailed enquiry should also be made regarding the effects of exposure to substances capable of producing allergic reactions, such as grass pollen, house dust, animal dander, foods and drugs. Exposure to allergens may occur only during the patient's working hours and it may not be recognised. In these circumstances the important clue is usually given by the temporal relationships between occupation and symptoms, and of improvement during weekends and holidays.

Previous radiological examination. If an abnormality is present on the chest radiograph, patients should be asked if they have been X-rayed in the past. Every effort should be made to obtain the earlier films, or at least the reports, since comparison with the current radiograph may be of diagnostic value.

Family and social history

The *family history* of patients with respiratory disease may be significant in three ways:

1. Certain *infections*, notably tuberculosis, may be transmitted from one person to another. Any history of contact with an infected person is, of

course, more important than the family relationship.

2. In *allergic disorders*, such as bronchial asthma, there is often an inherited predisposition, and a family history is not uncommon.

3. In *chronic bronchitis*, although an inherited predisposition cannot be excluded, the liability of several members of one family to develop the disease is more likely to be related to their living conditions, e.g. an overcrowded house situated in a district with a high level of atmospheric pollution.

Social problems, such as those of housing, finance and employment, loom large in the management of patients with all types of chronic respiratory disease and should be fully documented. Information which should be obtained from all patients with chronic breathlessness must include the nature of their employment and the physical effort it involves.

Cigarette smoking is the most important cause of bronchial carcinoma and chronic bronchitis. Indeed both are rare in non-smokers. A smoking history should include details such as the age when regular smoking started, the age when smoking was given up (where applicable), and the average consumption of tobacco (number of cigarettes or cigars per day, amount of pipe tobacco per week).

Obesity invariably causes an increase in exertional breathlessness, whatever the basic pulmonary pathology. Extreme obesity may rarely be responsible for respiratory and cardiac failure.

Occupational and other environmental hazards

Since both acute and chronic respiratory disease may be caused by the inhalation of certain inorganic and organic dusts and chemical substances, it is important to record a complete occupational history, covering both present and previous employment. Hazards may be encountered by workers in the coal, iron and steel, and pottery industries, by stonemasons and farmworkers, and by those who are liable to inhale asbestos dust and chemical substances, such as isocyanates, in the course of their work. Whenever such an occupational history is obtained, detailed information should be sought regarding the degree

and duration of exposure, and its time relationship to the onset of symptoms. This may establish a diagnosis of occupational asthma or allergic alveolitis.

Dust hazards may also be encountered in the patient's home environment. Persons in close contact with pigeons, parrots, budgerigars or canaries may develop extrinsic allergic alveolitis or psittacosis, while atopic subjects may develop allergic rhinitis or bronchial asthma when exposed to allergens such as pollen, house dust, feathers, animal dander or certain types of fungal spore. Legionnaires' disease is spread by water droplets and may be contracted from shower heads. The organism may contaminate water cooling systems and humidifiers.

THE PHYSICAL EXAMINATION

The external features of respiratory disease

Initial impression. A number of features may have become evident during the course of history-taking and should immediately cause the observer to suspect respiratory disease. These are cough, wheeze or stridor, and laboured breathing.

The frequency, severity and type of cough should be noted. The character of wheeze and the degree of respiratory distress should also be observed. The speed with which a patient can dress or undress is often a useful index of respiratory disability. Attention should be paid to any abnormality of the voice and to *fetor* of the breath, for which an anaerobic infection of the lung may be responsible if a local cause in the mouth can be excluded. The state of nutrition should be roughly assessed pending measurements of height and weight. Any suggestion of anaemia or polycythaemia should be noted, as these may be relevant findings in certain types of respiratory disease.

Cyanosis. The cardiac causes of cyanosis are described on page 88. Central cyanosis of respiratory origin is most frequently seen in chronic obstructive airways disease. In such cases peripheral vasodilatation due to carbon dioxide retention (Type II respiratory failure) leads to warm blue hands, but the colour of the tongue is a more reliable indicator of central cyanosis. This may also occur in pneumonia, bronchial asthma, pulmonary infarction, allergic alveolitis and in any disease which can give rise to extensive pulmonary fibrosis such as fibrosing alveolitis and sarcoidosis.

Peripheral cyanosis affecting the face and neck, and in some cases the upper limbs also, is one of the features of superior vena caval obstruction (see below). Severe chronic hypoxia of either pulmonary or cardiac origin is often associated with polycythaemia and an extreme degree of cyanosis, partly central and partly peripheral, may be seen.

Oedema. The presence of peripheral oedema in patients with chronic obstructive airways disease suggests right ventricular failure. Oedema of a different distribution is seen in *obstruction of the superior vena cava*. This condition is a complication of bronchial carcinoma, but may also occasionally be caused by benign lesions. When the superior vena cava is obstructed the external jugular veins become grossly distended but no venous pulsation is visible in the neck. After a week or two, dilated superficial veins and venules appear on the anterior and lateral aspects of the chest wall from the clavicles to below the costal margins. These veins convey blood from the territories of the subclavian and axillary veins to the drainage area of the inferior vena cava. The downward direction of blood flow can be demonstrated by emptying a vein between two finger tips and lifting each finger in turn. The face and neck appear swollen and puffy — although the tissues seldom pit on pressure — and conjunctival oedema (chemosis) is often present. Because of the collateral venous drainage the upper limbs are less frequently affected, but sometimes there is pitting oedema of the hands and forearms.

The hands. Examination of the hands in patients with suspected respiratory disease, apart from the observation of cyanosis, is chiefly concerned with the recognition of *clubbing of the fingers*. This phenomenon occurs in a variety of respiratory, cardiovascular and alimentary diseases (Table 6.3). The swelling of the terminal phalanges in clubbing, which usually, but less obviously, affects the toes also, is due to interstitial oedema and dilatation of the arterioles and capillaries. The early features of clubbing comprise loss of the normal angle between the nail and nail bed and fluctuation of the nail bed.

Table 6.3 Causes of finger clubbing

Respiratory	Bronchial carcinoma
	Intrathoracic suppuration
	Bronchiectasis
	Empyema
	Lung abscess
	Fibrosing alveolitis
Cardiovascular	Cyanotic congenital heart disease
	Bacterial endocarditis
Alimentary	Hepatic cirrhosis
	Ulcerative colitis
	Crohn's disease
	Coeliac disease
Congenital	Familial clubbing

To elicit fluctuation the finger is placed on the pulp of the examiner's two thumbs and held in this position by gentle pressure with the tips of the middle fingers on the proximal phalangeal joint. The patient's finger is then palpated over the base of the nail by the tips of the index fingers (Fig. 6.1). The test is positive when the sensation of movement of the nail is greater than the very slight degree of fluctuation which can be detected in normal fingers. When fluctuation is marked, palpation of the nail itself may give the impression that it is floating free on its bed.

With more advanced degrees of clubbing, various visible changes develop progressively (Fig. 4.1 p. 53):

1. Swelling of the subcutaneous tissues over the base of the nail causes the overlying skin to become tense, shiny and red, with obliteration of the skin creases.
2. Later, as the swelling involves the nail bed, the curvature of the nail, especially in its long axis, increases (Fig. 6.2).

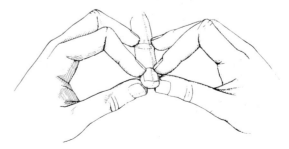

Fig. 6.1 Testing for fluctuation of the nail bed.

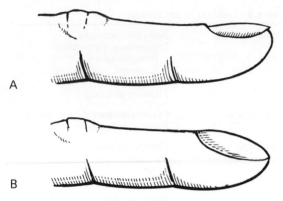

A

B

Fig. 6.2 Note the difference between normal (A) and clubbing (B) with loss of nail bed angle and increased curvature of the nail.

3. Finally, swelling of the pulp of the finger in all its dimensions occurs in fully developed clubbing. In a few cases there may also be hypertrophic pulmonary osteoarthropathy causing pain and swelling of the hands, wrists, knees, feet and ankles, with radiographic evidence of subperiosteal new bone formation.

Increased curvature of the finger nails is commonly seen in normal subjects and, as an isolated phenomenon without other evidence of clubbing, is of no significance.

The eyes. It is important to examine the eyes in patients suspected of having respiratory disease to look for conditions such as Horner's syndrome (p. 200), phlyctenular keratoconjunctivitis, which may be a manifestation of primary tuberculosis, and iridocyclitis, which may be seen in tuberculosis or sarcoidosis. Ophthalmoscopy is essential whenever a diagnosis of acute miliary tuberculosis is suspected since choroidal tubercles are a pathognomonic feature of that condition. Chemosis and dilatation of the conjunctival and retinal veins are very common in patients with hypercapnia secondary to chronic obstructive airways disease, and a few of these patients may develop papilloedema.

The neck. A systematic method of examining the neck has been described on page 65. In patients with possible respiratory disease the scalene lymph nodes require careful examination. These nodes are often involved when a

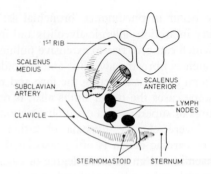

Fig. 6.3 Relation of lymph nodes to scalenus anterior.

pathological process, such as carcinoma, lymphoma, sarcoidosis or tuberculosis, affects the mediastinal nodes, and aspiration or biopsy of an enlarged scalene node may yield diagnostic information. This group of nodes is within a pad of fat on the surface of the scalenus anterior muscle, just in front of its insertion into the scalene tubercle of the first rib (Fig. 6.3). To reach this situation the palpating finger must dip behind the clavicle through the clavicular origin of sternomastoid. For the examination to be adequate all the anterior cervical muscles must be completely relaxed. This is best achieved by having the patient sitting in a chair with the hands resting on the thighs and the cervical spine partially flexed. The examination should be carried out from behind, one side at a time, and the whole of the supraclavicular and retroclavicular regions of the neck from the trachea to the anterior border of trapezius should be carefully palpated for enlarged nodes, special attention being directed to the scalene regions (Fig. 6.4). When a node is found it should be assessed as indicated on page 36. Nodes which are greater than 0.5 cm in diameter, firm in consistence and round in shape are usually pathological, many of

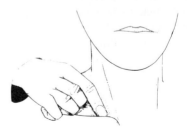

Fig. 6.4 Palpation of lymph nodes in scalene area.

them containing metastatic deposits from a bronchial carcinoma. Large, fixed masses are present in some of these cases. Hard, craggy nodes may, however, be caused by healed and calcified tuberculosis; in such cases calcification is visible on radiographic examination.

The skin. Examination of the skin may yield information of considerable value in the diagnosis of respiratory disease. Some of the cutaneous and subcutaneous lesions which may be relevant are:

1. Erythema nodosum (p. 77), which may be the initial clinical manifestation of a primary tuberculous infection or of sarcoidosis.
2. Metastatic tumour nodules, which may be derived from a primary bronchial carcinoma.
3. Cutaneous sarcoids and lupus pernio, which may occur in association with sarcoidosis involving the intrathoracic lymph nodes or the lungs.
4. The rash of lupus erythematosus (p. 77) which may accompany systemic, including pulmonary or pleural, manifestations of this connective tissue disorder.
5. Herpetic vesicles, which may identify the cause of unilateral chest pain.

THE UPPER RESPIRATORY TRACT

The upper respiratory tract extends from the external nares to the junction of the larynx with the trachea. It includes the nasal cavity, the nasopharynx, the nasal sinuses, the oropharynx and the larynx. Infective and allergic disorders of the upper respiratory tract are very common and infection may produce or aggravate disease of the bronchi and lungs. Oral sepsis, particularly suppurative gingivitis, may cause pulmonary disease, such as lung abscess. Clinical examination of the nose, throat and mouth is therefore an essential part of the investigation of all patients with respiratory disease (see p. 62–65).

The larynx

External examination of the larynx seldom yields any useful information, but swelling of the lips, the tongue, around the eyes and on the front of the neck caused by a hypersensitivity reaction (angio-oedema) is a relevant finding, since the oedema may involve the glottis and give rise to breathlessness and stridor, which may progress to complete respiratory obstruction.

Examination of the interior of the larynx by indirect or direct laryngoscopy is an essential step in the investigation of hoarseness. In indirect laryngoscopy, a small (demisted) mirror reflecting light from a head lamp or from the small electric bulb on the laryngoscopic attachment of a diagnostic set is placed just in front of the uvula and with a co-operative patient a clear view can be obtained of the epiglottis, the arytenoid region and the vocal cords (Fig. 6.5). The examination can often be facilitated by the use of an anaesthetic lozenge (benzocaine). Direct laryngoscopy, using a laryngoscope, is necessary in some cases, particularly if a biopsy has to be taken, but is an uncomfortable procedure which requires more extensive local or general anaesthesia. Lesions which can be detected by laryngoscopy include laryngeal tuberculosis, laryngeal tumours and vocal cord paralysis.

A paralysed vocal cord adopts a position midway between abduction and adduction and fails to adduct on phonation. Paralysis of abduction may precede complete paralysis of the cord.

The trachea

In normal subjects the upper 4–5 cm of the trachea can be felt in the neck between the cricoid cartilage and the suprasternal notch, but in thick-set or obese subjects it may be so deeply placed that it is difficult or impossible to feel.

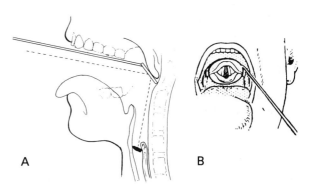

Fig. 6.5 Indirect laryngoscopy (A) position of mirror in relation to soft palate and larynx. (B) view of larynx in mirror.

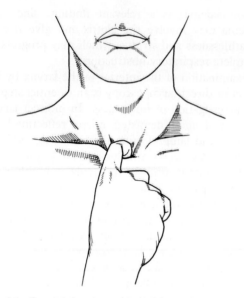

Fig. 6.6   Determining the position of the trachea.

The position of the trachea is determined by gently thrusting the tip of the index finger into the suprasternal notch, exactly in the midline (Fig. 6.6). By this manoeuvre any deviation of the trachea to either side can readily be detected. Thyroid enlargement may displace the trachea, and the thyroid gland should be examined before tracheal deviation is attributed to intrathoracic disease. In patients with chronic airflow obstruction there is a downward movement of the trachea during inspiration. This can be detected by placing a finger below the cricoid cartilage, when the distance from the suprasternal notch may be greatly reduced and the cricoid cartilage may be tugged down with sufficient force to squeeze the finger.

THE CHEST

Physical examination of the chest, like examination of the heart and abdomen, makes use of the techniques of inspection, palpation, percussion and auscultation.

In health the two sides of the chest move to an equal extent with respiration. The trachea is central and the apex beat is in the normal position. Percussion of the chest wall elicits a resonant note over the lungs. On auscultation the breath sounds are vesicular in type (p. 144). In diseases of the bronchi, lungs and pleura, various changes in these physical signs may be observed. It is convenient to first examine the front and sides of the chest and then the back. When the anterior and lateral aspects are being examined the patient should lie in a semi-recumbent position on a bed or couch, with the chest and upper abdomen fully exposed and evenly illuminated down to the level of the umbilicus, and with the arms sufficiently abducted to allow access to the axillary regions. When the posterior aspect of the chest is being examined all pillows should be removed to allow unimpeded access to the whole length of the back. The patient should sit upright with arms folded across the chest. Some patients are too weak to maintain this position and have to be held forward.

Examination from the front and from the back should begin with inspection and palpation of the chest wall followed by observation of respiratory movements and a comparison of the range of movement on the two sides during both normal and deep breathing. The position of the trachea and the apex beat (p. 99) should be determined. The percussion note on the two sides should be compared and any areas of dullness carefully delineated. Finally, by means of auscultation, the type and intensity of the breath sounds and voice sounds should be assessed and the nature of any added sounds identified.

Inspection and palpation

Abnormalities in the shape of the chest

Those of clinical importance are as follows:

1. The anteroposterior diameter may be increased relative to the lateral diameter. In normal subjects the ratio is usually about 5 : 7, and in flat-chested patients without respiratory disease, it may be as low as 1 : 2. In some patients with emphysema, however, the two measurements may approximate (barrel-chest). It should be remembered that an increase in the anteroposterior diameter may be due to thoracic kyphosis unrelated to respiratory disease. Chest deformity in emphysema is not a reliable guide to the severity of the functional defect.

2. Pectus carinatum (pigeon chest) is a common

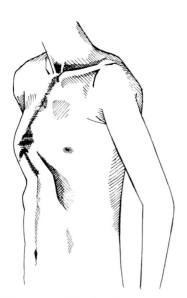

Fig. 6.7 Pigeon chest deformity (*Pectus carinatum*)

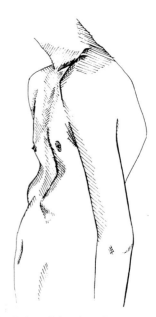

Fig. 6.8 Funnel chest deformity. (*Pectus excavatum*)

sequel to chronic respiratory disease in childhood. It consists of a localised prominence of the sternum and adjacent costal cartilages, often accompanied by indrawing of the ribs to form symmetrical horizontal grooves (*Harrison's sulci*) above the costal margins, which are themselves usually everted (Fig. 6.7). These deformities are thought to result from lung hyperinflation with repeated strong contractions of the diaphragm while the bony thorax is still in a pliable state. Pectus carinatum deformity may also be caused by rickets.

3. Pectus excavatum (funnel-chest) is a developmental defect in which there is either a localised depression of the lower end of the sternum (Fig. 6.8), or, less commonly, depression of the whole length of the body of the sternum and of the costal cartilages attached to it. Pectus excavatum is usually asymptomatic, but, when there is a very marked degree of depression of the sternum, the heart may be compressed between it and the vertebral bodies. This produces displacement of the apex beat to the left, and the ventilatory capacity of the lungs may be restricted.

4. Thoracic kyphoscoliosis. This ranges in degree from the minor changes in spinal curvature seen in many otherwise healthy subjects to grossly disfiguring and disabling deformities (Fig. 6.9).

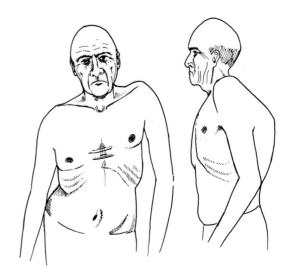

Fig. 6.9 Kyphoscoliosis

Thoracic scoliosis may alter the position of the mediastinum in relation to the anterior chest wall, with the result that abnormalities in the position of the trachea and the cardiac apex beat may be mistakenly attributed to cardiac or pulmonary disease. Severe kyphoscoliosis may have profound effects on pulmonary function, as the chest deformity reduces the ventilatory capacity of the lungs and increases the work of breathing. Many such patients develop hypoxaemia, hypercapnia and heart failure at an early age.

5. *Thoracic operations*, particularly thoracoplasty, may result in a considerable degree of chest deformity, of which scoliosis may be an important secondary feature.

Lesions of the chest wall

Abnormalities which may be detected by combined inspection and palpation of the chest wall include:

1. *Cutaneous lesions*, e.g. skin eruptions, sarcoid or other nodules, purpuric spots, bruises, scars, discharging sinuses.

2. *Subcutaneous lesions*, e.g. inflammatory swellings, metastatic tumour nodules, neurofibromas, lipomas. (The nature of certain cutaneous and subcutaneous lesions, e.g. sarcoid nodules and tumours, may require to be determined by aspiration or biopsy.)

3. *Subcutaneous emphysema* (air in the subcutaneous tissues) may cause diffuse swelling of the chest wall, the neck and, in some cases, the face. The condition is recognised by the characteristic crackling sensation elicited by palpation of the air-containing tissues. When subcutaneous emphysema is localised to the chest wall, it is usually derived from a pneumothorax, air having escaped along the track of a needle or intercostal catheter introduced into the pleural space. In other cases air extruded from the lungs as a result of interstitial rupture of the alveoli tracks into the mediastinum (*mediastinal emphysema*). The air usually escapes innocuously into the neck and produces subcutaneous emphysema of the neck, face and chest wall which in severe cases may be very gross but is not in itself dangerous. When air is present in the mediastinum the heart sounds may be replaced by a churning noise, accentuated during systole.

4. *Vascular anomalies*, e.g. spider telangiectases (p. 75), enlarged vascular channels (arterial in coarctation of aorta; venous in superior vena caval obstruction).

5. *Localised prominences and deformities*, involving clavicles, scapulae, sternum, ribs, costochondral junctions and spinous processes.

6. *Localised tenderness on palpation*, e.g. from a fractured rib, from tumour invading the chest wall, from spinal injury or disease, or in association with pleural or nerve root pain.

7. *Lesions of the breasts* (p. 69) and *enlargement of the axillary lymph nodes* (p. 67).

The observation of respiratory movements

1. **Respiratory frequency.** The number of breaths in a full minute is counted by surreptitiously observing the movements of the chest wall, with the fingers held on the pulse to avoid drawing the patient's attention to breathing. The normal frequency at rest in a healthy adult is about 14 respirations per minute. The rate is increased in a variety of pathological states, including pyrexia, acute pulmonary infections, particularly those accompanied by pleural pain, and conditions in which there is a sudden increase in the work of breathing, e.g. bronchial asthma and acute pulmonary oedema.

2. **Respiratory depth.** This is difficult to estimate clinically as the movements of the chest and diaphragm, on which it is dependent, cannot be accurately measured. It is usually possible with practice, however, to recognise marked degrees of overventilation and underventilation. The latter may be of considerable importance in the diagnosis of Type II respiratory failure.

In massive pulmonary embolism and in metabolic acidosis, usually due to diabetic ketoacidosis or uraemia, pulmonary ventilation at rest may be considerably raised. This can be recognised by an increase in the depth of respiration (*air hunger*) which may give rise to the subjective sensation of breathlessness. In *periodic* or *Cheyne-Stokes breathing* there is a cyclical variation in the depth of respiration, with periods of overventilation alternating with apnoea. It is believed to be caused by a decrease in the sensitivity of the respiratory centre to carbon dioxide. This occurs in certain neurological conditions, particularly those involving the medulla and in some patients with cardiac failure. The cycle usually lasts for less than two minutes and during the phase of overventilation the patient may experience respiratory distress.

Overventilation may also occur in patients who are unconscious as a result of severe brain damage caused by trauma, haemorrhage or infarction.

3. **Maximum chest expansion.** This is estimated by placing a tape measure round the lower

third of the chest and recording the maximum inspiratory/expiratory difference in the chest circumference. There is a considerable degree of observer variation with this measurement and it does not correlate well with vital capacity, probably because in some subjects breathing is predominantly diaphragmatic. A figure of above 5 cm can, however, be regarded as normal and one of 2 cm or less as definitely abnormal. Chest expansion is diminished in almost every type of diffuse broncho-pulmonary disease, e.g. bronchial asthma, emphysema and pulmonary fibrosis, and in conditions which restrict movement of the ribs, such as ankylosing spondylitis.

4. Mode of breathing. In normal subjects inspiration is effected by contraction of the intercostal muscles and the diaphragm, while expiration is a passive process dependent upon the elastic recoil of the lungs. Women make more use of the intercostal muscles than of the diaphragm and their respiratory movements are predominantly thoracic. Men rely more on the diaphragm and their respiratory movements at rest are mainly abdominal. Babies of both sexes are also diaphragmatic breathers. Any departure from the normal mode of breathing should receive close attention. If respiratory movements are exclusively thoracic this may indicate that diaphragmatic movement is inhibited by pain caused, for example, by peritoneal irritation, or restricted by increased intra-abdominal pressure in conditions such as ascites, gaseous distension of the bowel, a large ovarian cyst or pregnancy. If respiratory movements are exclusively abdominal, ankylosing spondylitis, intercostal paralysis or pleural pain may be responsible for the lack of chest expansion.

Although breathlessness is a subjective phenomenon it is usually accompanied by objective evidence of respiratory difficulty or distress. There is often an increase in respiratory frequency, which may be accompanied by dilatation of the alae nasi during inspiration, but as these features may be observed in the absence of breathlessness they are not reliable indices of respiratory distress. A much more useful criterion is the presence of abnormal respiratory movements of the following types:

a. Abnormal inspiratory movements produced by contraction of the cervical muscles (principally the sternomastoids, scaleni and trapezii), by which the whole thoracic cage is, in effect, lifted off the diaphragm with every inspiration. Patients breathe in this way if adequate pulmonary ventilation cannot be achieved by normal inspiratory efforts, for example, when there is gross overdistension of the lungs in advanced emphysema and severe bronchial asthma. More violent inspiratory movements of a similar character are observed in patients with obstruction of the larynx or trachea. Indrawing of the suprasternal and supraclavicular fossae, the intercostal spaces and the epigastrium with each inspiration invariably accompanies airways obstruction of this type and may also be seen, although it is usually less conspicuous, in chronic bronchitis and asthma.

A much more striking degree of indrawing of the chest wall is seen in patients who have sustained double fractures of a series of ribs or of the sternum. The portion of the thoracic cage between the fractures becomes mobile and, with the overlying soft tissues, is sucked in with every inspiration. *Paradoxical movement* of this type in-

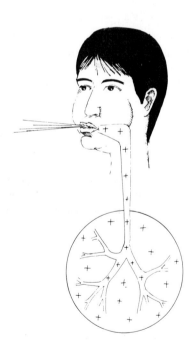

Fig. 6.10 Purse-lip breathing. This manoeuvre helps to keep the intrabronchial pressure above that within the surrounding alveoli and delays or prevents collapse of the bronchial wall which would otherwise result from the unopposed pressure of air trapped in the alveoli.

terferes seriously with pulmonary ventilation and may cause grave respiratory distress and hypoxaemia.

b. *Abnormal expiratory movements* produced by powerful contractions of the abdominal muscles and latissimus dorsi. These are observed if the elastic recoil of the lungs is insufficient to complete the expulsion of air from the alveoli, as in emphysema, or when expiratory airflow obstruction is present, as in bronchial asthma and some cases of chronic bronchitis. Patients with a severe degree of expiratory obstruction prefer to be upright, grasping a bed table or the back of a chair. This enables them to fix the shoulder girdle so that the latissimus dorsi can be used to augment the expiratory efforts. Many patients, especially those with emphysema and with acute exacerbations of chronic bronchitis, exhale through their mouths with pursed lips (Fig. 6.10).

c. *Localised impairment of respiratory movement* is usually caused by disease in the underlying lung or pleura, and is almost invariably associated with abnormal findings on percussion and auscultation.

Methods of comparing range of movement of the chest wall

The object of these procedures is to detect differences in the range of movement on the two sides of the chest. Unless such differences are gross they are difficult to detect, especially by palpation. More reliance should therefore be placed on inspection. There are indeed clinicians who believe that palpation is of such limited value that they do not perform it.

1. Respiratory movement in the infraclavicular regions is compared by inspecting the chest with the patient supine and the head resting on a pillow. Care must be taken to ensure that the head and trunk are in a straight line and that the shoulders are relaxed and in a symmetrical position. The observer views the infraclavicular regions tangentially and asks the patient to take steady deep breaths. By this technique unilateral impairment of chest wall movement can usually be recognised. Breathless patients should not be examined in this way because their distress is increased if they lie flat.

2. Respiratory movement at the costal margins can also be accurately gauged by inspection if the patient is thin. In other cases, however, palpation may be helpful. The sides of the chest are grasped with the fingers in such a way as to approximate the tips of the outstretched thumbs in the region of the xiphoid process. The hands should be adjusted to ensure that there is a loose fold of skin between the two thumbs so that they can move apart as the chest expands. The movement of the two thumbs with deep breathing can then be used to estimate the relative degree of movement on the two sides.

3. Respiratory movements of the lower ribs posteriorly are estimated by a similar technique (Fig. 6.11). With the patient sitting erect, the chest is grasped from behind with the two hands and the tips of the outstretched thumbs are brought together in the region of the tenth thoracic spine. Again it should be ensured that there is a loose fold of skin between the thumbs, the movement of which can then be used to estimate the relative degree of chest expansion on the two sides.

The significance of reduced movement. Unilateral reduction of chest wall movement occurs in many types of respiratory disease. In pleural effusion (Fig. 6.12) and empyema, movement may be absent, and if the lesion has persisted for some weeks retraction of the ribs and intercostal spaces may produce flattening of the affected side of the chest. The term 'frozen chest' is some-

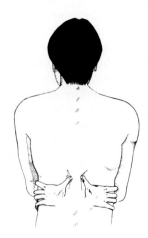

Fig. 6.11 Estimation of respiratory movements of the lower ribs posteriorly.

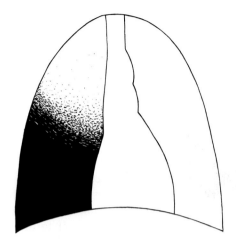

Fig. 6.12 Right pleural effusion.
Chest expansion — reduced
Percussion note — stony dull
Breath sounds — absent or decreased
(occasionally bronchial)
Added sounds — none
Vocal resonance — absent or decreased

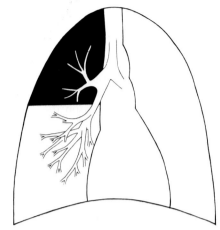

Fig. 6.13 Right upper lobe consolidation
Chest expansion — reduced
Percussion note — dull
Breath sounds — bronchial
Added sounds — crepitations
Vocal resonance — increased (whispering
pectoriloquy)

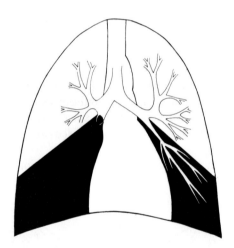

Fig. 6.14 Collapse of the lower lobes. Right lower lobe
bronchus obstructed, left lower lobe bronchi patent (rare).

	Right	Left
Chest expansion —	reduced	reduced
Percussion note —	dull	dull
Breath sounds —	absent or decreased	bronchial
Added sounds —	none	crepitations ± rhonchi
Vocal resonance —	absent or decreased	increasing (whispering pectoriloquy)

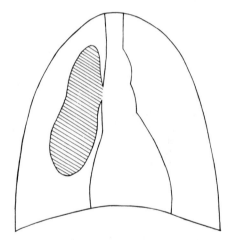

Fig. 6.15 Large right pneumothorax.
Chest expansion — reduced
Percussion note — hyperresonant
Breath sounds — absent or decreased
Added sounds — usually none
Vocal resonance — decreased

times applied to this condition. Less marked
reduction of movement occurs in pulmonary consolidation (Fig. 6.13) and collapse (Fig. 6.14). In
pneumothorax (Fig. 6.15) the limitation of movement is related to the amount of air in the pleural
space; in tension pneumothorax the affected side
of the chest may be immobilised in a position of
almost full inspiration. In pulmonary tuberculosis
even extensive lesions may have little effect on
chest wall movement during the early stages of the
disease, but later, when fibrosis develops, there

may be severe restriction of movement, with flattening of the affected side of the chest.

In bronchial asthma, emphysema and diffuse pulmonary fibrosis movements of the chest wall are symmetrically reduced. In the first two conditions this results from overinflation of the lungs. In diffuse pulmonary fibrosis, on the other hand, inspiratory movement is restricted by the reduced distensibility of the lungs. In severe cases this may bring each inspiration to an abrupt halt and produce the phenomenon of 'door stop' breathing.

Vocal fremitus

This crude test provides no information that is not obtained by vocal resonance. It is performed by placing the palm of the hand on equivalent areas of the chest wall and asking the patient to say 'one, one, one'.

Palpable accompaniments

The vibrations from a low-pitched rhonchus or a coarse pleural rub can occasionally be detected by a hand placed on the chest wall. In such cases an unusually loud rhonchus or rub is invariably present on auscultation and there is seldom any difficulty in distinguishing between the two. A palpable rhonchus generally has its origin in a large bronchus and, if persistent and unilateral suggests partial bronchial obstruction by a tumour or foreign body. A palpable pleural rub, which may be recognised by the patient as a grating sensation within the chest, has no specific significance, but is more often encountered in chronic than in acute pleurisy, and is not always accompanied by pain.

Percussion

The object of percussion is to compare the degree of resonance over equivalent areas on the two sides of the chest, and to map out any area in which the percussion note is abnormal. The percussion note loses its normal resonance whenever aerated lung tissue is separated from the chest wall by pleural fluid or thickening, or when lung tissue is rendered airless by consolidation, collapse or fibrosis. Over such lesions the percussion note is impaired or dull. The most marked degree of dullness on percussion is found over a large pleural effusion.

A hyperresonant percussion note may be found over a large thin-walled pulmonary cavity, over a pneumothorax, particularly if the pleural pressure is above atmospheric level, and also over lung which is markedly emphysematous. An apparent finding of generalised hyperresonance must, however, be accepted with reserve, since a change in the absolute pitch of a percussion note is always difficult to recognise and may depend mainly upon the thickness of the chest wall. For that reason it is not usually advisable to attempt to distinguish between normal resonance and hyperresonance when the percussion note is equally resonant on the two sides. The sound produced by percussion over a hollow viscus is described as tympanitic.

Anatomical considerations

The regions of the thorax over which a resonant percussion note is normally found correspond approximately with the surface marking of the lungs (Fig. 6.16). Percussion over the heart or the liver will elicit a dull note, but the area of dullness is always less extensive than would be expected from anatomical surface marking, since aerated lung is interposed between part of the viscus and the chest wall.

When an abnormality of the percussion note is

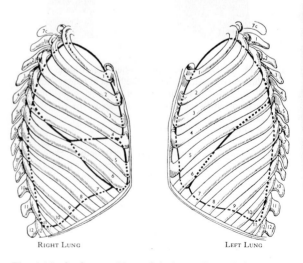

RIGHT LUNG   LEFT LUNG

Fig. 6.16 Surface markings of the lungs (Lateral views)

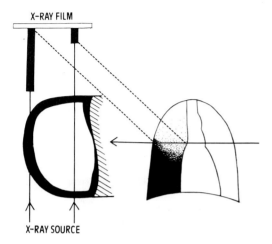

Fig. 6.17 Radiographic appearances of a left pleural effusion. A horizontal section of hemithorax close to the upper margin of the effusion (represented by the horizontal arrow) shows that there is at this site a similar amount of liquid anteriorly, posteriorly and laterally. However, because of the shape of the hemithorax the X-ray beams traverse more fluid laterally than they do centrally. This produces the characteristic radiographic shape of a pleural effusion shadow with a curved upper margin ascending towards the axilla.

due to pulmonary consolidation or collapse it is usually possible to identify the lobe or lobes involved by reference to the surface marking of the fissures but, unless a lobe is totally consolidated, the area over which the percussion note is impaired is often much smaller than would be expected from its surface marking. This is even more striking when a lobe is collapsed. With a pleural effusion the area of dullness on percussion is unrelated to the surface anatomy of the lobes. Except with loculated effusions, it is situated over the lower part of the hemithorax if the patient is examined in the upright position. When there are no pleural adhesions the radiograph shows an effusion to have a curved upper border which misleadingly suggests more fluid being present laterally (Fig. 6.17)

In localising the position of a pulmonary or pleural lesion the observer should make use of the breath sounds and voice sounds in addition to the percussion note. However, small lesions such as areas of segmental consolidation or collapse, may not produce any abnormal physical signs. Even with larger lesions the signs may be partly or completely obscured if the lungs are emphysematous.

Technique of percussion

The basic technique of percussion for a right-handed clinician is as follows:

1. The left hand is placed on the chest wall, palm downwards and with the fingers slightly separated, so that the second phalanx of the middle finger is precisely over the area to be percussed.

2. The middle finger of the left hand is then pressed firmly against the chest wall and the centre of its second phalanx is struck sharply with the tip of the right middle finger. In order to produce a satisfactory percussion note the right middle finger must be held at a right angle (to produce a 'hammer' effect) and the entire movement must come from the wrist joint (Fig. 6.18)

The positions in which the percussion note on the two sides should be compared are as follows:

Anterior chest wall. (a) Clavicle. (b) infra-clavicular region (Fig. 6.19). (c) Second to sixth intercostal spaces (Fig. 6.19).

Lateral chest wall. Fourth to seventh intercostal spaces (Fig. 6.19)

Posterior chest wall. (a) Trapezius, percussing downwards on lung apex (Fig. 6.20). (b) Above spine of scapula (Fig. 6.20) (c) At intervals of 4–5 cm from below spine of scapula down to eleventh rib (Fig. 6.20).

The technique of clavicular percussion which may be of value in detecting lesions of the upper lobes, differs from that used elsewhere in that the

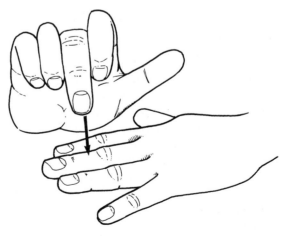

Fig. 6.18 Technique of percussion

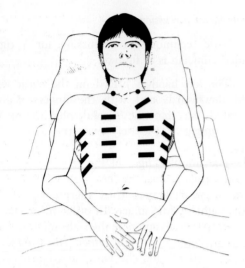

Fig. 6.19 Sites for percussion — anterior and lateral chest wall.

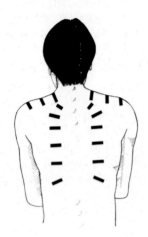

Fig. 6.20 Sites for percussion — posterior chest wall.

Table 6.4 Percussion note

Type	Lesions by which produced
Tympanitic	Hollow viscus
Hyperresonant	Pneumothorax
Resonant	Normal lung
Impaired	Pulmonary consolidation Pulmonary collapse Pulmonary fibrosis
Dull	Pulmonary consolidation Pulmonary collapse Pleural thickening
Stony dull	Pleural effusion

When an area of impaired resonance is discovered, its boundaries should be mapped out by percussing from a zone of normal resonance towards the suspected abnormality. The same technique should be used to determine the boundaries of cardiac dullness (p. 100) and hepatic dullness (p. 173).

A crude impression of the range of diaphragmatic movement can be obtained by measuring the distance between the lower borders of pulmonary resonance at the back of the chest in full inspiration and forced expiration, but this procedure (*tidal percussion*) is of little practical value.

The terms used to describe different types of percussion note are shown on Table 6.4.

Auscultation

Auscultation of the lungs is important in the diagnosis of certain respiratory diseases, but is of little or no value in others. In bronchial asthma and pleurisy, for example, the stethoscope provides diagnostic information which cannot be obtained in any other way. In contrast, auscultation is unhelpful in the early diagnosis of pulmonary tuberculosis, which may reach an advanced stage before any abnormality can be detected.

Breath sounds and voice sounds

Breath sounds are produced by vibrations of the vocal cords caused by the turbulent flow of air through the larynx during inspiration and expir-

clavicles can be percussed directly with the right middle finger or, if preferred, with the right index, middle and ring fingers held closely together. The correct situation for percussion is within the medial third of the clavicle, just lateral to its expanded medial end. Percussion more laterally will merely elicit the dullness produced by the muscle masses of the shoulder. The lung apices are percussed by placing the left middle finger across the anterior border of the trapezius muscle, overlapping the supraclavicular fossa, and directing the percussion downwards.

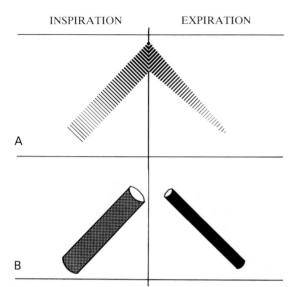

INSPIRATION   EXPIRATION

A

B

Fig. 6.21 Diagrammatic representation of breath sounds. (A) vesicular. (B) bronchial.

ation. The sounds so produced are transmitted along the trachea and bronchi and through the lungs to the chest wall. In their passage through normal lungs the intensity and frequency-pattern of the sounds are altered. When they are heard through a stethoscope on the chest wall they have a characteristic rustling quality to which the term *vesicular* is applied. The intensity of the sounds increases steadily during inspiration and then quickly fades away during the first one-third of expiration (Fig. 6.21). Disease of the bronchi, lungs and pleura may alter the breath sounds in three main ways:

1. Diminished vesicular breath sounds. If the conduction of the breath sounds to the chest wall is attenuated by airflow limitation (either general, as in bronchial asthma, or local, as when a large bronchus is obstructed by a tumour) or by a shallow pneumothorax, a small pleural effusion or pleural thickening, they remain vesicular but are diminished in amplitude. This change in the breath sounds is invariably accompanied by a reduction in the amplitude of the conducted voice sounds.

2. Bronchial breath sounds. If the lung tissue through which the breath sounds are transmitted from the air passages to the chest wall has lost its normal spongy consistence and has become firm or solid, e.g. in consolidation or fibrosis, the

sounds picked up by the stethoscope resemble more closely those produced at the larynx than those heard over normal lung. Such *bronchial breath sounds* are found whenever: (a) normal lung tissue is replaced by a uniform conducting medium, be it consolidation, fibrosis, collapse or air and (b) the relevant major bronchus remains patent.

The pathological processes which produce these criteria are detailed in Table 6.5 (p. 148).

Bronchial breath sounds resemble more closely those produced at the larynx than those heard over normal lung. The criteria for the recognition of bronchial breathing must be strict and unambiguous. Three conditions must be satisfied:

a. both the inspiratory and expiratory sounds must be blowing, sometimes called tubular, in character;
b. the expiratory sound must be as long and as loud as the inspiratory sound; and
c. there must be a pause between the end of the inspiratory sound and the beginning of the expiratory sound (Fig. 6.21).

Voice sounds (vocal resonance) conducted through consolidated lung tissue also resemble more closely those produced at the larynx than those heard over normal lungs, in that they are louder and more distinct. In some cases the whispered voice may be transmitted almost without distortion, so that individual syllables can be clearly recognised (*whispering pectoriloquy*).

The pitch of bronchial breath sounds varies according to the nature of the pulmonary changes. As high-frequency sounds are selectively conducted through consolidated lung tissue, high-pitched bronchial breath sounds are heard in lobar or segmental pneumonia (Fig. 6.13). Fibrotic lung tissue, on the other hand, transmits sounds of lower frequency and thus produces low-pitched bronchial breath sounds. With voice sounds, there is a similar selective conduction of certain frequencies. High-pitched bronchial breath sounds are associated with voice sounds of a bleating high-pitched quality, (*aegophony*), a phenomenon less often observed in the presence of low-pitched bronchial breath sounds.

When bronchial breath sounds traverse air-containing cavities in their passage to the chest wall, they may occasionally acquire a resonating *amphoric* quality, resembling the sound produced by blowing across the top of a bottle.

3. Intermediate breath sounds. Breath sounds may be intermediate in type between vesicular and bronchial, for example, vesicular with prolonged expiration. This type is heard commonly in the presence of diffuse pulmonary fibrosis, chronic bronchitis and emphysema. Other variants, such as bronchovesicular breath sounds in which the inspiratory component is bronchial in type and the expiratory sound is vesicular, have no specific significance.

Added sounds

For many years the terminology of added sounds has been confused by the ambiguity which has surrounded the use of the word râle. Translated literally from the French it means rattle, but Laënnec wrongly regarded it as equivalent to the Latin term 'rhonchus'. In fact, rhonchus is a latinised version of the Greek rhonchos, meaning wheezing, and its use should logically be restricted to the musical sounds produced in narrowed bronchi. The word crepitation, derived from the latin *crepitare*, to crack or rattle, is an unambiguous term which can be appropriately used to describe all non-musical crackling sounds. The adoption of the terms rhonchus and crepitation, as defined below, allows the term râle to be discarded and for the sake of clarity this policy has been followed.

It has been suggested that the terms wheezes and crackles should replace rhonchi and crepitations. The word wheeze is, however, usually used to describe the sound heard without a stethoscope in patients with generalized expiratory airflow obstruction. The substitution of wheezes for rhonchi may thus give rise to confusion and the traditional terms are preferable.

Added sounds heard on auscultation of the chest are therefore of three types: rhonchi, crepitations and pleural sounds.

1. Rhonchi (wheezes). These are musical sounds of high, medium or low pitch produced by the passage of air through narrowed bronchi. Rhonchi caused by mucosal oedema or spasm of the bronchial musculature are usually super-imposed upon the expiratory phase of the respiratory murmur, which is always prolonged when rhonchi are present. Rhonchi heard during inspiration are more often due to secretion in the large bronchi and may disappear, or at least become less numerous, after coughing. A constant low-pitched rhonchus (fixed rhonchus) usually indicates partial obstruction of a major bronchus by a local lesion, such as a tumour or an inhaled foreign body.

2. Crepitations (crackles). These are non-musical sounds mainly audible during inspiration. At one time they were attributed to the bubbling of air through secretions in the bronchi and alveoli, but that view is no longer tenable, except when the sounds originate in the major bronchi, dilated bronchi (bronchiectasis) and pulmonary cavities. In these circumstances the presence of secretions is confirmed by the observation that the crepitations either decrease in number or disappear temporarily after coughing.

A much more frequent cause of crepitations in lung disease is the explosive reopening, during inspiration, of peripheral small airways which have become occluded during expiration. These crepitations are most numerous during the second half of inspiration and in some cases confined to the last part of the breath in (end-inspiratory crepitations). Such crepitations are not influenced by coughing, and are more conspicuous over the lower parts of the lungs because in the upright position small airway closure is more liable to occur there than in the upper lobes.

3. Pleural sounds. A *pleural rub* is a leathery or creaking sound produced by movement of the visceral pleura over the parietal pleura, when both surfaces are roughened as by fibrinous exudate. It is usually heard at two separate stages in the respiratory cycle, towards the end of inspiration and just after the beginning of expiration. A pleural rub may be inaudible during normal breating but can be heard when the patient is asked to breathe deeply.

It is sometimes difficult to distinguish between a low-pitched rhonchus, coarse crepitations and a pleural rub. If there is any doubt auscultation should be repeated after a forceful cough, when rhonchi or crepitations will usually alter in character or disappear, while a pleural rub will remain unchanged.

A *pneumothorax click* is a rhythmical sound, synchronous with cardiac systole, which may be heard with or without the aid of a stethoscope. It is produced by a shallow left pneumothorax between the two layers of pleura overlying the heart.

Technique of auscultation

The design of stethoscope recommended for routine clinical use provides the choice of a bell or diaphragm. As most of the sounds reaching the chest wall from the bronchi and lungs are in the low-frequency range, the bell should normally be used in preference to the diaphragm. Another reason for selecting the bell is that stretching of the skin and hairs under the diaphragm during deep breathing is apt to produce sounds which may be difficult to distinguish from a pleural rub and/or crepitations.

Auscultation should be carried out with the patient relaxed, breathing deeply and fairly rapidly. The mouth should be kept wide open and the patient should be specifically asked not to purse the lips during expiration. It should be borne in mind that prolonged deep breathing may cause giddiness or even tetany.

The following information can be obtained from auscultation:

1. The type and amplitude of the breath sounds
2. The type and number of any added sounds and their position in the respiratory cycle
3. The quality and amplitude of the conducted voice sounds.

To ensure that small localised lesions are not overlooked, auscultation must be performed over a large number of positions. It is important to compare the findings in equivalent positions on the two sides, anteriorly from above and then just below the clavicle down to the sixth rib, laterally from the axilla down to the eighth rib, and posteriorly from above the level of the spine of the scapula down to the eleventh rib. Auscultation on the two sides alternately is essential for comparing the amplitude of breath sounds and vocal resonance. Auscultation within 2–3 cm of the midline, either anteriorly or posteriorly, may give misleading information in regard to the type of breath sounds and voice sounds, particularly in the upper half of the chest, where the stethoscope may pick up sounds transmitted directly from the trachea and main bronchi to the chest wall. Bronchial breath sounds heard in these situations should be disregarded in the absence of other pathological signs.

Auscultation should be carried out in two stages. In the first, attention should be directed to breath sounds and added sounds, and in the second to the voice sounds. A systematic method of listening to the breath sounds and added sounds is essential. With the patient breathing regularly and fairly deeply, the observer should concentrate separately on the inspiratory and expiratory phases, on their quality and amplitude, and also on the type, number and position of any added sounds. It should also be noted if there is any gap between the end of the inspiratory murmur and the beginning of the expiratory phase. Finally, it may be necessary to repeat auscultation during and after coughing.

The quality and amplitude of the vocal resonance should be assessed and compared in the same positions as the breath sounds by asking the patient to say 'one, one, one'. Where there is an increase in the amplitude and clarity of the voice sounds or an alteration in their quality the examiner should test for whispering pectoriloquy.

The technique of auscultation may have to be modified to meet the needs of individual cases. Examples of this are:

1. When abnormal breath sounds are heard, the extent of the lesion should be mapped out by moving the chest piece of the stethoscope with each breath from the normal towards the abnormal zone and noting the level at which the breath sounds change.
2. A patient with severe pleural pain should not be asked to take frequent deep breaths. It is preferable to test the vocal resonance first. If an area is found in which the voice sounds are increased, the patient should be asked to take one or two deep breaths and bronchial breath sounds will usually be heard in the same area.
3. Auscultation after coughing is often a useful procedure. It may resolve doubt as to whether an added sound is a low-pitched rhonchus, a series of coarse crepitations or a pleural rub. When the breath sounds are diminished or absent over a lobe

or segment thought to be involved in pneumonia, this may be due to bronchial obstruction by secretions, and bronchial breath sounds often become audible when these secretions are dislodged by coughing.

The interpretation of auscultatory findings

Cause of bronchial breath sounds and diminished or absent breath sounds are given in Table 6.5. When bronchial breath sounds are audible the voice sounds are louder than normal and whispering pectoriloquy is usually present. When breath sounds are diminished vocal resonance is decreased in amplitude to the same degree as the breath sounds are diminished.

Rhonchi (wheezes) are heard diffusely over both lungs in bronchial asthma and in most cases of acute and chronic bronchitis. In asthma the rhonchi are medium- or high-pitched and are mainly heard during expiration which is prolonged. In bronchitis they are usually low- or medium-pitched and both inspiratory and expiratory. A localised rhonchus may be heard over a partially obstructed large bronchus. If the obstruction is caused by a fixed lesion, such as a tumour or foreign body in a large bronchus, the rhonchus is usually louder during inspiration, is not altered by coughing and is often accompanied by stridor. If due to secretions, these are usually removed by coughing, which causes the rhonchus to disappear.

Forced expiratory time (FET) is measured by placing the chest piece of a stethoscope over the trachea and timing the duration of forced expiration following a full inspiration. This is normally less than four seconds. A prolonged FET is indicative of diffuse airflow limitation, and is a feature of chronic bronchitis, emphysema and bronchial asthma.

Crepitations (crackles) caused by secretions within the large bronchi in acute or chronic bronchitis, or in resolving bronchopneumonia, are widespread and bilateral, while those audible over resolving lobar or segmental pneumonic consolidation, dilated bronchi (bronchiectasis), lung abscesses or tuberculous cavities are localised to the site of the lesions. In all these conditions they are audible throughout inspiration, and alter after coughing (p. 146). Crepitations in other parenchymal lung conditions, such as interstitial pulmonary oedema, allergic and fibrosing alveolitis, and perhaps early pneumonic consolidation and miliary tuberculosis, are in contrast audible mainly during the second half of inspiration, and are uninfluenced by coughing. No useful purpose is served by trying to distinguish between moist and dry, and between fine, medium and coarse crepitations. It is much more important to note their timing in the respiratory cycle and how they are affected by coughing.

A pleural rub is heard over areas of pleurisy. It disappears as soon as the visceral and parietal pleura are separated by fluid, but often remains audible above an effusion. If pleurisy involves the pleura adjacent to the pericardium, a pleuropericardial rub may also be heard. This is a rather misleading term since the pericardial element in the sound is not due to pericarditis. It is caused merely by roughened pleural surfaces adjacent to the pericardium being moved across one another by cardiac pulsation. A pleuro-pericardial rub may, in some cases, be impossible to distinguish from a pericardial rub.

Table 6.5 Bronchial, diminished or absent breath sounds

Auscultatory findings	Disease process
High-pitched bronchial breath sounds	Pneumonic consolidation (Fig. 6.13) Large superficial pulmonary cavity Collapsed lung or lobe when large bronchi are patent (Fig. 6.14) Lung compressed by pleural effusion (sometimes) Tension pneumothorax (sometimes)
Low-pitched bronchial breath sounds	Localised areas of pulmonary fibrosis e.g. chronic pulmonary tuberculosis chronic suppurative pneumonia
Diminished or absent breath sounds	Pleural effusion (Fig. 6.12) Thickened pleura (if gross) Collapsed lung or lobe when large bronchi occluded (Fig. 6.14) Pneumothorax (Fig. 6.15) Emphysema (symmetrical diminution over both lungs)

Integration of physical signs

Certain groups of physical signs are typically associated with certain pathological changes in the lungs and pleura. Such changes are not necessarily specific for one particular disease. For example, the physical signs of consolidation may occur in pneumonia or tuberculosis and those of pleural effusion may be present in malignant disease, empyema or cardiac failure. Each group of physical signs therefore gives an indication only of the gross pathology of the lesion, and not of its precise nature, the diagnosis of which depends on an analysis of all the clinical and other evidence. The characteristic physical signs of the more common lesions are shown in Figures 6.12–6.15, namely pleural effusion, consolidation, collapse and pneumothorax. It must be emphasised that these signs are not necessarily present in every case. An area of consolidation or collapse may, for example, be too small to give rise to the classical pattern of physical signs. Furthermore, the picture may be confused by the coincidence of two groups of signs, as when consolidation or collapse is accompanied by pleural effusion. Difficulties are also apt to arise when the differential diagnosis rests on the observer's estimate of the position of the mediastinum. In patients with pulmonary collapse or pleural effusion mediastinal displacement is an inconstant feature and, even when present, may be difficult to detect since the trachea and apex beat are not always readily palpable.

FURTHER INVESTIGATION

From the history and clinical examination it is possible in many cases to make a reliable diagnosis. This applies, for example, to conditions such as bronchial asthma, chronic obstructive airways disease and to some cases of pneumonia and pulmonary infarction. At other times clinical examination fails to reveal any abnormality and the diagnosis depends entirely on specialised investigations, particularly radiology. Pulmonary tuberculosis and bronchial carcinoma are two important diseases which may not give rise to any clinical abnormality in the early stages. It is therefore essential to advise radiological examination of the chest whenever one of these conditions is suspected from the history. By means of radiology the precise anatomical position of a lesion can be determined, and from this and other features its pathology may be deduced. Microbiological and cytological examination of sputum and pleural fluid may provide specific data, by means of which a clinical diagnosis can be elaborated into an aetiological diagnosis, for example by the identification of the organism responsible for an acute pneumonia or by the finding of malignant cells in sputum or in pleural fluid. In a few cases the diagnosis cannot be completed without more formidable investigations, such as bronchoscopy, bronchography, pleural biopsy, thoracoscopy, mediastinoscopy and even thoracotomy.

Even when a precise diagnosis has been made, it is usually desirable to measure the effect the disease is having on respiratory function. This is useful for the assessment of fitness for work and suitability for certain forms of treatment, such as surgery for bronchial carcinoma.

A full account of all the special methods of investigation cannot be given here, nor is it possible to indicate in any detail the information they can be expected to provide. The summary which follows is therefore intended to serve only as a guide to the value of each investigation and the indications for its use.

Radiological examination. 1. *Radiographs* (postero-anterior) should be obtained whenever pulmonary or pleural disease is suspected. It is not possible to determine accurately the site of most abnormalities visible on postero-anterior or antero-posterior X-rays and a lateral should be used to elucidate any abnormality shown on PA film (Fig. 6.22). A comparison between current and previous films, if they can be obtained, may provide vital diagnostic information (a) if a pulmonary opacity has not increased in size over a period of a year or longer, a diagnosis of bronchial carcinoma is highly improbable, (b) if an opacity has become smaller or less dense in the course of a few days or weeks, pneumonia is its most likely cause; and (c) if a lesion was not present on an earlier film, or has become larger, it is almost certainly a tumour or an active tuberculous infection.

Radiographic examination of the nasal sinuses is an integral part of the investigation of chronic infection of the upper respiratory tract.

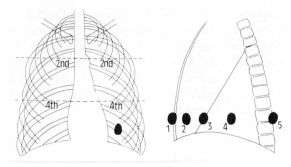

Fig. 6.22 Chest radiographs. For descriptive purposes the straight X-ray is divided into zones — upper, mid and lower — separated by imaginary horizontal lines between the anterior ends of the second and fourth ribs. There is a round shadow in the left lower zones of the straight X-ray. The lateral view shows five possible sites of the abnormality: (1) anterior chest wall or pleura (2) left upper lobe (3) fissure between the lobes (4) left lower lobe (5) posterior chest wall or pleura.

2. Screening provides information about the movement of the diaphragm and the position and outline of the oesophagus. It is indicated particularly in patients with bronchial carcinoma. Unilateral diaphragmatic paralysis or a localised displacement of the barium-distended oesophagus would, by demonstrating mediastinal invasion, contraindicate an attempt at surgical treatment.

3. Tomography is a special radiographic technique by means of which an opacity or part of an opacity lying in one particular plane can be visualised clearly, even when there are superimposed opacities in different planes. This technique is of value in the detection of pulmonary cavities and in demonstrating local variations in density (e.g. calcification) within a pulmonary lesion. It can thus be helpful in distinguishing between a tumour and a tuberculous lesion.

Computed tomography provides much more accurate information on the position and nature of localised pulmonary lesions and can detect others which may not be visible on conventional radiographs. It is also valuable in the investigation of mediastinal abnormalities.

4. Pulmonary angiography can be used to detect vascular abnormalities in the lung. A series of chest radiographs is taken in rapid succession after the injection of contrast medium into the main pulmonary artery. This is of particular value in the confirmation and delineation of the extent of a large pulmonary embolism.

Radionuclide scanning. Perfusion scanning of the lungs following the intravenous injection of isotope-labelled macro-aggregated albumin can be used to detect and delineate underperfused areas of lung. This technique is of value in the diagnosis of pulmonary embolism, particularly if combined with ventilation scanning following the inhalation of an isotope-labelled gas.

Examination of the sputum. This examination is an important diagnostic measure in all suspected bronchopulmonary infections, particularly pneumonia and tuberculosis. In all such cases a direct film, appropriately stained, should be examined microscopically and suitable culture media inoculated. Large numbers of eosinophils or haemosiderin-containing macrophages may be found in pulmonary eosinophilia and pulmonary haemosiderosis respectively. Sputum should also be examined for malignant cells if bronchial carcinoma is suspected.

Intradermal tests. The *tuberculin test* is chiefly of value in excluding present or past tuberculous infection. A positive test is of definite diagnostic significance only in children. A positive *Kviem test* confirms a diagnosis of sarcoidosis. *Skin sensitivity tests* indicate the presence or absence of atopy, and may help to identify the cause of allergic rhinitis or asthma.

Examination of the blood. The *total and differential white cell counts* may give guidance as to the nature of a radiographic abnormality, e.g. whether it is an area of acute pneumonic consolidation or an eosinophilic infiltrate. *Blood culture* and *examination of serum for viral and other antibodies* may be of value in determining the aetiology of a pneumonic illness. A positive Coombs' test is found in mycoplasma pneumonia.

Bronchoscopy. With a rigid bronchoscope the bronchi can be inspected as far as the segmental orifices. A flexible (fibreoptic) bronchoscope is of value in the diagnosis of more peripheral lesions and can also be used to obtain specimens of lung tissue for histological examination in patients with diffuse pulmonary disease (transbronchial lung biopsy). Bronchoscopy is an essential investigation whenever bronchial carcinoma is suspected, and often the diagnosis can be confirmed histologically by biopsy. It is also a valuable method of investigating other causes of bronchial obstruction, e.g. inhaled foreign body, tuberculous lymph nodes.

Bronchoalveolar lavage. This is performed during fibreoptic bronchoscopy. Saline is introduced through the bronchoscope and re-aspirated to provide fluid that can be subjected to cytological and microbiological examination. In addition to its value in the investigation of some patients with peripheral pulmonary tumours or infections, it may also be of use in the diagnosis of conditions which give rise to diffuse X-ray abnormalities such as allergic and fibrosing alveolitis and sarcoidosis.

Bronchography. In this examination radiographs are taken after the bronchial tree has been outlined by a contrast medium. Its main value is in the diagnosis of bronchiectasis and the precise determination of its degree and distribution.

Pleural aspiration and biopsy. Cytological and bacteriological examination of pleural fluid often provides information which reveals the cause of the effusion. Pleural biopsy taken from the site of aspiration is of particular value in the diagnosis of tuberculous and malignant effusions.

Thoracoscopy. The examination of the pleural surfaces with a telescope, after air has been introduced into the pleural space, may show pleural abnormalities from which tissue can be removed for histological examination. This technique is used only when examination of pleural fluid and pleural biopsy by the ordinary method are unhelpful.

Lymph node biopsy. Removal or needle aspiration of a supraclavicular, particularly a scalene lymph node, or less frequently an axillary lymph node, may provide histological or cytological proof of the diagnosis in bronchial carcinoma, lymphoma, sarcoidosis and, occasionally, tuberculosis. A lymph node can also be removed from the vicinity of the trachea and main bronchi by the technique of *mediastinoscopy*.

Mediastinoscopy. The examination of the structures of the anterior mediastinum with an instrument inserted behind the sternum through an incision in the neck.

Lung biopsy. If the nature of a diffuse pulmonary abnormality cannot be determined by other methods, a histological diagnosis can be made by transbronchial or transthoracic needle biopsy of lung. A similar technique can be used for the diagnosis of localised peripheral pulmonary lesions. Thoracotomy may be required for the diagnosis of pulmonary or mediastinal lesions if the results of all other investigations are negative or inconclusive.

Tests of respiratory function. Disturbances of ventilation, distribution, diffusion and lung compliance can be measured, but many of these tests require complex facilities, which are not generally available. For practical purposes, respiratory function can be adequately investigated by the following procedures:

1. The measurement of the partial pressure of *oxygen* (Pa_{O_2}) and of *carbon dioxide* (Pa_{CO_2}) in a sample of arterial blood obtained from the radial, brachial or femoral artery. Pa_{CO_2} is normally 4.8–6.0 kPa (36–45 mmHg), and is always increased when there is inadequate alveolar ventilation. The hydrogen ion concentration (normal range: 36–44 nmol/l) should be measured on the same sample to determine the patient's acid-base status. Where blood gas monitoring is indicated, transcutaneous oximetry provides a useful alternative to arterial blood sampling.

2. The measurement of *forced expiratory volume* (FEV_1) and *forced vital capacity* (FVC). This requires either a recording spirometer, or a standard spirometer incorporating an electronic timing device. The FEV_1 is the largest volume which can be expired, from full inspiration, in one second, and provides information about ventilatory capacity. In health the FEV_1 amounts to at least 75% of the FVC. In diseases such as bronchial asthma and emphysema, which produce narrowing of the air passages during expiration, both FEV_1 and FVC are reduced but the reduction in FEV_1 is proportionately greater, i.e. the FEV_1/FVC ratio is reduced. In restrictive lung disease and ankylosing spondylitis, which render the lungs or chest wall more rigid, the FEV_1 and FVC are reduced proportionately and the normal FEV_1/FVC ratio is preserved or even increased. These simple measurements are thus of value in distinguishing between one type of respiratory disorder and another, as well as in providing an index of its severity. Serial measurements can be used to assess improvement or deterioration and also the

response to bronchodilator drugs or corticosteroids in patients with reversible airways obstruction.

The *peak expiratory flow* (PEF), which correlates closely with the FEV_1, can also be used to assess the degree of airflow obstruction. The device employed for this measurement (a peak flow meter or gauge) is portable and easy to operate, and is eminently suitable for use in general practice. The normal range of PEF in healthy adults is 400–650 litres per minute.

3. Transfer factor. The diffusing capacity of lung tissue can be assessed by measuring the transfer factor of carbon monoxide which provides a useful index of the severity of restrictive lung conditions such as fibrosing alveolitis.

THE METHODS IN PRACTICE

THE EXAMINATION OF THE INJURED CHEST

In patients suffering from severe multiple injuries in which there is damage to the chest, routine clinical methods of examination may be difficult to apply and their results may be misleading. Furthermore, the examination must be performed expeditiously since many of the patients urgently require resuscitation either because of respiratory insufficiency, blood loss, or injury to other systems.

Manifestations of respiratory inadequacy, such as breathlessness or central cyanosis, may be the first indication that the chest has been injured. These may on occasions be misinterpreted as, for example, when panic causes hyperventilation, and the first object of the physical examination must be to determine whether or not organic damage has occurred. The next step is to discover whether the chest wall, the lungs or the air passages are involved and whether a pneumothorax or a haemothorax is present. Finally, it will be essential to assess the severity of respiratory insufficiency and decide how urgent is the need for resuscitation in this respect.

The upper respiratory tract

The first part of the examination should be directed towards ensuring that the airway is ade-

quate and that there is no obstruction to the oropharynx, larynx or trachea by the tongue, by damaged tissues or by blood.

The chest

The examination of the chest follows the sequence that has been described, but must not be unnecessarily detailed or time consuming. Signs of particular importance should be sought, such as paradoxical movement of a segment of the chest wall or subcutaneous emphysema.

Inspection. Breathlessness and central cyanosis must be assessed in the usual way. Paradoxical movement of the chest wall is seen in patients who have sustained double fractures of a series of ribs or of the sternum. The portion of the thoracic cage between the fractures becomes mobile and, with the overlying soft tissue, is sucked in during inspiration. This causes compression of the underlying area of lung during inspiration and seriously interferes with pulmonary ventilation and perfusion. Subcutaneous emphysema develops when the trachea, bronchi or lungs have been damaged and air escapes into the adjacent tissues; in some cases, the resultant swelling may be visible. Haemopericardium causes tamponade which should be suspected when the jugular venous pressure is increased after injury.

Palpation. The neck and chest should be palpated for the presence of subcutaneous emphysema. Deviation of the trachea from the mid-line, indicating displacement of the mediastinum by lesions such as haemothorax, pneumothorax or collapse, should be noted. The apex beat, which may also be displaced in these circumstances, is usually difficult to locate if there is hypotension, tachycardia, subcutaneous emphysema or bruising of the chest wall. The extent of any paradoxical movement can be assessed by gently laying the palms on the injured and uninjured segments of the chest wall and observing how one hand moves inwards and the other one outwards with each respiration.

Percussion. This is of value only in helping to establish the presence of a gross haemothorax or pneumothorax. It should be carried out very gently.

Auscultation. This is also of little value when

the chest is extensively injured, as the multiplicity of added sounds arising from lung, pleura and chest wall mitigates against their accurate interpretation.

Further investigation

Radiographs taken in the erect position must be obtained at the earliest possible moment whenever a chest injury is suspected. In the severely injured a portable apparatus may have to be used. Because of the technical difficulties with this method in distressed patients, radiographs are frequently of poor quality, but a pneumothorax, a haemothorax, severe lung damage or collapse and rupture of the diaphragm can usually be recognised.

Tests of respiratory function in the form of serial studies of arterial blood gases should be carried out whenever respiratory insufficiency is suspected. These measurements will indicate whether resuscitation by intermittent positive-pressure ventilation is required, and can also be used to monitor the patient's response to this form of treatment.

FURTHER READING

Clark T J H 1981 Clinical investigation of respiratory disease. Chapman and Hall, London
Crompton G K 1987 Diagnosis and management of respiratory disease, 2nd edn. Blackwell Scientific, Oxford
Crompton G K, McHardy G J R In: Macleod J, Edwards C, Bouchier I (eds) Davidson's principles and practice of medicine, 15th edn. Churchill Livingstone, Edinburgh
Forgacs P 1978 Lung sounds. Bailliere Tindall, London
James D G, Studdy P R 1981 A colour atlas of respiratory disease. Wolfe, London

7. The alimentary and genitourinary systems

D. W. Hamer-Hodges   J. F. Munro

The diagnosis of abdominal diseases is often dependent more upon a careful history than the presence of physical signs. Pain is prominent among the symptoms encountered in the alimentary and genitourinary systems. When present interrogation is essential before complicated investigations are initiated. If this is neglected, the clinician may arrange for unnecessary tests which may reveal a symptomless abnormality such as a hiatus hernia or gallstones. This may result in inappropriate management and even unnecessary surgery.

THE HISTORY

SYMPTOMS OF ALIMENTARY DISEASE

Complaints in alimentary disease include abdominal pain, difficulty in swallowing, indigestion, heartburn, loss of appetite, decrease in weight, vomiting, jaundice, abdominal distension, alteration in bowel habit and bleeding per rectum. Sometimes, organic disease may be suspected only from the development of a secondary feature such as anaemia. Occasionally patients may conceal important symptoms such as bleeding per rectum because of embarrassment, a belief that the cause is trivial, or fear of serious disease. The clinician must not only listen carefully to the patient's presenting complaints but also systematically enquire about the other principal symptoms of abdominal disease. It must also be remembered that the emotional state of a patient may produce symptoms in the absence of an organic cause.

Abdominal pain

This is a very frequent symptom of disorders of the alimentary system. After listening to the patient's history, additional questions should be framed in the manner described on page 25. Pain from unpaired structures is usually central. The patient should be asked to demonstrate the exact site and also any areas to which the pain may radiate. The type of pain should be listed, e.g. 'stitch-like'. Frequency, duration and timing of attacks may be of diagnostic significance as may be associated factors and those which relieve or aggravate the pain. In Table 7.1 the principal features of four common disorders are listed to illustrate the value of analysis along these lines.

Abdominal pain, sometimes of great intensity, may result from disorders outwith the alimentary system. Pain arising from retroperitoneal structures may be felt anterior-abdominally as well as in the back. Such conditions include renal and ureteric colic, aortic aneurysmal dissection and pancreatitis. Anterior abdominal pain may also be caused by vertebral collapse or other diseases of the spine. Unilateral disease of the vertebra, collapsed intravertebral disc or tumour affecting a nerve, may give rise to pain on one side of the abdomen. Associated features such as aggravation by certain movements and coughing are usually present to indicate the source of the pain. Table 7.2. illustrates some non alimentary conditions which can cause abdominal pain.

Difficulty in swallowing (Dysphagia)

Initiation of swallowing is a conscious action followed by reflex oesophageal peristalsis. Difficulty in initiating swallowing may be due to a painful lesion of the mouth or throat or to a neurological or neuromuscular disorder such as pseudobulbar

Table 7.1   Examples of the analysis of acute abdominal pain

	Peptic Ulcer	Acute Cholecystitis	Acute Pancreatitis	Ureteric Colic
Main site	Epigastric	Epigastric or R. hypochondrical	Epigastric	From loin to groin
Radiation	Into the back	Beneath R. scapula R. shoulder tip	Into the back May become generalised	Into genitalia
Character	Gnawing	Constant	Sudden onset	Constant
Severity	Mild to moderate	Severe	Very severe	Very severe
Duration	½–3 hours	3–24 hour	Usually more than 24 hours	Usually hours
Frequency and Periodicity	Remissions for weeks or months	Unpredictable	Unpredictable	—
Special times of occurrence	Nocturnal Between meals	—	—	—
Aggravating factors	Irregular meals Smoking Alcohol Aspirin	Sometimes food	After alcohol or heavy meals	Dehydration Previous urinary infections
Relieving factors	Food, antacids Vomiting	—	May be eased by sitting upright	—
Associated phenomena	Family history GI haemorrhage Perforation	Restless and vomiting Jaundice Fever with rigors	Gallstones Produces vomiting Jaundice and paralytic ileus are common	Restless and vomiting Haematuria

palsy or myasthenia gravis. Sticking of food is an important symptom of oesophageal disease for which an explanation must be sought. At the level of the cricoid cartilage this may be due to a growth, a stricture, a pharyngo-oesophageal pouch or as a reflex effect from some disorder further down the gullet. Food felt to be held up behind the xiphisternum implies a lesion at the lower end of the oesophagus, either a tumour, achalasia of the cardia or a stricture resulting from peptic oesphagitis. The sensation may be intermittent and occur only with large lumps of food such as meat or potato. Later, any solid may be responsible and symptoms may become acute with its impaction at the area of narrowing. Discomfort may be relieved when food is regurgitated, though the patient may describe this as vomiting. In patients with a pharyngo-oesophageal pouch or lower oesophageal obstruction recognisable food may be brought back long after it was eaten. Achalasia of the cardia in particular may lead to nocturnal coughing or dyspnoea due to spillage from the gullet into the trachea.

Dysphagia should not be confused with globus hystericus, a psychogenic symptom in which there is a feeling of a lump in the throat which needs to be swallowed; the latter is present between meals and there is no difficulty in swallowing food.

Vomiting

Although vomiting suggests disease of the stomach, it can also be a feature of a wide variety of local and systemic disorder. Instances include functional and organic disorders of the nervous system, for example, fear, motion sickness, labyrinthine disorders, migraine, meningitis or intracranial tumour. Vomiting may also result from severe pain, as in renal colic or myocardial infarction. Amongst systemic conditions are renal failure, pregnancy, and metabolic disorders such as diabetic ketoacidosis or hyperparathyroidism.

Table 7.2 Examples of non-alimentary causes of abdominal pain

Condition	Clinical features
Myocardial Infarction	Epigastric pain without tenderness Angor animi May exhibit the cardiovascular signs of myocardial infarction (hypotension, third heart sound, cardiac arrhythmias etc.)
Dissecting Aortic Aneurysm	Tearing epigastric/interscapular pain Angor animi Hypotension Asymmetry of femoral pulses
Acute Vertebral Collapse/Cord Compression	Lateralised pain restricting movement Pain on percussion of thoracic spine Dermatomal hyperaesthesia and spinal cord signs
Pleurisy	Lateralised pain on coughing Chest signs of consolidation pleural rub
Herpes Zoster	Dermatomal hyperaesthesia Vesicular eruption (may be limited to back)
Tabes Dorsalis	Paroxysmal severe girdle pain Vomiting Sensory ataxia Urinary retention Charcoat's joints Absence of deep pain, sensation and leg reflexes Argyll Robertson pupils and ptosis of tabo-paresis
Diabetic Ketoacidosis	Cramp-like pain Vomiting Tachycardia Air hunger Ketones in breath & urine
Acute Porphyria	Colicky pain Constipation Confusion Tachycardia Hypertension Peripheral neuropathy Porphobilinogen in urine

Many drugs are also prone to cause vomiting, some such as digoxin or morphine due to a central action, and others such as aminophylline or potassium chloride as a result of gastric irritation.

Vomiting may be induced by the patient suffering from bulimia nervosa or to relieve the pain of peptic ulceration. Gastric outlet obstruction is associated with copious vomiting. More distal obstruction also leads to vomiting but the lower the level of the obstruction, the more marked are the accompanying symptoms of abdominal distension and intestinal colic. Vomiting also occurs in such diverse conditions as acute gastritis, acute cholecystitis, acute pancreatitis and hepatitis. In most instances, vomiting is preceded by nausea but in some cases of intracranial tumour, the vomiting may be without warning and may be projectile.

Enquiry should be made about the frequency of the vomiting, the time of day at which it occurs and also about the taste, colour, quantity and smell of the vomitus. If the taste and smell are inconspicuous, this suggests either the presence of achlorhydria or that the 'vomit' has been regurgitated from the oesophagus. Foul smelling vomitus occurs in ulcerating carcinoma of the stomach or in pyloric obstruction. Faecal vomiting may occur in low intestinal obstruction or with a gastro-colic fistula. A yellow colour and bitter taste indicate the presence of bile and means that there has been regurgitation of duodenal content into the stomach.

Special attention should be paid to the presence of blood in the vomit (*haematemesis*). Bright red blood usually arises from an oesophageal lesion. A dark red vomit, sometimes containing liver-like clots of blood, is due to profuse bleeding such as may occur from a peptic ulcer. In less acute haematemesis the vomit is often blackish or dark brown and can contain sediment like 'coffee grounds', due to the conversion of the haemoglobin to acid haematin by the gastric acid.

Whenever possible, the patient's description should be supplemented by inspection of the vomitus.

Heartburn

This refers to a burning retrosternal discomfort or pain. It is very common and often occurs after meals. It is particularly frequent during pregnancy and when a patient with a hiatus hernia bends or lies down.

Jaundice

The clinical features are described on page 47. The principal complaints of patients with hepatocel-

ask about:

past history
family & contact history
travel abroad
alcohol consumption
drug usage
injections & blood transfusions
sexual activity
weight change
change in bowel
   habit
pruritus
gastrointestinal
haemorrhage

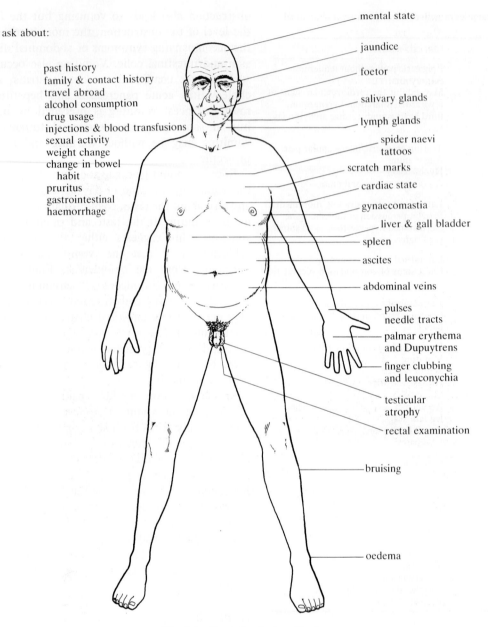

mental state

jaundice

foetor

salivary glands

lymph glands

spider naevi
tattoos

scratch marks

cardiac state

gynaecomastia

liver & gall bladder

spleen

ascites

abdominal veins

pulses
needle tracts

palmar erythema
and Dupuytrens

finger clubbing
and leuconychia

testicular
atrophy

rectal examination

bruising

oedema

Fig. 7.1 Check list for jaundice in a man.

lular jaundice are anorexia and nausea, even at the thought of food, sometimes associated with right sub-costal tenderness. Common causes include viral infections of the liver and damage by alcohol. The history should enquire about possible contacts and travel abroad (hepatitis A), consumption of alcohol and drugs, and any injections, blood transfusions or tattooing during the previous six months (hepatitis B). Hepatitis B is common in homosexuals and in drug addicts. See Fig. 7.1.

The two common causes of jaundice due to large duct obstruction are gallstones and carcinoma of the head of the pancreas. There is usually, but not always, a history of one or more attacks of biliary colic if the cause is gallstones. There is often a persistent pain in the back made worse by recumbency when carcinoma of the pancreas is responsible and the gall bladder may be palpably enlarged (p. 171). Biliary obstruction is frequently associated with fever, rigors and itching.

Important causes of jaundice due to small duct obstruction are drugs or alcohol, and biliary cirrhosis which affects middle-aged women and is often preceded by months of itching.

Jaundice due to extensive metastases occurs occasionally, and the cause is usually obvious on abdominal palpation.

Alteration in bowel habit

Normal habit varies between several evacuations

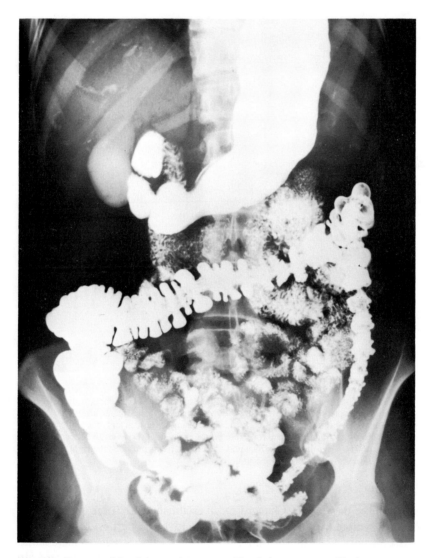

Fig. 7.2 Contents of the abdomen demonstrated by cholecystogram and barium examination. Note the stomach with peristaltic waves most marked in the gastric antrum which is surmounted by the duodenal cap; the feathery jejunal pattern in the left hypochondrium and the ileum in the hypogastrium; the caecum, appendix, and colon. Note the gall bladder alongside the duodenal cap and the calcification in the costal cartilages superimposed on the liver shadow. (Courtesy of Dr W A Copland.)

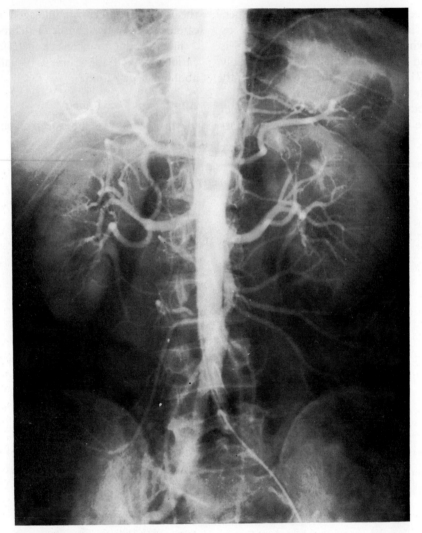

Fig. 7.3   Contents of abdomen demonstrated by aortography. Note on the left side from above downwards, the left phrenic artery immediately below the diaphragm, translucency from air in the splenic flexure overlying the splenic shadow; the splenic artery; the left renal artery; the left kidney and ureter; the superior mesenteric artery; the catheter in the left iliac artery passing into the aorta. Note on the right side, the liver; the hepatic artery; the right renal artery; the right kidney and ureter; the psoas muscles; the right iliac artery. (Courtesy of Professor Eric Samuel.)

per day to one every three days or so. Changes in habit may be the first symptom of serious underlying disease. It is necessary not only to find out the frequency of stools but also if motions are occurring at special times of the day or night and if they are associated with abdominal discomfort or a feeling of urgency. The nature of any medication, prescribed or self-administered, should be

established as some patients are unaware of the laxative properties of household remedies, and some drugs, such as mefenamic acid, may alter bowel habit. Diarrhoea may alternate with constipation, and faecal incontinence and constipation may coexist, especially from impacted faeces in the elderly.

A common cause of variability in bowel function

Table 7.3 Stool appearance in various conditions

Black	Upper gastrointestinal haemorrhage, oral iron, bismuth
Tarry black	Severe upper gastrointestinal haemorrhage
Pale, bulky and offensive	Small bowel malabsorption
Silvery pale	Pancreatic disease
Liquid, of uniform consistency	Small bowel diarrhoea
Admixed with blood & mucus	Usually colonic as in inflammatory bowel disease

is the irritable bowel syndrome in which periods of constipation and diarrhoea may alternate. Intermittent abdominal pain is another feature of this syndrome for which there is no organic explanation.

Tenesmus is the term used to describe a feeling of incomplete evacuation which may accompany bacillary dysentery or acute proctitis. It also results from a mass in the rectum, especially impacted faeces or a carcinoma.

Appearance of the stool. The patient should be asked to describe the consistency and colour of the stool. Examples of abnormal stools are illustrated in Table 7.3. Many patients do not normally inspect their faeces and therefore only positive observations can be accepted. If necessary, the clinician should confirm the description by observation. Sometimes words like 'stool' or 'faeces' are not understood, especially by children, and if there is doubt it is best to use a colloquial phrase.

Abnormalities such as threadworms, roundworms or segments of tapeworms may be present and special enquiry should be made about the presence of blood and about pus or mucus, often described by the patient as slime.

Bleeding per rectum

The cause of this important symptom should always be determined. The commonest is haemorrhoids but even though these occur frequently their presence in a patient with bleeding should not lead to the assumption that they are responsible. The important differential diagnosis is from carcinoma of the colon and rectum. Other

causes include inflammatory bowel disease, diverticular disease and anal fissure.

Bleeding from the anal canal is bright red. It is often clearly separate from the stool and may be seen only on the toilet paper. Coming from haemorrhoids, it may also splash the toilet bowl or drip into the pan after a motion is passed, whereas an anal fissure may be associated with severe anal pain which persists after defecation. In inflammatory disease of the colon, the stool may be unformed and accompanied by blood, mucus and pus. Both polyps and carcinoma may also cause excessive production of mucus. Bleeding from the upper gastrointestinal tract may present as haematemesis, melaena, circulatory collapse or with the symptoms of chronic anaemia. (see Fig. 7.4).

Loss of weight and loss of appetite

A decrease in weight may be the first indication of disease. In assessing its significance, the duration and extent of the weight loss should be established. It should be known whether it has been associated with loss of appetite (anorexia) or due to deliberate reduction in food intake. Weight loss accompanied by severe anorexia or other alimentary symptoms may not necessarily be due to intra-abdominal disease; such findings may occur, for example, in endogenous depression. Weight loss without reduction in food intake may be due to diabetes mellitus, hyperthyroidism or a malabsorption syndrome.

Abdominal distension

Increasing abdominal girth is usually due to adiposity. Its development in a patient who is otherwise becoming thinner suggests intra-abdominal disease. *Ascites*, the accumulation of fluid in the peritoneal cavity, is usually due to either cirrhosis of the liver, malignancy, tuberculous peritonitis or heart disease. The acute development of tense ascites suggests intra-abdominal malignancy, infective peritonitis or the onset of portal vein obstruction. Abdominal distension may also be the presenting complaint with an ovarian cyst which sometimes achieves an enormous size. In women of reproductive age, unadmitted pregnancy is a possibility that must be remembered.

ask about:

past history
family history
bleeding tendency
drug/alcohol use
dyspeptic symptoms
vomiting/diarrhoea
anorexia/weight loss
dizziness or fainting

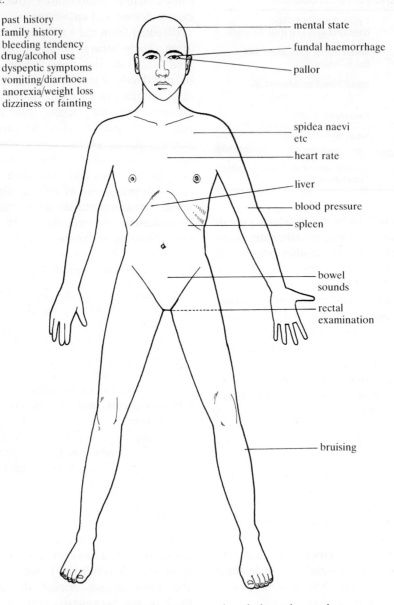

mental state

fundal haemorrhage

pallor

spidea naevi
etc

heart rate

liver

blood pressure

spleen

bowel
sounds

rectal
examination

bruising

Fig. 7.4 Check list for upper gastrointestinal tract haemorrhage.

Intestinal obstruction will cause acute abdominal swelling, usually associated with intestinal colic. Chronic constipation may result in sufficient faecal retention to cause distension. In children, the possibility of Hirschsprung's disease must be considered and the history should determine if bowel habit has ever been normal and whether soiling occurs.

Fluctuating abdominal swelling which develops during the day but resolves overnight is not uncommon, especially in women. This is caused by contraction of the diaphragm and lumbar muscles. It is never due to organic disease.

Wind

To the patient this may mean repeated belching, excessive or offensive flatus per rectum, abdominal discomfort or even borborygmi. Belched wind is often swallowed (aerophagy) without the patient's awareness. Belching itself is of no significance and is often a feature of anxiety but sometimes occurs in an attempt to relieve abdominal pain or discomfort.

The normal volume of flatus per rectum varies greatly from person to person in the range of 200 to 2000 ml per day. It consists of a mixture of gases mainly produced by bacterial action in the lower bowel. Offensive flatus is common. It is persistent and particularly unpleasant in association with intestinal malabsorption. Absence of flatus occurs in intestinal obstruction.

Borborygmi are audible bowel sounds caused by movements of gas through the bowel. Though usually nothing more than a cause for embarrassment, they may be a feature of small bowel disease.

Dyspepsia and/or indigestion

These vague terms are common complaints. Their usage is of value in obtaining a history but it is essential that the patient explains in detail what is meant. Thus 'indigestion' might describe nausea, heartburn, epigastric discomfort, abdominal pain or distension, or a feeling of post-prandial bloating. It may even be used to describe angina pectoris.

SYMPTOMS OF DISEASE OF THE GENITOURINARY SYSTEM

All patients, irrespective of the presenting complaint, should be asked about the principal symptoms of genitourinary disease which they might otherwise fail to volunteer for a variety of reasons, including embarrassment.

These are dysuria, frequency, polyuria, nocturia, haematuria, alteration in the force of micturition, incontinence, pain, and changes in sexual function. Sometimes renal disease may come to light only as the result of complaints of weakness or lethargy due to uraemia or following the discovery of proteinuria or arterial hypertension.

Dysuria, frequency and urgency

Dysuria means pain on passing urine rather than difficulty in doing so. Frequency implies the urine is passed more often than normal without there necessarily being an increase in the total volume. Urgency is a strong desire to pass urine which may be followed by incontinence if the opportunity to void is not available. Dysuria, urgency and frequency are associated with irritation of the bladder and urethra by infections, tumour or stones. Dysuria alone may be due to infection of the urethra as in gonorrhoea. Urgency alone may be a feature of anatomical change as in gynaecological prolapse or neurological disease affecting the motor control of the bladder. Frequency alone may be caused by anxiety.

Polyuria

This means an increase in urinary output and must be distinguished from frequency of micturition. It may be due to an increase in solute load as in uncontrolled diabetes mellitus. Other examples include the osmotic diuresis caused by urea in chronic renal failure and by sodium from the use of diuretics. Polyuria will also occur in diabetes insipidus where there is lack of anti-diuretic hormone (ADH) or if the renal tubules are non-responsive to ADH (nephrogenic diabetes insipidus). It may also result from psychogenic polydipsia. A patient's assessment of increased volume may be misleading and should be confirmed by performing a twenty-four hour urinary collection. Severe polyuria will cause thirst which may be the presenting symptom.

Oliguria and anuria

Oliguria means a diminution in the quantity of urine excreted. It is a feature of acute renal failure. The minimum quantity of urine which is necessary

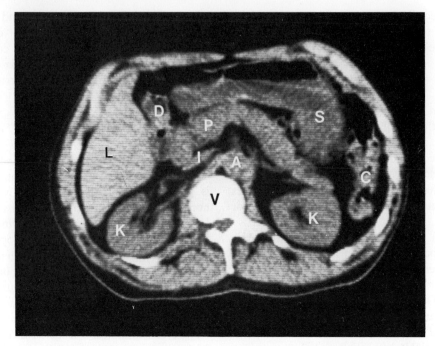

Fig. 7.5 Contents of abdomen as shown by CT scan; A: Aorta and renal arteries. C: Colon and faeces. D: Duodenum. I: Inferior vena cava. K: Kidney. L: Liver. P: Pancreas. S: Stomach. V: Vertebra, the apparent deformity of which is due to the scan passing through the pedicle and lamina on the left side and through the foramen on the right.

to maintain the constancy of the 'milieu intérieur' varies with diet, physical activity and metabolic rate as well as renal function: Thus about 200 ml might be sufficient for a healthy man at rest on a protein free diet, whereas 2000 ml might be insufficient when chronic renal failure is present. Indeed, non-oliguric renal failure is relatively common and frequently unrecognised. The uraemic patient should be questioned about possible aetiological factors such as a preceding sore throat in post-streptococcal glomerulo-nephritis.

Anuria means a complete cessation of urine production; this occurs infrequently. More commonly the complaint of 'failure to make urine' arises from urinary retention within the bladder for which a mechanical, neurological or psychological explanation should be sought.

Haematuria

Like bleeding per rectum or haemoptysis, an explanation of this serious symptom is mandatory.

The history often indicates the probable source of bleeding. When haematuria is painless, the most likely causes include papilloma of the bladder, carcinoma of the kidney or bladder, schistosomiasis or bleeding from the prostate. Haematuria associated with severe loin pain indicates a renal or ureteric origin — commonly the passage of a calculus. When frequency or dysuria accompany the bleeding, its source is usually in the bladder. Haematuria that clears during micturition arises from the urethra. Sometimes other causes of urinary discolouration may be confused with haematuria. These include the ingestion of beetroot and of various drugs such as rifampicin.

Pneumaturia

This bizarre and rare symptom is usually accurately described as a sensation of passing bubbles in the urine. It is almost always caused by a vesico-colic fistula.

Alteration in the force of micturition

A poor urinary stream is particularly common in elderly men developing obstruction from prostatic hypertrophy. The force of the stream can be assessed roughly by asking the patient to demonstrate how near he has to stand to an imaginary toilet. Other features of obstructed micturition include hesitancy, urinary spray, post-micturition dribbling, and frequency with nocturia due to incomplete emptying of the bladder.

Nocturia

The need to pass urine during the sleeping hours may be a life-long habit. As a newly developing symptom, it may be due to insomnia or to a number of organic causes including polyuria or prostatic obstruction. Nocturia is also a common symptom of cardiac failure, the diuresis resulting from the excretion of oedema fluid due to the improved renal blood flow which occurs with rest in bed.

Incontinence of urine

This is a deceptively difficult symptom to assess. It may help to ask the patient what protection, if any, is required. Many females, especially the parous, suffer from urinary incontinence provoked by the stress of laughing, sneezing or lifting. This is due to the development of a cystocele, a weakness of the anterior wall of the vagina, often accompanied by some prolapse of the uterus. Incontinence may also arise from neurological disturbances of bladder function. With a primary sensory disturbance, dribbling incontinence will result from painless over-distension of the bladder as in diabetic autonomic neuropathy. Loss of motor control results in urgency and the desire to pass urine must be obeyed at once or incontinence will occur. Multiple sclerosis is the most common neurological cause of urgency in Britain. Combined motor and sensory damage occurs in spinal cord lesions. The bladder fills to a certain pressure and then empties reflexly. The patient may be able to control bladder emptying by raising the intravesical pressure at regular intervals by manual compression of the lower abdomen.

Urogenital pain

The renal parenchyma is pain free and renal pain is associated with conditions affecting the pelvis of the kidney or causing stretching of the renal capsule. A dull aching discomfort in the renal angle may occur in such conditions as staghorn calculus and hydronephrosis. Intermittent pain can occur in polycystic disease from spontaneous bleeding into a cyst. In acute pyelonephritis the pain is more acute and is often accompanied by rigors and dysuria. Even more severe pain is caused by acute distension of the renal pelvis and kidney due to obstruction of the ureter by calculus or other causes such as blood clot. Patients with renal colic are restless, feel nauseated and often vomit. The pain may radiate to the hypochondrium or down to the groin and into the genitalia. Once a stone reaches the bladder, it is usually asymptomatic unless it enters the urethra to cause dysuria. In patients with renal colic specific questions should be asked to try and determine the cause. (see Fig 7.6). Conditions causing urinary bladder pain also produce frequency. Prostatic pain is felt in the perineum, may be caused by prostatitis and is usually associated with other features of bladder neck obstruction. Testicular and epididymal pain may be felt in the groin and lower abdomen to such an intensity that its testicular origin is obscured. Pain due to torsion of the testis usually occurs in pubertal boys or young men. It frequently develops at night and starts with pain in the iliac fossa. Tender swelling of the testis may require to be distinguished from a strangulated hernia or acute epididymo-orchitis. Ovarian pain is also felt in the iliac fossa and may be episodic as in endometriosis or more constant as in malignant tumours. Uterine pain is felt centrally, low in the abdomen and may radiate through to the lumbosacral area, for example in labour pains and dysmenorrhoea.

Sexual activity

Sexual activity may require to be assessed, for example, if there is a possibility of sexually transmitted diseases such as HIV or hepatitis B infection. Questions should be asked objectively and without prejudice; for example, 'How many

ask about:

family history of renal disease
work environment
haematuria/polyuria
previous urinary infections
joint/bone pain
indigestion
milk/alkali consumption
vitamin D medication
analgesic abuse
immobilisation

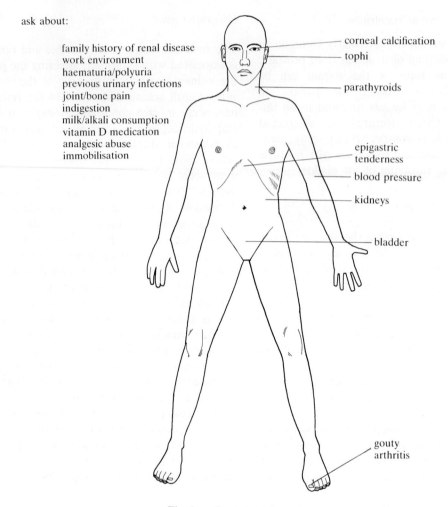

corneal calcification
tophi
parathyroids
epigastric tenderness
blood pressure
kidneys
bladder
gouty arthritis

Fig. 7.6   Check list for renal colic.

sexual partners have you had in the last twelve months and how many have been male and how many female?'; 'Do you use a condom?'.

Male sexual problems

The three principal symptoms are lack of libido, inability to achieve or maintain an erection and trouble with ejaculation. It is necessary to obtain precise information about such matters. Sexual problems are, however, difficult to assess for three main reasons: (1) the patient is often embarrassed and may not be forthcoming with a full history at the initial interview; (2) there may be a large

psychiatric component to the complaint requiring expert analysis and help; (3) physical examination at the time the patient is sexually aroused is usually impossible.

One method of overcoming the patient's initial embarrassment is to use a sexual problems questionnaire which is sent to the patient for completion before attendance at the clinic. It contains the explicit questions that must be asked. It allows the doctor to identify the main problem and to achieve rapport quickly at the initial interview; then the individual's difficulties can be clearly defined. Examples are given on page 358 of the questions asked when the problem is concerned with erection or ejaculation and an illustrative case of impotence is described on page 185.

Female sexual problems

The menstrual history should include a note of the age of the menarche or the menopause and details of the menstrual cycle. These are the frequency, regularity and duration of menses and whether blood loss is small, normal or excessive. The presence of clots suggests heavy menstrual losses. Menstrual blood loss can also be assessed by the number of pads or tampons required. The date of the last menstrual period should be noted. Secondary amenorrhoea is common and often psychological, but the possibility of an organic cause such as hyperprolactinaemia, androgen excess or post-partum hypopituitarism should be considered. Primary amenorrhoea demands a gynaecological or endocrinological explanation. The occurrence and the nature of any vaginal discharge must be assessed while a complaint of intermenstrual, postcoital or post-menopausal bleeding requires a gynaecological examination.

Dyspareunia (pain related to sexual intercourse) or failure to achieve an orgasm often occurs and is frequently due to, or may lead to, psychological difficulties. The longer these symptoms persist, the more difficult they are to eradicate. These topics may be avoided by the patient (or the doctor) because of embarrassment but if there is any indication of a difficulty, the patient should be encouraged to speak about it. Opportunity can be provided, once rapport has been established, by asking if sexual intercourse is satisfactory. Thereafter, any problem must be discussed frankly as indicated on page 8. Questionnaires can also be helpful as, for example in cases of infertility; they can be answered at leisure and in privacy, in conjunction with the partner.

THE PHYSICAL EXAMINATION

MOUTH AND THROAT

The examination of the mouth and throat is described on page 62. It is important to know whether the teeth provide an adequate chewing surface or, if the patient is edentulous, whether dentures are used for eating.

OESOPHAGUS

When there is a complaint of dysphagia it can be helpful to watch the act of swallowing solids and liquids. The reproduction of the symptom may confirm the organic nature and the site of the lesion. If swallowing is immediately followed by a distressing bout of coughing, this suggests either a neuromuscular disturbance as in bulbar or pseudobulbar palsy, or rarely a fistula between the trachea and the oesophagus.

ABDOMEN

The contents of the abdomen are illustrated in Figures 7.2, 7.3 and 7.5.

For purposes of description it has been customary to divide the abdomen into nine regions by the intersection of imaginary planes, two horizontal and two sagittal. The upper horizontal plane (transpyloric) lies at a level midway between the suprasternal notch and the symphysis pubis. The lower plane passes through the upper borders of the iliac crests. The sagittal planes are indicated on the surface by lines drawn vertically through points midway between the pubis and the anterior superior iliac spines (Fig 7.7). The resultant

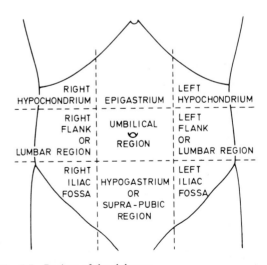

Fig. 7.7 Regions of the abdomen.

regions are artificial and though useful guides are less satisfactory in localising border lesions. An alternative description is to refer to the right and left upper and lower quadrants of the abdomen.

Whenever possible patients should be examined in a good light and in warm surroundings. The patient should lie comfortably supine with the head resting on one or two pillows in order to relax the muscles of the abdominal wall. Extra pillows may be necessary to prop up a patient with a kyphosis, or with severe breathlessness but the examination should be repeated in the optimum position once the dyspnoea has settled. Clothes must be removed so that there is complete exposure from the xiphisternum to the pubis. The chest and the legs should be suitably covered. For the examination of patients in bed, the bedclothing except for the sheet should be pulled down. The sheet can then be folded back to the pubis and the night clothes drawn up to the chest. The examination then follows the routine sequence of inspection, palpation, percussion and auscultation.

Inspection

Skin lesions. Any abnormality of the skin should be noted and the reasons for scars ascertained if these have not already been divulged. In elderly patients seborrhoeic warts, ranging from pink to brown or black, and haemangiomas (Campbell de Morgan spots) are so common that they could be considered as normal changes. The presence of striae requires explanation (p. 74).

Hair. Secondary sexual hair appears at puberty; its absence after this time should lead to a search for signs of hypopituitarism, or hypogonadism (p. 57). Virilism in the female leads to a male distribution of pubic hair, whereas cirrhosis in the male may produce a female distribution.

Veins. Collateral veins may be visible if the inferior vena cava is obstructed or if there is portal hypertension. These are usually tortuous dilatations of the superficial epigastric veins in which the blood flows upwards instead of down towards the groins. Rarely in the presence of hepatic cirrhosis, dilated collateral veins may also radiate from the umbilicus (caput Medusae) as a result of blood flowing from the portal vein through collateral vessels along the falciform ligament.

Movements and contour. In males particularly, quiet respiration is predominantly diaphragmatic, so that the abdominal wall moves out during inspiration. Respiratory movements of the abdomen usually cease in the presence of acute peritonitis.

Pulsation in the epigastrium is usually transmitted from the abdominal aorta (p. 99). Less frequently it is caused by the right ventricle, the liver or an abdominal aneurysm. It may sometimes be difficult to distinguish between pulsation of the aorta transmitted through an abdominal mass from an aneurysm. Expansile pulsation favours the latter. The distinction can be made by ultrasonography (Fig. 7.18).

The shape and symmetry of the abdomen should be observed. A sunken abdomen may be due to starvation or wasting diseases. Protuberance may be due to obesity, gaseous distension, ascites, pregnancy or other swellings. In obesity the umbilicus is usually sunken, whereas in these other conditions it is flat or even projecting. Visible enlargement of the bladder, uterus or ovary shows a characteristic shape as these structures rise out of the pelvis, the swelling being predominantly central in contrast to the bulging of the flanks in ascites. Visible bulges may also be due to gross enlargement of the liver, spleen or kidneys, or to large tumours.

Distension of the stomach due to pyloric obstruction causes bulging of the upper part of the abdomen; tangential inspection is the best means of seeing the slow waves of gastric peristalsis passing from the rib margin on the left, across the midline, and subsiding beneath the right upper rectus. Activity may be stimulated by a gassy drink or by flicking the skin over the area. Confirmation may be obtained by placing the examiner's hands over the lower ribs, and giving the patient a quick shake from side to side, when a sound like that due to shaking a hot-water bottle which contains water and air is heard and is known as a *succussion splash*. Similar sounds can be produced from a normal stomach for an hour or two after food or drink.

Small intestinal peristalsis may be seen through a thin abdominal wall, or if there is divarication of the recti abdominis or an incisional hernia. It may become unduly prominent in the presence of in-

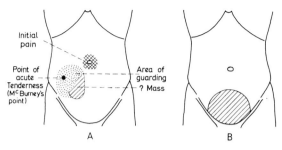

Fig. 7.8 The use of diagrams in case recording. (A) Pain, tenderness, guarding and mass in patient with acute appendicitis and appendix abscess. (B) Tumour arising from the pelvis. This could be a bladder, uterine or ovarian swelling. Note also that McBurney's point is situated one-third of the distance along a line from the anterior superior iliac spine to the umbilicus.

testinal obstruction. It is recognised as writhing movements in the centre of the abdomen.

Hernias are frequent causes of local swellings. An *umbilical hernia* bulges through the navel. It is very common in babies and usually disappears spontaneously. Divarication of the recti is also common in the multiparous and becomes evident immediately the supine patient attempts to sit; the intra-abdominal pressure rises and the region of the linea alba bulges between the recti abdominis.

An *epigastric hernia* is visible as a small swelling usually not more than 1 cm in diameter. It is due to a piece of extraperitoneal fat bulging through a defect in the linea alba. By gentle massage with the finger-tip it is often possible to reduce such a hernia and then the small defect can be felt.

Incisional hernias may form at the site of any operation on the abdomen, especially if the wound has been complicated by sepsis.

Femoral and *inguinal hernias* and their examination are described on page 174.

Palpation

If the patient is in a low bed, it may be necessary to sit on, or kneel beside the bed. The examiner's hands must be warm. An assessment of obesity can be made by grasping a double thickness of skin and subcutaneous tissue between the fingers and thumb. The elasticity of the skin provides a rough index of the degree of hydration and redundant skin folds are evidence of weight loss. The patient

should be asked to place the arms alongside the body, as this helps to relax the abdomen, and to report any tenderness elicited during the examination. In addition, the patient's face should be observed for any grimace indicative of local discomfort. Palpation can be conveniently divided into three phases; light, deep and palpation during respiration.

Light palpation. The examiner's hand should remain in continuous contact with the patient's abdomen. Muscle tone should be tested by light dipping movements over symmetrical areas commencing at a point remote from the site of any pain. Generalised tenderness of abdominal muscles is commonly due to an anxious patient's inability to relax. This can be suspected by the circumstances and confirmed by variability in resistance during the early phase of expiration. The tendency may be reduced by ensuring the patient is warm and comfortable, that the examiner's hand is not cold and by gaining the patient's confidence with a gentle approach. Resistance due to increased muscle tone accompanies organic lesions, particularly when pain is present. It may be restricted to one side or region, according to the organ affected and the extent of peritoneal involvement, for example, at McBurney's point in acute appendicitis. Deep-seated inflammation, not causing localised guarding, may be revealed by rebound tenderness elicited by the sudden release of pressure by the examining hand. Generalised 'board-like' rigidity implies peritonitis; the abdomen does move on respiration and bowel sounds cease. Attempts to elicit other signs such as rebound tenderness are unnecessary. It should however be remembered that pelvic peritonitis may be advanced before the signs are apparent on abdominal examination and may be revealed only by rectal examination.

Deep palpation. The abdomen should now be palpated more deeply with the flat of the hand. The predominant use of finger tips is apt to induce muscular resistance. Each region should be palpated deeply, starting remote from any area of tenderness. In the normal patient, it may be possible to feel the descending colon in the right iliac fossa; the caecum and sometimes the transverse colon may also be palpable, especially if they contain faeces. The aorta, the liver edge and the lower

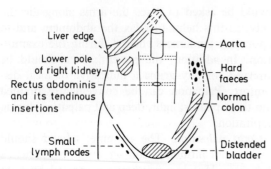

Fig. 7.9 Palpation of the abdomen. Diagrammatic representation of some findings which may be normal and are often misinterpreted.

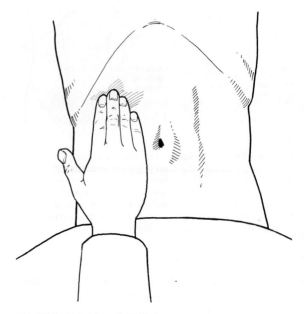

Fig. 7.10 Palpation of the liver.

pole of the right kidney are often palpable (see Fig 7.9). Faeces are commonly palpable in the sigmoid colon but in severe constipation can be felt in any part of the lower bowel. Indentation of a lump by finger pressure is evidence that it is faecal. Sometimes however, a hard, craggy lump of faeces can only be distinguished from malignancy by re-examination after a bowel action. Enlargement of the bladder, ovary or uterus often suspected from inspection, may be confirmed as a dome-shaped swelling rising above the pubis. An upper abdominal mass which does not move on respiration, either arises from or has become attached to the abdominal wall. Masses which are superficially situated within the abdominal wall, continue to be palpable when the muscles are contracted, for example, raising the head off the pillow. Tightening muscles in this way identifies the intersections of the recti abdominis (Fig 7.9). An intersection may mislead the beginner into believing that a tumour or the liver edge has been felt. Masses situated more deeply within the abdominal cavity, are less easily palpable when the muscles are contracted. Characteristics of any mass should be assessed (p. 36) and illustrated diagrammatically (see Fig 7.9).

Palpation during inspiration. The liver, spleen and kidneys should now be examined in turn during deep inspiration. The secret of success is to keep the examining hand or hands, still and wait for the diaphragm to push the organ down onto the hands.

Palpation of the liver. The hand should be placed flat with the fingers pointing upwards and positioned so that the sensing fingers (index and middle) are lateral to the rectus muscle (Fig. 7.10). The hand should be firmly pressed inwards and upwards and it should be kept steady while the patient takes a deep breath through the mouth. At the height of inspiration the inward pressure on the front hand is released while the upward pressure is maintained. With this movement the tips of the fingers should slip over the edge of a palpable liver. It should be noted whether the edge is sharp as is normal, or whether it is rounded, firm, irregular or tender. The surface and edge of a palpable liver should then be traced across the abdomen and examined for irregularities using the fingertips and keeping them steady in a new position each time the patient takes a deep breath. Irregularities may be felt as the liver slides under the fingertips with each respiration. Two common errors should be avoided. One is to feel for the liver with the hand placed horizontally. In this position the palm of the hand may press backwards the edge which it is desired to feel. The second error is to start feeling too high up.

In the presence of ascites, enlargement of the liver may be detected by the dipping technique (p. 173).

As the liver descends 1–3 cm on inspiration, it can normally be palpated in adults below the right

Table 7.4 Common causes for hepatic enlargement

Condition	Features
Infectious mononucleosis	Tender, sharp edge. Associated splenomegaly
Viral hepatitis (type A)	Tender, sharp edge. No spleen palpable
Acute cardiac failure	Tender, sharp edge. Raised JVP
Chronic cardiac failure	Less tender. Edge is firm and sharp
Hepatic cirrhosis	Rounded edge, sometimes irregular; very hard. Signs of hepatocellular damage (spleen may become palpable)
Carcinomatsis	Hard, sometimes irregular. Edge may be rounded or nodular. Sometimes tender

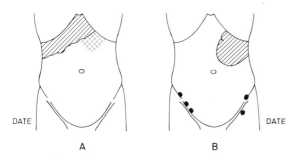

Fig. 7.11 The use of diagrams in case recording. (A) Abdominal mass and enlarged liver in patient with gastric carcinoma and hepatic metastases. (B) Splenomegaly and lymphadenopathy in a patient with Hodgkin's lymphoma.

costal margin during deep inspiration. Common causes of enlargement of the liver in the adult in Britain are shown in Table 7.4.

Palpation of the gall bladder. Gallstones occur very commonly with advancing years, especially in women. These are not palpable. Stones, however, may be associated with attacks of acute cholecystitis, with tenderness below the right costal margin midway between the xiphisternum and the flank. If the examiner's fingers are placed over this point and the patient is asked to take a deep breath, inspiration may be sharply arrested due to a sudden accentuation of pain (*Murphy's sign*).

A palpable gall bladder implies its enlargement. In the absence of jaundice this is due to obstruction of the cystic duct leading to mucocele or empyema. Obstruction of the common bile duct

produces jaundice; if the gall bladder is also enlarged, the obstruction will usually be due to causes other than gallstones since in most cases of cholelithiasis the wall of the gall bladder is so thickened that it cannot stretch (*Courvoisier's law*). Carcinoma of the head of the pancreas is the most common cause of palpable enlargement of the gall bladder in the presence of obstructive jaundice.

Palpation of the spleen. The normal spleen lies against the postero-lateral wall of the abdominal cavity, beneath the ninth, tenth and eleventh ribs with its anterior border reaching the mid-axillary line. As it enlarges, it expands forwards, downwards and eventually medially, the tip emerging somewhere beneath the left costal margin. One hand supports the tissues in the left lower costal area and the other is placed flat with the fingers at right angles to the left costal margin, pressing inwards and upwards (Fig. 7.12A). A very large spleen can be easily detected as a quick movement forwards with the back hand will bump the spleen against the other hand. The spleen is examined during inspiration when it will bump against the tips of the index and middle fingers. At the height of inspiration, the pressure on the anterior hand is released so that the finger tips slip over the pole of the spleen confirming its presence and feeling its surface and consistency. An enlarged spleen retains its shape. Therefore, if a lump is felt below the left costal margin which is not smooth and rounded, it should be regarded as something other than spleen. If the spleen is not palpable, the anterior hand is moved upwards after each inspiration until the finger tips are under the costal margin. This should be repeated along the entire rib margin as the position of the enlarging splenic tip is variable. Sometimes it is easier to feel the tip of the spleen with the patient lying on the right side and with the left hip and knee flexed at a right angle. Alternatively, a spleen which is just palpable may be more easily felt by standing to the left of the patient's chest, placing the left hand on the lower chest and 'hooking' the examining fingers round the costal margin while the patient breathes in deeply (see Fig 7.12B).

Even when the spleen is large enough to be felt in the groin, it should not be mistaken for a large kidney. The examining fingers can usually be pushed deep to the lower pole and anterior edge

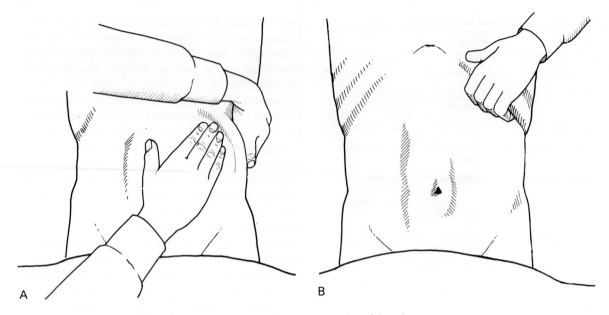

Fig. 7.12 (A) Palpation of the spleen. (B) Alternative method for palpation of the spleen.

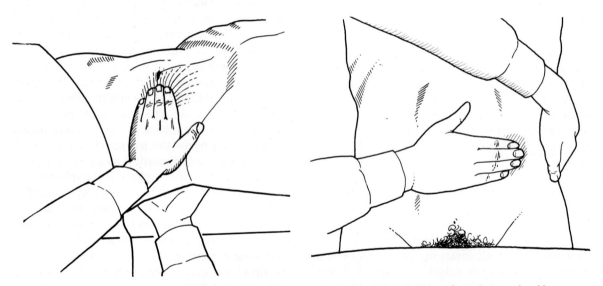

Fig. 7.13 (A) Palpation of the left kidney from the same side. (B) Palpation of the left kidney from the opposite side.

of the spleen and one or two notches may be felt on the edge (Fig. 7.11). It will not be possible to insert the fingers between the spleen and the costal margin. In addition, a very large spleen tends to point towards the right iliac fossa and may cross the mid-line. In contrast, an enlarged kidney rarely crosses the mid-line; it fills the loin diffusely, and unless a lump projects from it, the fingers

cannot be inserted deep to the mass at any point, but can usually be inserted between the kidney and the costal margin. In addition, the kidney is much more readily appreciated bimanually than the spleen.

A palpable spleen is always pathological. Common causes of splenomegaly are various infections including glandular fever and malaria, hepatic cirrhosis, the leukaemias and the myeloproliferative disorders.

Palpation of the kidneys. A bimanual technique should be employed. (Fig. 7.13). The two hands are firmly but gently pushed together as the patient breathes out. During deep inspiration, the lower pole of the descending kidney may now be felt to bump into the hands. Sometimes if the pressure is postponed until the end of inspiration, it may be possible to trap the kidney between the two hands. Then when the pressure is reduced on expiration, the kidney can be felt to slide back above the hands thereby providing an excellent idea of its size and consistency. Although the left kidney can be examined from the opposite side (Fig. 7.13A), it is most readily palpated from the same side (Fig. 7.13B).

A normal kidney has a very firm consistency and the surface is smooth. The lower half of the normal right kidney is often palpable, especially in slim women. The normal left kidney is less often palpable. Owing to the varying thickness of the parietes, enlargement of a kidney, unless it is gross, is difficult to judge without a good deal of practice. Irregularity of the surface or an abnormally hard consistency may be appreciated quite easily. When the liver is readily palpable, it may be difficult to decide whether the right kidney can also be felt. Tenderness of the kidney is usually greatest posteriorly and is readily elicited by tapping the renal angle with the patient sitting forward.

Percussion of the abdomen

The basic technique has been described (p. 143). Three additional principles can be applied to abdominal percussion:

1. Percuss from resonant to dull
2. Place the finger used for percussion on the abdomen parallel to the direction of the anticipated note change
3. Percuss softly for superficial structure, such as the lower border of the liver and more firmly for deeper structures.

The main value of abdominal percussion is to find out whether distension is due to gas, ascites, a fluid filled cyst or solid tumour. Gaseous disten-

sion is resonant. Large ovarian cysts and other solid pelvic masses extending into the abdomen cause dullness in the centre of the abdomen and resonance due to any gas in the gut is arranged around it.

Ascites. A moderate accumulation of ascites should be suspected from inspection and palpation but is confirmed on percussion. In the presence of ascites, the gas containing gut floats uppermost. The liquid gravitates to the dependent part of the peritoneal cavity. The presence of *shifting dullness* provides confirmation of ascites. It is usually simplest to detect it by examining the patient supine and by percussing from the centre of the abdomen into the left flank until a dull note is obtained. The finger is kept in place while the patient rolls on to the right side. After pausing for a few seconds, the presence of ascites is suggested if the note has become resonant and established by obtaining a dull note while percussing back towards the umbilicus. The presence of small quantities of free fluid in the peritoneal cavity cannot be determined with certainty, for slight changes in percussion note may be due to gravitational shift of normal bowel.

An additional useful sign in ascites is *dipping* over the upper abdomen to determine if the liver or spleen is enlarged. The examiner's hand is laid over the abdomen, and quick dipping movements are made. The sudden displacement of liquid gives a tapping sensation over the surface of the liver or spleen comparable to the patellar tap (p. 285). By this manoeuvre it may also be possible to detect and to map the outlines of enlarged organs or of tumours which cannot be felt in the ordinary way because the abdomen is so distended.

Percussion of the spleen. Percussion is a poor method of seeking for enlargement of the spleen, but may be helpful if it is doubtful whether the tip can be felt. The patient should be asked to take in a deep breath and hold it while the area below and then just above the costal margin is percussed. The position of the underlying spleen may be detected by impairment of the percussion note.

Percussion of the liver. Heavy percussion from above and a light percussion from below in the mid-clavicular line can give only a rough estimate of the size of the liver, particularly in regard to the upper border. Although this may be raised above the level of the fifth rib by a greatly enlarged liver, the percussion note is largely dependent upon the state of the lung and pleura.

The apparent level of the lower border of the liver varies with the amount of gas in the colon and a palpable lower border may be 3 or 4 cm below the edge detected by percussion. However, a positive finding on percussion implies that the borders of the liver extend at least as far as the level of impairment. Absence of liver dullness may be detected when gas has leaked from a perforated peptic ulcer.

Auscultation of the abdomen

Activity of the gut creates characteristic gurgling sounds which may be heard from time to time by the unaided ear. Through the stethoscope they can be heard every 5–10 seconds, though the interval varies greatly in relationship to meals. Bowel sounds disappear in paralytic ileus. They increase in frequency and intensity in association with malabsorptive disorders of the small intestine, and when there is much blood in the bowel from upper alimentary haemorrhage; the noise may be so loud in the rare carcinoid syndrome as to cause social embarrassment. When mechanical obstruction is present, not only are sounds increased in frequency and intensity, but gaseous distension of the gut adds a tinkling quality to the sounds.

Most arterial bruits in the abdomen arise from the aorta. Systolic murmurs due to stenoses of mesenteric or renal arteries may be audible but owing to the distracting effects of the bowel sounds, a conscious effort must be made to listen for them. An arterial bruit may be heard over a hepatoma. A venous hum is occasionally audible between the xiphisternum and the umbilicus due to turbulence in a well-developed collateral circulation from portal hypertension. Friction sounds resembling those of pleurisy may be present over an area of perisplenitis or perihepatitis.

Examination of the groins

Groins should be examined for hernias, femoral pulses (p. 89) and for lymph nodes (p. 67) which in health vary considerably in size and consistency.

The examination of hernias. Hernias occur at the site of operation scars and at points of anatomical weakness. All hernias bulge more when the pressure within them is raised. Hernias of the abdominal wall are therefore more prominent in the erect position, and an impulse can be felt in the hernia when the patient coughs. Both of these features also apply to a saphenous varix. After the identification of a hernia, an attempt should be made to replace the contents by the application of a gentle sustained pressure. A hernia may be irreducible but a strangulated hernia is tense and tender and shows no impulse on coughing.

A *femoral hernia* lies in the femoral canal below the inguinal ligament and is therefore below and lateral to the pubic tubercle.

An *inguinal hernia* emerges from the abdominal wall through the external inguinal ring and is therefore above and medial to the pubic tubercle.

It is customary to attempt to differentiate direct from indirect (oblique) inguinal hernias. An indirect inguinal hernia occurs into a persistent remnant of the processus vaginalis. It occurs in young men and may extend to the testes. Following reduction, control will be obtained by pressure over the internal inguinal ring, just above the midpoint of the inguinal ligament.

Direct inguinal hernia occurs directly through the weakened posterior wall of the inguinal canal medial to the inferior epigastric artery and lateral to the rectus muscle. It is more common in older men and does not reach the testes. It will not be controlled by pressure over the internal inguinal ring.

Examination of the male genitalia

The stages of physical sexual development in relation to age are given on page 355. In the male, examination of the genitalia conveniently follows palpation of the groins. Enlargement of the groin lymph nodes should raise the possibility of sexually transmitted disease. The penis and scrotum are inspected and the testes, epididymes and vasa deferentia palpated. The left testis usually lies in a lower position in the scrotum than the right. Minor degrees of hypospadias occur once in every 300 boys. Both testes are atrophic in hypogonadism and one may atrophy after orchitis

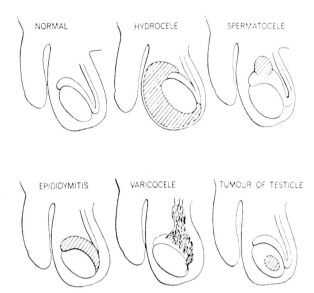

Fig. 7.14 Swellings of the scrotum.

due to mumps. An empty scrotum on one or both sides should lead to a search for incompletely descended testes in the inguinal canal or for ectopic testes in sites such as the groin.

Examination of a scrotal swelling should follow the principles laid down on page 36. It is necessary to confirm that any swelling originates in the scrotum and is not an inguinal hernia. By careful palpation of both testes, the exact site of most swellings can be determined. Swellings within the scrotum commonly contain a clear liquid, a finding which can be confirmed by transillumination (p. 39). A hydrocele, a spermatocele and a cyst of the epididymis are differentiated by their relationships to the testis (Figure 7.14). The possibility that a hydrocele may obscure a testicular tumour must not be overlooked and in each case the testis must be palpated with care. Infections other than syphilis and mumps affect primarily the epididymis and tuberculosis produces a characteristic nodular change within the epididymis accompanied by thickening of the cord. Shortening of the cord is a characteristic of torsion of the testis.

Examination of the genital organs in the female is described on page 177. It is not a routine procedure.

Examination of the rectum

Digital examination of the rectum should be part of any general medical examination and the student must become familiar with the feel of the normal structures. Because this simple procedure is disagreeable to the patient, and a little extra trouble for the doctor, it is often inappropriately omitted. It is recommended that a third person should always be present. Rectal examination should never be omitted in the following circumstances:

1. *Alimentary problems*
   Suspected appendicitis, pelvic abscess, peritonitis.
   Lower abdominal pain.
   Diarrhoea or constipation; mucus or blood in the stools.
   Anal irritation or pain; tenesmus or rectal pain.
   Bimanual examination of a lower abdominal mass.
   In the search for tumours of transperitoneal metastases either diagnostically or in making a decision about treatment.
2. *Genitourinary problems*
   Dysuria; haematuria; haematospermia; epididymo-orchitis. In lieu of gynaecological examination in virgins.
3. *Miscellaneous problems*
   In the search for a cause of backache, root pains in the legs, unexplained bone pain or iron deficiency anaemia.
   In all cases of pyrexia of unknown origin or unexplained weight loss.

Digital examination. The patient should be informed that it is necessary to examine the back passage. If the examiner is right-handed, the patient should lie in the left lateral position with a maximal degree of flexion of the spine and legs consistent with comfort. The buttocks should be at the edge of the couch or bed. The patient should be encouraged to relax and be reassured that the examination should not be painful. The clinician's right forefinger, protected by a suitable glove, should be smeared with a lubricant. In a good light the perianal skin should be examined for intertrigo or for evidence of scratching, throm-

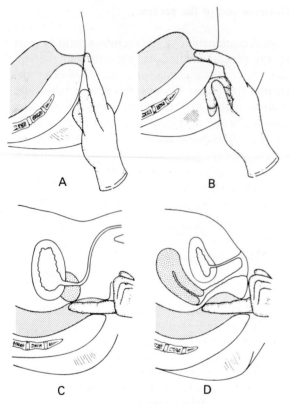

A   B

C   D

Fig. 7.15 Examination of the rectum. The finger is inserted as shown in (A) and (B). The hand is then rotated and the most prominent features are the prostate in the male (C) and the cervix in the female (D).

bosed external piles, fissure or fistulae as in inflammatory bowel disease. The possibility of sexually transmitted disease must also be borne in mind.

The forefinger tip is placed on the anterior anal margin and with steady pressure on the sphincter is moved backwards. The finger then slides gently through the anal canal into the rectum (Fig. 7.15). Resistance at the anus is commonly due to spasm induced by anxiety, and this can sometimes be overcome by asking the patient to strain down in an attempt to defaecate. If spasm is associated with local pain, an anal fissure is the common cause but more sinister lesions must be excluded; a local anaesthetic suppository may be required before a satisfactory examination can be made. The upper end of the anal canal is marked by the pubo-rectalis muscle which should be easily palpable and which will be felt to contract reflexly on

coughing or on conscious contraction by the patient. Any weakness of the sphincter should be noted as a possible indication of sexual activity.

Beyond the anal canal, the direction of the rectum is upwards and backwards along the curve of the coccyx and the sacrum. The exploring finger should then feel round the whole extent of the rectum. The normal rectum should be empty and the wall should be smooth and soft. In cases of habitual constipation the rectum is full of firm faeces. An obstructing carcinoma of the upper rectum will produce a ballooning of the empty cavity below. Posteriorly the coccyx and sacrum can be felt through the rectal wall, while anteriorly from below upwards, the membranous urethra, the prostate and often the base of the bladder may be felt in the male, while the firm round cervix uteri can be felt projecting backwards in the female (Fig. 7.15). The normal prostate is smooth and has a fairly firm consistency with the lateral lobes and a median groove between them. Prostatic hyperplasia in the adult, which is a common cause of urinary obstruction, often produces a palpable enlargement but may not do so if the hyperplasia is confined to the median lobe. The prostate is abnormally small in hypogonadism. Tenderness, accompanied by other local and systemic symptoms and by a change in the consistency of the gland, may be due to prostatitis or an abscess. A hard, irregular gland, which may be fixed to the mucosa or the surrounding structures, and usually without a detectable median groove, is characteristic of carcinoma. Piles which are not thrombosed and normal seminal vesicles cannot be felt.

Any deviation from normal should be noted, and lumps in particular should be examined systematically (see p. 36) Bimanual palpation is sometimes helpful with the other hand laid flat over the abdomen. A faecal mass is commonly palpable and this should be movable and may be indented. If several masses are present, the examination should be repeated after the patient has defaecated. Metastases or a tumour in a loop of colon lying in the lower part of the peritoneal cavity may otherwise be mistaken for faeces. In lesions palpable within the rectum the percentage of the rectal circumference involved and the distance of the upper and lower edges from the anal margin should be recorded. After withdrawal, the finger should be examined for blood, the colour of the faeces noted and a sample tested chemically for occult blood (p. 178).

Protoscopy. Visual examination of the rectum and anal canal complements the digital method. Proctoscopy should always be preceded by digital examination. Through the proctoscope it is possible to inspect haemorrhoids and other lesions, to remove polypi and to take specimens for biopsy. With the patient in the left lateral position the forefinger and thumb of one hand separate the buttocks, while with the other, a warmed and well-lubricated proctoscope is gently inserted in the same directions as described for digital examination. The surface of the normal rectum is similar to the appearance of the buccal mucosa – clean, shiny, smooth, reddish pink with clearly visible submucosal veins. For the detection of piles the patient should be asked to strain down as the proctoscope is gradually withdrawn. Under these conditions the piles will be distended with blood and their extent can be fully appreciated.

Gynaecological examination

The contents of the female pelvis are illustrated in Figure 7.16.

The intimate nature of a gynaecological examination makes it difficult to combine with routine abdominal examination and may raise medico-legal problems. The patient's consent must be obtained, and a third person should be present during the examination.

For the comfort of the patient and for ease of interpretation of the examination, the bowel and bladder should be empty. The patient should lie comfortably on her back with her head on a pillow to relax the abdominal muscles. The trunk is covered with a sheet. The hips and knees should be flexed, the thighs abducted, and illumination arranged so that a good light falls upon the vulva. The examiner should wear gloves. The labia minora are separated by the forefinger and thumb of the left hand, bringing into view the clitoris anteriorly, then the urethra, the vagina and finally the anus posteriorly. Any discharge from the urethra or vagina should be swabbed; one specimen should be sent for culture and another smeared on to a glass slide for microscopical examination. Direct miscroscopy of a smear is particularly useful in the confirmation of infection due to *Trichomonas vaginalis*; a smear, promptly stained, may also give conclusive evidence of gonorrhoea or thrush.

The lateral walls of the vulva on either side of the lower third of the vagina should be palpated

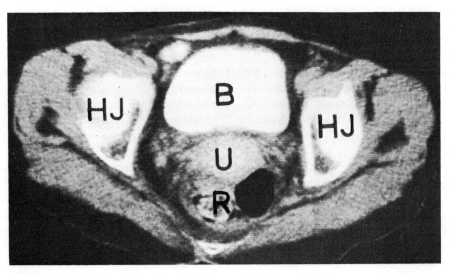

Fig. 7.16 Contents of pelvis as shown by CT scan. B: Bladder outlined by contrast medium. HJ: Hip joint. R: Rectum. U: Uterus. (Courtesy of Professor Ian Isherwood.)

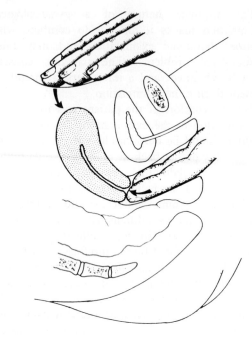

Fig. 7.17   Vaginal examination.

with the right hand for abnormalities of Bartholin's glands. In parous women two fingers should then be turned palmar surface down and spread, to test for laxity of the superficial muscles, and to allow inspection of the vaginal walls for prolapse when the patient is asked to strain down. The index finger of the right hand smeared with a lubricant and in most cases the middle finger too should then be inserted into the vagina (Fig. 7.17). The cervix uteri is readily felt, being circular, with a small central os in the nulliparous patient. The normal cervix points downwards and slightly backwards. In parous women, the cervix is usually larger and the os a good deal bigger and often palpable as a transverse slit.

Bimanual palpation is now made. With the middle finger of the right hand at the os and the forefinger in the anterior fornix, the left hand is placed flat on the abdomen and worked down towards the pubis. The position and other characteristics of the uterus can then be identified between the hands. Each fornix should now be palpated in turn with particular regard to tenderness and swellings of the Fallopian tubes and

ovaries. The bladder lies immediately anteriorly. In the posterior fornix, abnormalities may be appreciated in the pouch of Douglas.

Digital examination should be supplemented by inspection of the vagina and uterine cervix through a vaginal speculum. Using a spatula a smear is taken from the cervix for cytological examination. This important screening procedure should be performed at regular intervals for the early detection of cancer of the cervix.

Vaginal examination of virgins should if possible be avoided, and minors should not be examined without the consent of a parent or guardian. In these circumstances adequate information can often be obtained by digital examination of the rectum.

FURTHER INVESTIGATION

In many cases it will be possible to make a satisfactory diagnosis by clinical examination. Further investigation will then be required only for confirmation. When the diagnosis is uncertain, the clinician must decide which investigations should be performed and in which order because an indiscriminate series of tests is a burden on the patient, costly and time consuming.

ALIMENTARY TRACT

Examination of the faeces

Inspection of the consistency and colour of the faeces is often of diagnostic value (p. 161). Supplementary investigations include stool culture, microscopic examination especially for parasites, their cysts and for ova, and testing for occult blood.

Occult blood in the faeces. The chemical detection of occult blood in the stools is an important investigation of gastrointestinal and haematological problems. It may be an early manifestation of carcinoma of the colon or the rectum. Since bleeding may be intermittent, samples should be tested from three stools over several days. If one is positive, further investigation is indicated. When difficulty is encountered in obtaining specimens, sufficient material for testing can usually be obtained on the gloved finger at rectal examination. In patients with haemorrhoids it may be necessary to obtain the stool samples through a proctoscope above the pile-bearing area if bleeding from the upper gastrointestinal tract is suspected. The test employed should not be too sensitive because there is a 'normal' daily faecal blood loss of about 2.5 ml.

The *Hemocult test* is recommended. In this commercial preparation guaiac is oxidised to a blue colour by the peroxidase-like activity of haemoglobin. Neither barium nor medicinal iron interferes with the test.

Gastrointestinal radiology

A good quality radiograph will show the outline of the kidneys, the liver and, sometimes, the spleen. Radio-opaque stones may be present in the renal or more rarely in the biliary tract. Calcification may often be seen in lymph nodes, in phleboliths and, in older patients, in the aorta and its major branches. It may also occur within the kidneys, adrenal glands, pancreas or uterine fibroids. Faeces are seen as a stippled pattern within the colon. Large amounts of faeces in the right side of colon are an indication of delayed intestinal transit and although this may be caused by disease in the distal large bowel, it is often due to constipation.

Plain radiographs of the whole abdomen can be taken in the erect and supine positions. The supine view is a useful film for examination of the abdomen giving a good impression of gas distribution within the gastrointestinal tract. The erect film is required to show fluid levels. It is only indicated in suspected obstruction as an adjunct to a supine film. A small air/fluid level is normal in the gastric fundus but fluid levels elsewhere may indicate an obstructive or paralytic ileus. The presence of gas beneath the diaphragm in acute perforation of a hollow viscus is best seen on the erect chest film. A chest radiograph may also show mediastinal widening and the absence of air in the gastric fundus due to achalasia of the cardia, or a fluid level seen through the heart shadow may be caused by a paraoesophageal hernia. A raised right diaphragm with pleural effusion may suggest the diagnosis of liver abscess.

Contrast radiography can outline the whole of the gastrointestinal tract (Fig. 7.2). In all cases, the radiologist must be given adequate details to understand the clinical problems so that the best examination can be undertaken for the particular patient. A barium swallow delineates the oesophagus. Hold-up of barium can be due to a failure of the lower oesophageal sphincter to relax in achalasia of the cardia or to oesophageal narrowing due to either a benign or malignant stricture. Other lesions that can be identified include mucosal ulceration and oesophageal varices which are best seen by a special technique. Barium meal involves examination of the stomach and the duodenum. It may reveal such lesions as peptic ulceration or gastric carcinoma. Water soluble contrast should be used if there is any possibility of perforation. Displacement of the stomach or widening of the duodenal loop may be seen in disease within the pancreas. The further progress of barium through the small bowel may be studied in the course of a 'follow through' examination. Better quality pictures are obtained when this investigation is performed as a separate examination. An abnormal small bowel pattern may be due to malabsorption or to an inflammatory lesion such as Crohn's disease.

The colon is examined by barium enema in which the contrast medium is run in through an anal catheter and which will outline tumours, polyps, diverticula and inflammatory disease of the colon. Preparation for a barium enema consists of complete evacuation of faeces by purgation and/or enemas. Sometimes this is inadvisable, for example in ulcerative colitis, and preparation may be restricted to diet and washout or avoided completely as when there is established lower bowel obstruction. Digital examination of the rectum, supplemented by proctoscopy, must always be done before a barium enema.

Occasionally, for example in extensive Crohn's disease, both barium meal and enema examinations are required. The enema should be performed first as the barium should be evacuated quite quickly and enable the meal to be performed without undue delay. Both examinations may be enhanced by the double contrast technique of introducing air as well as contrast medium.

Angiography is sometimes of value in diagnosing the source of obscure gastrointestinal bleeding as in angiodysplasia.

Endoscopic examination

The development of flexible fibreoptic instruments has made it possible to diagnose lesions of the oesophagus, stomach and duodenum by visual inspection supplemented where necessary with small but adequate biopsies. The rectum and lower sigmoid colon are visualised during rigid sigmoidoscopy. Particular attention must be paid to passing the sigmoidoscope around the rectosigmoid junction as this is where lesions are missed during a barium enema. The colon may also be examined by flexible fibreoptic endoscopy. During this procedure not only can biopsies be taken from any point in the colon but also polyps of quite large size can be removed by snaring them with a diathermy loop, thereby avoiding the need for laparotomy. Sigmoidoscopy may result in trauma to the mucosa and even perforation.

Choice of investigation: endoscopy or contrast radiology. Barium examination and upper alimentary endoscopy should be regarded as complementary. The initial choice will depend upon various factors, such as the degree of urgency, the age of the patient and the availability of facilities. In general, a radiograph is cheaper but sometimes, for example in acute upper gastrointestinal bleeding, an early endoscopy may give information that radiology cannot provide. Sometimes both may be required; for example when the diagnosis is elusive, in the investigation of dysphagia, and when pathological samples are required from a lesion detected by radiography.

Sigmoidoscopy usually precedes barium enema examination. The latter should be avoided for several days after sigmoidoscopy and for a week if a biopsy has been taken. A repeat sigmoidoscopy may be impossible until the barium has been completely evacuated and these factors must be considered when planning colonic investigations. Fibreoptic colonoscopy is time consuming and is undertaken only if there remains an indication for it after barium enema and rigid endoscopy examinations.

Ultrasonography

Ultrasound imaging provides a two-dimensional picture which is built up to give the impression of a 'cut' through the body. Transverse cuts are

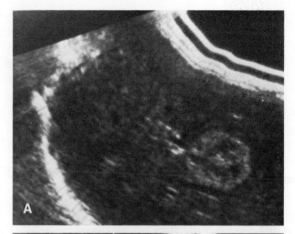
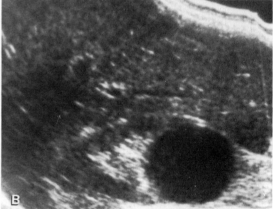
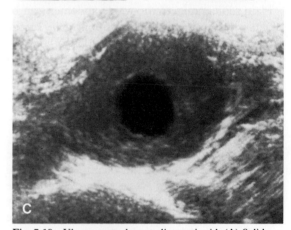

Fig. 7.18 Ultrasonography as a diagnostic aid. (A) Solid tumour in liver (longitudinal scan through right lobe of liver towards diaphragm which is seen as a curved white line). (B) Renal cyst (anterior longitudinal scan of right kidney through liver). (C) Aneurysm of aorta the lumen of which is reduced by mural thrombus. The vertebral body is seen as the curved white area towards the lower left (transverse scan). Note (1) A, B and C are at different magnification. (2) Best results are obtained if the abdomen is not obese, scarred or flatulent. (Courtesy of Dr S R Wild.)

usually viewed, like CT scans, as though looking up from a patient's feet. Examination is non-invasive and requires no special preparation. The investigation is useful in assessing abdominal and pelvic masses and in distinguishing between solid and cystic lesions (Fig. 7.18). Pelvic ultrasonography should be performed when the bladder is full. Aspiration of cysts may be performed under ultrasound guidance and biopsy of solid tumours directed by ultrasound control. The quality of the examination may be restricted by adiposity, intestinal gas and abdominal scars.

Computed tomography (CT Scan)

This provides an alternative non-invasive method of investigation. It is particularly of value in assessing the presence or absence of deep-seated intra-abdominal malignancy; for example, carcinoma of the pancreas, metastatic seminoma of the testis and when ultrasound imaging has been unhelpful.

Tests of gastrointestinal function

The pentagastrin secretion test may be of value in the assessment of the patient with peptic ulceration and the insulin secretion test is used to determine the effectiveness of surgical vagotomy. Several tests are usually employed to investigate intestinal absorption. Blood may be tested for a rise in the concentration of a substance, such as glucose or iron given by mouth. Urine may be collected for the estimation of substances which, after absorption are largely excreted by the kidneys, e.g. xylose. Folic acid assays and vitamin B_{12} absorption tests may help to differentiate between disease of the jejunum and ileum as hydroxocobalamin is absorbed solely in the ileum. Examination of stools may reveal evidence of failure to absorb food, especially fat. The hydrogen ion breath test provides a method of assessing small bowel bacterial colonisation.

Tests of motility

Intra-oesophageal pressure and motility studies occasionally supply diagnostic information in difficult problems such as the differentiation of atypical chest pain of oesophageal origin from myocardial ischaemia. It is also a straighforward procedure to insert catheters into the anus and rectum to measure pressures but the clinical application is confined to those few patients with sphincter problems in which some form of surgery is contemplated.

THE LIVER AND BILIARY TRACT

General assessment

The commonest problem is to distinguish between hepatocellular and obstructive jaundice. This is established partly by chemical investigations based on the excretory and synthetic functions of the liver and on enzymes released by cell damage. None of these tests is specific so several are done in conjunction and the results must be interpreted in the light of the clinical features. Other tests and investigative procedures are indicated for specific reasons.

Hepatitis B surface antigen

In any case of possible viral hepatitis, this antigen should be looked for as soon as possible, and preferably before performing any other blood tests. A positive result is not only of diagnostic value but should also alert those dealing with the patient or handling the blood in the laboratory to the danger of infection and may raise the possibility of coexistent infection with AIDS virus.

Biochemical tests

Bilirubin. Clinical jaundice is not evident until the serum level has risen to about 50 μmol/l (normal range 5–17 μmol/l). A rise in conjugated bilirubin occurs in obstructive jaundice or hepatitis. Unconjugated hyperbilirubinaemia indicates haemolysis or an abnormality of bilirubin transport or metabolism such as Gilbert's disease. Some increase in unconjugated bilirubin in the plasma also occurs in the early and recovery stages of acute hepatitis in which the jaundice is largely due to conjugated bilirubin.

Alkaline phosphatase. This is increased much more in obstructive than in hepatocellular jaundice.

As the enzyme occurs in most tissues an isolated rise is usually not due to liver disease; electrophoretic separation of the isoenzymes can distinguish that derived from bone which is the other common source.

Plasma proteins. Albumin is synthetised in the liver. In chronic liver disease its concentration is frequently below normal and electrophoresis may show a concomitant rise in the gammaglobulin peak.

Prothrombin time. The concentration of coagulation factors II, VII and X of liver origin falls in a matter of days in severe hepatitis, and the one stage prothrombin time gives a good guide to prognosis. In obstructive jaundice there is malabsorption of vitamin K which results in prolongation of the prothrombin time.

Serum transferases. The principal value in estimating the activity of these enzymes is to test the integrity of liver cells, thus helping to distinguish obstructive from hepatocellular jaundice. Elevation of the αGT is a sensitive index of hepatocellular disease and elevated aspartate and alanine amino transferases (AST and ALT) may also indicate hepatic damage. Neither enzyme is specific to the liver and results must be interpreted in the clinical context. As ALT occurs in much higher concentration in the liver than in other organs, an increase in its activity is a more specific indication of hepatic damage.

Other tests of liver disease.

Autoantibodies. Anti-nuclear, smooth muscle or mitochondrial antibodies may be of diagnostic value in chronic liver disease; for example the last is positive in primary biliary cirrhosis.

Alpha-fetoprotein. The reappearance of this fetal alpha-globulin in adult life is almost always due to a hepatoma, although the test is often negative in the presence of a hepatoma.

Investigative procedures in liver and biliary disease.

Scanning. Ultrasonography is the examination of choice in the investigation of jaundice. It will show whether or not the jaundice is obstructive and may demonstrate the cause of obstruction. Ultrasound may also show the presence of diffuse liver disease such as cirrhosis or focal lesions within the liver exceeding 2 cm in diameter. Radionuclide scanning is complementary to ultrasound as each may detect lesions missed by the other.

Radiological examination. Cholecystography may demonstrate stones in a functioning gall bladder and cholangiography may reveal dilatation of the common bile duct and suggest a cause for the obstruction. The latter has been replaced by ultrasonography. Endoscopic retrograde cholangio-pancreatography (ERCP) permits retrograde filling of the biliary and pancreatic tracts to define the cause for obstruction. It can be combined with therapeutic features such as sphincterotomy thereby sometimes avoiding the need for open surgery.

A barium swallow may give evidence of portal venous hypertension by showing evidence of oesophageal varices. Selective angiography via the hepatic artery, hepatic vein or portal vein can define the site of local lesions and portal pressures can be measured.

Biopsy. Focal lesions should be investigated by liver aspiration or biopsy under ultrasound control. The choice depends upon the skill and interest of the cytopathologist. Blind percutaneous liver biopsy should be reserved for diffuse liver disease.

Paracentesis abdominis. Diagnostic paracentesis allows examination for protein and cell count and cytology for malignant cells and culture for bacteria including tuberculosis.

PANCREAS

Tests of exocrine secretion can be made by collecting pancreatic juice through a tube passed via the mouth or nose into the duodenum. The pancreas can be stimulated either indirectly by a test meal containing carbohydrate, protein and fat or directly by secretin and/or cholecystokinin. Following stimulation the duodenal aspirate is collected for 30 min and the volume of aspirate and the concentrations of bicarbonate, amylase, trypsin and lipase are estimated.

Extensive disease of the pancreas may damage its endocrine function with the development of overt or latent diabetes. A glucose tolerance test may help to distinguish between malabsorption due to pancreatic disease, in which there may be a diabetic type of curve, and that due to diffuse disease of the small intestine in which there may be an abnormally small and sustained rise in the blood sugar.

Acute pancreatitis is accompanied by a transient but often marked increase in serum amylase, although this may also rise in other abdominal crises such as a perforated duodenal ulcer.

Radiological examination may indicate that the pancreas is swollen by showing displacement of the stomach and duodenum and absence of gas in the middle of the transverse colon. Ultrasonography of the pancreas may show features of a pancreatic tumour or of acute pancreatitis and is a useful method of detecting pancreatic pseudocysts. Computed tomography (CT scanning) targeted on the pancreas is the method of choice for looking for occult pancreatic tumours.

URINARY SYSTEM

In renal disease accurate collection of the urine, biochemical testing and microscopic and bacteriological examination are essential. These procedures are described in Chapter 12.

Estimation of blood urea and creatinine will indicate the degree of renal failure and a creatinine clearance determination provides an estimation of the glomerular filtration rate.

A plain radiograph of the abdomen may show the presence of renal calculi or indicate renal size. Ultrasonography is non-invasive and can distinguish solid from cystic lesions (Fig. 7.18). Radionuclide studies provide renal scans and renography. The former gives information of renal function and also of the size of the kidneys and the definition of the renal outlines. Symmetrically small kidneys suggest either congenital hypoplasia or chronic parenchymal disease. Renography also assesses renal function and is most useful in urinary tract obstruction and sometimes in the investigation of hypertension. An excretory urogram (IVU) will also delineate the kidneys and the pelvicalyceal system. This can be distorted in chronic pyelonephritis and destruction of papillae can occur in analgesic abuse and diabetes. After

the pyelogram, the ureters and bladder will also be shown.

The urethra can be inspected through a urethroscope and the bladder and ureteric orifices can be examined by means of a cystoscope. Antegrade or retrograde pyelography can demonstrate ureteric obstruction and give more precise definition of the renal pelvis. The former does not require general anaesthesia and is gaining wider acceptance.

The renal arteries may be outlined by aortography. In this way stenosis of a renal artery or the abnormal circulation in a tumour can be demonstrated. In selected cases, renal artery angiography can be combined with transluminal angioplasty for renal artery stenosis. The use of digital computer techniques for vascular imaging during angiography is being evaluated.

Histological examination of the kidney can be carried out by percutaneous renal biopsy. Specimens are examined under the light microscope, electron microscope and also by immunofluorescent techniques.

GENITAL SYSTEM

Appropriate specimens may be required to confirm the diagnosis of sexually transmitted infection or to identify the cause of discharges.

Pregnancy can be confirmed by immunological and other tests whereby the presence of chorionic gonadotrophin in the patient's urine is demonstrated. The diagnosis can be made at a much earlier stage than by clinical means but positive results are also obtained when a hydatidiform mole or a chorionepithelioma is present. Ultrasonic examination can be very helpful in detecting and dating pregnancy and assessing foetal wellbeing. It will also distinguish between a healthy foetus, an early abortion and a hydatid mole.

The investigation of infertility involves a detailed endocrine assessment of both partners. In addition seminal analysis or testicular biopsy may be required in the male. Venography may be indicated to assess varices and angiography to detect undescended testes. Ultrasonic examination may help when there is a possibility that a hydrocoele is obscuring a testicular tumour. In the female ultrasound examination of the ovaries is not only useful in investigating infertility but also for detecting ovarian disease and other pelvic masses. Hysterosalpingography or laparoscopy are other methods of investigating female infertility.

Miscroscopical examination of the lining of the uterus after dilatation of the cervix and curettage (D & C) is a routine procedure in the investigation of abnormal vaginal bleeding, and the cytological examination of cervical smears, supplemented if necessary by biopsy of the cervix, is invaluable in the early detection of carcinoma. The laparoscope is particularly useful in the elucidation of the cause of lower abdominal pain of gynaecological origin.

THE METHODS IN PRACTICE

Two contrasting examples have been chosen.

THE EXAMINATION OF THE ACUTE ABDOMEN

The term 'acute abdomen' is applied to disorders of sudden onset which may involve surgical intervention. Correct diagnosis may be lifesaving and will depend primarily upon an accurate history and careful physical examination.

The history. Pain is often the presenting feature and care should be taken to obtain a full description (p. 25). Pain of sudden onset in a patient who was well a few moments before may indicate a free perforation of a hollow viscus whereas pain of more gradual onset may suggest an inflammatory lesion such as appendicitis, salpingitis or diverticular disease. Changes in the character of the pain should be sought. Thus, the pain of appendicitis may start in the periumbilical area and later move to the right iliac fossa as the local peritoneal inflammation develops. Similarly the onset of a constant pain in a patient who has been experiencing small bowel colic implies the development of an ischaemic loop. It is important to enquire about drug treatment. For example, systemic corticosteroid therapy may not only increase the risk of a perforation but also mask the clinical features.

The physical examination. Some patients will be very ill, and a prolonged history and examin-

ation will be displaced by the need for resuscitation. Shock may be due to concealed haemorrhage as in a leaking aortic aneurysm or ruptured ectopic pregnancy. It can also be associated with septicaemia due to infection in the biliary or urogenital systems and may also be a feature of pancreatitis. In others a full general assessment must be made as abdominal symptoms may be prominent in disorders such as myocardial infarction, pneumonia or even diabetic ketoacidosis. Examination commences while the patient recounts the symptoms and includes recording the temperature, pulse and respiratory rates and blood pressure.

Examination of the abdomen follows the usual pattern of inspection, palpation, percussion and auscultation. All abdominal scars should be accounted for and the patient's story should be verified from the original operation notes when available. Palpation may reveal the special features found in the acute abdomen: tenderness, rebound tenderness, guarding and rigidity. Generalised board-like rigidity implies peritonitis and attempts to elicit other signs such as rebound tenderness are then unnecessary. Guarding, the reflex spasm of the abdominal wall muscles over an area of peritonitis, must be differentiated from contraction of the abdominal muscles due to the patient's anxiety or the examiner's cold hands. Deep-seated inflammation not causing localised guarding may be revealed by rebound tenderness. Pelvic peritonitis may be advanced before signs are apparent on abdominal palpation and a rectal examination must never be omitted. The groins should be carefully examined for small hernias and the external genitalia palpated in the male.

Percussion may be useful; for example the presence of free gas may be suspected by the absence of normal liver dullness.

Auscultation may reveal the active bowel sounds of intestinal obstruction and these may develop a 'tinkling' quality when bowel is distended. A 'silent' abdomen implies paralysis of the intestines.

Further investigation. A urinary specimen should be examined microscopically and tested routinely for blood, glucose, ketones and bile. Porphobilinogen should be sought if acute intermittent porphyria is a possibility. A faecal sample obtained during the rectal examination should be inspected and tested for occult blood.

Laboratory studies of value include a white cell count; a leucocytosis supports a diagnosis of an inflammmatory lesion. If pancreatitis is a possibility, the serum amylase should be estimated.

Routine radiographs of the abdomen are not required to diagnose such disorders as appendicitis and the need for any films should always be questioned in women of child-bearing age. A supine film may show radiopaque calculi in the biliary or renal tracts. Erect and supine views are required in assessing patients with suspected obstruction of the bowel. An erect chest X-ray should be obtained if perforation is a possibility.

Management. Further treatment may involve surgery. If an operation is not required, suitable medication including analgesia should be given but it must be borne in mind that the initial diagnosis may be wrong; the patient will need continued observation and reassessment.

IMPOTENCE

An illustrative case

A 50-year-old barman gave a history of impotence which had not responded to an empirical course of mesterolone — a synthetic androgen which does not depress the pituitary. The sexual problem questionnaire (p. 358) revealed no suggestion of neurological disease, diabetes or hypertension and the man was on no medication. There was however a history of regular drinking with episodic heavy drinking. The sexual history of partial erections was not enough to allow intercourse although morning erections were present. He had stopped trying to have intercourse because of worry about further failure.

Physical examination showed a normal male physique with no evidence of gynaecomastia and the penis and both testes were normal. Gentle pressure on the testes produced normal testicular pain — a simple test to help to exclude autonomic neuropathy. Neurological examination was normal and in particular, sensation around the anus was unimpaired and the tone of the anal sphincter was normal on rectal examination. The prostate gland was slighty enlarged but was not hard or tender. The blood pressure was normal.

A urine sample was tested for glucose and protein with negative results. Blood estimations of urea, haemoglobin, testosterone, follicular stimulating hormone and liver function tests were all normal. If there had been gynaecomastia or uraemia a prolactin estimation would also have been performed as male hyperprolactinaemia is associated with impotence and sometimes renal failure.

The history of full erections in the morning suggested that there was nothing wrong with the vascular or neurological mechanisms of erection and it was concluded that the patient's libido and performance were simply diminished by his excessive consumption of alcohol. Initial advice from the clinical psychologist attached to the psychosexual clinic was followed by further guidance from an alcoholism unit before the drinking problem was brought under control. Libido then returned to normal.

REFERENCES

Shearman D J C, Finlayson N 1989 Diseases of the gastro-intestinal tract and liver, 2nd edn. Churchill Livingstone, Edinburgh
Sherlock S, Summerfield J A 1980 A colour atlas of liver disease. Wolfe Medical Publications, Chicago
Smith D R 1984 General urology, 11th edn. Lange Medical Publications, Los Altos, California

8. The nervous system

R. E. Cull

The study of neurology is founded on those principles of clinical medicine which are outlined in Chapter 1. No other clinical discipline offers so exemplary an illustration of the logical and scientific foundations on which medicine is based. Deviations from normal neural function are observed. The nerve pathways and tracts whose interruption would cause such functional disturbances are inferred. Where possible the precise anatomical sites of lesions are then determined. In the light of the distribution of lesions, the history of the patient's illness and collateral evidence of disease in other systems, the causal pathological process is deduced. This diagnostic process constitutes a logical sequence which should always be followed. Though increasing facility will enable the steps to be made more rapidly, there are no short cuts; few signs are pathognomonic of disease processes.

The nervous system is organised functionally in a hierarchical fashion. Peripheral effectors and receptors are supplied by nerves whose function is restricted, which originate from the spinal cord and dorsal root ganglia and which are arranged in a segmental fashion. Connections within a spinal cord segment between afferent and efferent nerve fibres enable reflex motor responses to occur as a result of certain sensory stimuli. Activities within the spinal cord are modified by influences deriving from 'higher' levels such as the basal ganglia or cerebellum which function as coordinating centres. The highest level of activity is represented in the cerebral cortex which is concerned with the elaboration of ideas, with the complex patterns of learned movements and with the integration and interpretation of sensory information. This organisational pattern is of fundamental clinical importance. Dissolution of neural activity at dif-ferent levels produces different patterns of disability.

Neurological lesions may affect normal function in three ways:

(1) 'negative' features result from the loss of normal neural functions as, for example, the muscle paralysis and impaired sensation which follow damage to a peripheral nerve,

(2) they may give rise to positive phenomena, i.e. there may be overaction of part of the nervous system, as for instance in Jacksonian epilepsy where convulsive movements of a limb result from an irritative lesion affecting the motor cortex;

(3) abnormal function may occur because of a 'release' of lower levels of nervous activity from restraints or inhibitions which in normal circumstances are imposed by the functions of higher levels. A common example of this is the increased tone seen in limbs after damage to the pyramidal pathway.

Sometimes damage to nerve pathways will concurrently cause patterns of positive, release and negative phenomena which are distinctive, as, for example, the tremor, rigidity and hypokinesis of the parkinsonian syndrome.

The significance of some signs may be difficult to interpret because the results of examination often depend on the patient's cooperation and subjective responses to stimuli. Some signs are less reliable than others. There are 'soft' and 'hard' neurological signs. An extensor plantar response is an obvious example of a 'hard' neurological sign. In contrast the assessment of deep pain sensation by pinching the patient's calf depends on the patient's reaction and personality and, little reliance can be placed on this sign in isolation. It is however rarely necessary to base interpretation on single signs. Several abnormalities elicited during the examination will add weight to each other. It it important, however, that this process of assessing signs in combination in order to localise lesions should not lead to a false importance being given to indeterminate observations. It is even more dangerous to attribute significance to findings in order to complete a pattern which is 'typical' of a disease. For example when a young patient presents with paralysis of the legs (paraparesis), it must not be assumed that the diagnosis is multiple sclerosis. Examination of the optic discs may reveal pallor of the temporal halves of the discs relative to their nasal halves which is a normal phenomenon. If, however, this is recorded as 'bitemporal pallor', a spurious significance is given to a normal finding. A diagnosis of multiple sclerosis may be made on false grounds and a potentially remediable lesion such as a spinal cord tumour may be missed.

Clinicians must appraise each of their observations in the light of their knowledge of normal variations and then decide whether a given finding is abnormal. There is little point in saying that a patient's optic discs look pale; the observer must try to decide whether the discs are abnormally pale or not. When there is real doubt, the clinician should ask a more experienced doctor to assess the findings.

THE HISTORY

Many neurological symptoms are both frightening and mysterious to the patient who will often find them difficult to describe and may use words which are inappropriate and misleading. Each symptom must therefore be carefully analysed; this can be a time consuming process needing patience on the part of the clinician and of the patient. For example, most physicians equate a complaint of 'numbness' with a disturbance of sensation, whereas some patients may use this term to describe weakness. The nature of an altered sensation is hard to communicate to a listener who has not experienced it. Terms like 'pins and needles' are generally understood because everyone has occasionally felt them. More complex

sensory disturbances lead to profound difficulties of description, particularly if the patient is relatively inarticulate. The clinician should allow patients time to elaborate their descriptions, encouraging them to try alternative phrases until they find one which they think most apt. It is often advisable to record the patient's actual words rather than to translate them into potentially misleading jargon.

Some words are thought by laymen to have a precise meaning. Thus pain is considered by many to be self-explanatory and indeed patients may be confused and even resentful if asked to elaborate on the nature of their pain. It is sometimes helpful to offer several adjectives such as 'stabbing', 'throbbing', 'pressing', 'burning' and then asking the patient to choose one which most closely fits. The distribution of the pain, its time relationships and precipitants should also be delineated (p. 25). Dizziness is a term in common usage. It will sometimes describe a hallucination of movement which we call vertigo, but it is also used for such varying conditions as syncope, hypoglycaemia, epilepsy and episodes of anxiety. As a symptom it required clarification. It is often helpful to ask patients to distinguish between a sensation of movement of themselves or their surrounding (vertigo) from a fainting sensation and lack of balance. Likewise complaints of 'blackouts' or 'fits' need to be critically analysed (p. 29).

In contrast, double vision is a phenomenon easily understood by both patients and doctors. However this complaint becomes much more informative if the directions of displacement of the two images, the direction of gaze in which they are maximally separated, and the variation, if any, of the diplopia are established (p. 200).

The object of taking a neurological history should be to determine the course of the patient's illness in terms of its severity and time relationships; the process of interpretation by the clinician should be applied while doing so in terms of the possible physiological and anatomical implications of previous or present symptoms.

Physical examination will often enable lesions of the nervous system to be localised with precision, but the pathological nature of the lesion can be intelligently surmised only in the light of the development of the illness. In general, lesions which suddenly affect the nervous system cause maximal disability within a few hours and after a static period of days or weeks then show a tendency to improve, are due to vascular disturbances. Lesions of insidious onset and slow but inexorable progression are often due to degenerative disorders or to tumours of the central nervous system. A remittent history, wherein episodes of disability are followed by periods of marked improvement and wellbeing, with later recurrence of symptoms elsewhere in the nervous system, suggests a diagnosis of multiple sclerosis.

Interrogation. After evaluation and recording of the patient's history, specific questions should routinely be asked about headache, fits, intellectual impairment, changes in mood, visual difficulties, weakness, tingling or numbness of the limbs and disturbances of micturition or defecation. Details of birth, illness in early life, previous injuries of the head and spine, and current or previous medication should be obtained. A family history of epilepsy, migraine, and neuromuscular disorders is worth specific enquiry.

THE PHYSICAL EXAMINATION

The technique and the order of the physical examination is highly variable. Many neurologists begin at the head and work down to the feet; some do the converse. The examination of the central nervous system can be interspersed with that of other systems. Though the order in which the examination is carried out may be varied, the findings should be recorded in a systematic way (p. 359).

General observations

Whilst a patient is giving the history, observation should be made of those features which are outlined in Chapter 4. Signs of disease of other systems may be relevant to a patient's neurological disorder. During the course of listening to the history, observation of the patient's face will often suggest the nature of neurological disabilities. There may be cranial nerve palsies such as ptosis, squint or facial weakness. The cheeks may show the typical pigmented papules of adenoma

sebaceum and hence point to tuberous sclerosis as the cause of epilepsy in a child. Poverty of facial expression observed during the diagnostic interview may be due to depression or to the hypokinesis of parkinsonism. Facial grimacing may point to a diagnosis of chorea. A facial weakness which develops during the course of the patient's history may be a direct diagnostic pointer to myasthenia gravis. The pouting lips and transverse smile of myopathic weakness may indicate the presence of one of the primary diseases of muscle. The detailed examination of specific nerve functions should be preceded by assessment of the patient's mood and personality (see Ch. 2) intellectual function, speech and gait.

Intellectual function

Usually the history will indicate whether intellectual function is within normal limits and in many cases a formal clinical assessment is unnecessary. However when the patient's narrative or conduct, or evidence from relatives suggests that there may be intellectual deterioration, an assessment should be made as described in the examination of the mental state (p. 19). Attention should therefore be paid to the patient's orientation, memory, attention and concentration, fund of general information and powers of abstraction. The examiner's approach must be flexible and tailored to the patient's previous level of intellectual function and educational background. A mathematician, although demented, may still possess a facility for calculation which is greater than the examiner's. In contrast, a patient whose inherent intellectual gifts were poor should not be expected to perform well during testing.

Speech

It is first necessary to determine whether the patient suffers from a defect of language or of speech production. Impairment of language functions is manifest by inappropriate usage of words or by a disturbance of the understanding of words. This may occur as part of a generalised intellectual disturbance (p. 22). Such a defect should be perceived when taking the history and the associated intellectual impairment would become apparent during the testing of general intellectual function. Specific difficulty with language function is called dysphasia. It may be that words are used appropriatedly but that speech production is impaired either because of a defect in articulation (dysarthria) or because of alternation in the quality or reduction of volume of speech (dysphonia). A total inability to fulfil these functions is denoted by the prefix 'a' — (Gr. α = without) hence aphasia, anarthria and aphonia respectively.

Dysphasia

This results from a lesion affecting the speech areas in the dominant hemisphere. The examination of speech function should be preceded by an assessment of the likely side of the dominant hemisphere. Many left-handed people were forced to write with the right hand at school. The patient should be asked not only which hand is used for writing but also for such activities as cutting bread or catching a ball and which foot would normally be used for kicking. Since hand preference, in most instances, is congruous with the side of the dominant eye, the patient can be asked which eye would be used for sighting a rifle or to look through a rolled-up newspaper as if it were a telescope. This will almost always be put to the dominant eye. This eye dominance is invalidated if there be a marked discrepancy of visual acuity in the two eyes. In many clinical circumstances, these problems of dominance are self-evident. If the patient has a dysphasic defect accompanied by a right hemiplegia, it is clear that the left hemisphere is affected and that is dominant for speech. Sometimes, however, it may be a matter of importance to determine which is the hemisphere concerned with speech if surgical removal of part of a hemisphere is contemplated.

In the vast majority of right-handed people language function is represented in the left hemisphere. The situation is more complicated in those who preferentially use the left hand, in at least half of whom language functions are served by the left hemisphere. In others who are genetically determined left-handers, the right hemisphere is concerned with language. Such patients often give a family history of left-handedness.

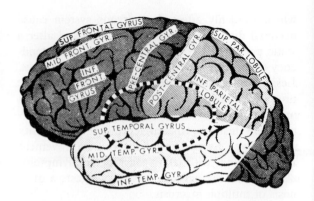

Fig. 8.1 The cerebrum. The dotted line indicates the approximate extent of the 'speech area' in the dominant hemisphere.

Those areas which are principally concerned with speech function are shown in Figure 8.1 and include the inferior frontal, superior temporal, and inferior parietal regions of the dominant hemisphere. The simplest clinical classification divides dysphasia into motor (expressive) and sensory (receptive) categories.

In *motor or expressive dysphasia* internal speech is preserved intact and patients comprehend language satisfactorily. They know what they wish to say but are unable to say it although the peripheral speech apparatus is intact. The number of words used is reduced; errors of articulation and grammar are common and speech may take on a 'telegraphic' quality. This type of disturbance (Broca's dysphasia) arises from discrete lesions in the inferior part of the frontal lobe (Broca's area).

Sensory or receptive dysphasia. This is the term used when comprehension of speech is impaired. It is always accompanied by derangement of the patient's use of language. Although the output of words may be normal or increased and their pronounciation and fluency intact, much of the patient's speech is irrelevant in content and often contains incorrectly substituted words (verbal paraphasia) or letters (literal paraphasia), or entirely new words (neologisms). Dysphasia of this type is called Wernicke's dysphasia and arises from lesions in the temporo-parietal area (Wernicke's area). It is usually associated with an impaired ability to read (*dyslexia*).

Conduction dysphasia. This disorder may contain elements of both Broca's and Wernicke's dysphasia, but is characterised by a marked impairment in ability to repeat words or phrases spoken by the examiner. The lesion responsible lies between Wernicke's and Broca's areas in the perisylvian region.

Global dysphasia. This term is used to describe a severe form of dysphasia in which there is little or no intelligible speech as well as marked deficits of comprehension. Global dysphasia is usually due to a large lesion in the region of the Sylvian fissure, involving both the anterior and the posterior speech areas.

Examination of language function. This should include careful attention to the patient's speech when giving the history and responding to questions. Inappropriate usage of words, the use of nonsense words or the formulation of sentences in which the word order is unconventional reveal an underlying defect of language function. Very well known or automatic speech is often surprisingly well preserved even in the presence of severe dysphasia. Patients may be able to count fairly well, may be able to say 'yes' and 'no' quickly and confidently and they may be able to swear with fluency.

Comprehension of spoken speech is tested by asking patients to carry out commands. The level of difficulty of these commands can gradually be raised. The clinician may start by asking the patient to close the eyes or raise an arm and go on to make the command more difficult by asking the patient consecutively to touch the nose with the left thumb and thereafter to bow the head. The examiner should avoid giving visual cues. Verbal instructions for arranging a small collection of coins may reveal more subtle defects of comprehension. The responses to commands will often reveal the presence of deficits of comprehension in patients apparently suffering from a purely motor dysphasia.

The assessment of language function is supplemented by tests of the patient's reading ability. Impaired ability to read (*dyslexia*) often results from a lesion in the dominant parietal lobe. This may be associated with an inability to write (*dysgraphia*) which may result from lesions of the frontal or parietal lobes.

Dysarthria

Speech may be normal in its use of language but may be difficult to comprehend because of defective articulation (dysarthria). The impaired intelligibility is largely due to the imprecise enunciation of consonants. The production of clearly defined consonants requires precise, coordinated movements of the lips, tongue and palate. Before assessing the neurological cause for dysarthria, the mechanical integrity of all these structures should be established. Ill-fitting false teeth commonly cause slurring of consonants; a cleft palate will give rise to a nasal speech quality similar to that produced by a palatal palsy.

It is sometimes possible to define which speech organ is primarily affected. A rapidly vibrating tongue is required to produce the rolled 'R' and impairment of tongue movements cause a lisp due to imperfect pronunciation of 'R'. The enunciation of 'P', 'B' and 'M' demands finely coordinated movements of the lips. Normal speech requires the soft palate to elevate and prevent air escaping through the nose during the generation of explosive consonants (e.g. 'B' and 'G'). Failure of palatal closure results in 'nasal' speech where 'rub' becomes 'rum', and 'egg' becomes 'eng'. Asking the patient to puff out the cheeks may reveal nasal air escape.

Dysarthric difficulties vary in severity from complete inability to articulate (*anarthria*) to very minor slurring of consonants. In the latter case attention to the patient's spontaneous speech may leave the examiner in doubt as to whether dysarthria is present. The patient should be asked to repeat such well known tongue-twisters as 'Royal Irish Constabulary', 'The Leith police dismisseth us', 'Red leather, yellow leather'. Slurring of speech, even when of minor degree, is easily recognised by others but the patient is often unaware of the problem even when the speech is badly affected.

Having established the presence of dysarthria the clinician must then determine the site of the neural lesions responsible. The possibilities include;

1. Intrinsic weakness of the articulating muscles due to myopathy;
2. Lesions at the neuromuscular junction in

myasthenia gravis where characteristically the dysarthria becomes more marked as the patient continues to speak.

3. Diffuse lesions of the lower brain stem leading to bulbar palsy;
4. Bilateral upper motor neurone lesions causing supranuclear bulbar palsy;
5. Parkinsonism; impairment of voluntary movements may affect speech as it does other motor functions.
6. Cerebellar defects which may cause a distinctive type of dysarthria in which the slurring of consonants is accompanied by a staccato, interrupted cadence of speech referred to as 'scanning' dysarthria.

Dysphonia

Normal speech not only involves the articulation of learned language but also requires a method of sound production or phonation. Phonation depends on an adequate flow of air passing from the lungs through the glottis, causing vibration of the vocal cords. Impairment of phonation (dysphonia) may result from disordered function of the vocal cords or from respiratory dysfunction leading to inadequate expiratory air flow. Lesions of both vocal cords and respiratory musculature may be combined. Dysphonia is characterised by an alteration in quality (often a hoarseness) of the voice or by a loss of voice volume or both features may be evident.

Dysphonia is the result of neurological disease in only a minority of cases; other more common causes are described on page 47. Dysphonia may rarely result from primary diseases of muscles or may be due to myasthenia gravis when it tends to be variable. More often it results from damage to neural structures, such as bilateral lesions of the vagus nerve in bulbar palsy or bilateral upper motor neurone lesions above the level of origin of the vagus nerve causing supranuclear bulbar palsy. Dysphonia may be a manifestation of impaired movements in parkinsonism wherein speech tends to be low in volume and monotonous.

Miscellaneous disorders of speech

Though most speech disorders will fit into the broad categories outlined above, the examination should also include a detailed analysis of the rhythm and cadence of speech.

Stammering or stuttering. This comprises an abrupt halt to the flow of speech together with repetitive utterance of sounds or syllables or of the initial consonants of words. This disorder usually arises in childhood and is more common in boys. It is not associated with organic neurological disease but can be mimicked occasionally by patients with expressive dysphasia and sometimes the delayed initiation of speech seen in parkinsonism may superficially resemble a stammer.

Bradylalia. Undue slowness of speech occurs in some patients with depression, parkinsonism or hypothyroidism. The rate of verbal utterance varies greatly from individual to individual and only profound slowness of speech should be regarded as of pathological significance. Likewise a rapid delivery of speech is more often a manifestation of temperament rather than of organic disease. It may be noticeable in some patients with hypomania.

Echolalia. Echolalia is a term used to describe the automatic repetition by the patient of the examiner's utterances. This is a normal stage of development of language in childhood. When it occurs in adults, it is usually a manifestation of widespead cortical disease.

Palilalia. This rare disorder of speech differs from echolalia in that patients here repeat the terminal parts of their own utterances. Either the last sentence, the last phrase, or even the last word may be reiterated again and again, often at an increasing rate. It can be exemplified in 'My father was a gramophone maker but it hasn't affected me, affected me, affected me'. The disorders of neural function which produce this speech phenomenon are ill understood. It tends to occur in widespread cerebrovascular disease but is also found in patients suffering from post-encephalitic parkinsonism.

Summary of assessment of speech

A comprehensive assessment should pay attention to :

1. Spontaneous speech — fluency, articulation, content;

2. Naming of objects — e.g. pen, cup, comb;
3. Comprehension of spoken and written commands;
4. Repetition of words and phrases;
5. Reading aloud;
6. Handwriting — form, grammar, syntax.

Spontaneous speech should be listened to attentively and, if necessary, language or articulatory function should be tested. The appraisal of speech defects should first determine the type of disturbance, whether it be due to dysphasia, dysarthria or dysphonia or to one of the miscellaneous disorders discussed above. These categories are not exclusive. Some patients may exhibit several types of speech disturbance concurrently. Patients suffering from diffuse cerebrovascular disease may exhibit generalised intellectual deterioration as well as dysphasia and may also be dysarthric. Patients with parkinsonism are frequently dysphonic, often dysarthric and they may show the features of bradylalia or palilalia.

Having assessed the nature of the speech disturbance, the clinician should then determine the level in the central nervous system at which a lesion might cause such a disorder.

Gait

Inspection of a patient's gait is an integral part of the neurological examination and should never be omitted if the patient can walk. Normal walking depends on an intact motor system, proprioceptive and vestibular information, and also normally functioning higher centres such as the cerebellum and the extrapyramidal system. A careful examination of gait will often lead to an accurate deduction of the nature of a patient's neurological deficit (p. 258). Observation of the gait is readily combined with testing of the proprioceptive and vestibular systems by Romberg's test (p. 229).

THE EXAMINATION OF THE CRANIAL NERVES

Initially it may be helpful to examine the cranial nerves individually and in consecutive order. With practice, this rigid approach can be replaced by a more flexible technique which minimises repetition — for example, testing tongue sensation, if indicated, is undertaken after assessing tongue movements.

In order to test cranial nerves effectively a knowledge of their functions and their anatomy as well as their connections with higher levels of the central nervous system is essential. These features will be outlined for each cranial nerve, the tests of function described and then an interpretation given of the findings.

The olfactory (first cranial) nerve.

The olfactory nerve subserves the sense of smell. Its receptors are situated high in the nasal cavity from whence thin filaments pass centrally, through the cribriform plate, where they are extremely vulnerable to injury, to the olfactory bulbs. Second order neurones arise here, run through the olfactory tract and divide into the medial and lateral olfactory striae. Some of the medial group cross to the opposite side; the remainder pass to the medial surface of the cerebral hemisphere. The lateral striae pass to the temporal lobe. The sense of smell is essential for the appreciation of flavours and hence a patient whose sense of smell is impaired may complain of a loss of taste.

Disturbances of function of the first cranial nerve are uncommon, but the sense of smell should be meticulously examined whenever a patient's history suggests a lesion in the anterior cranial fossa.

Testing the sense of smell

Loss of sense of smell is much more commonly due to nasal disease than to neurological causes. Before examining the sense of smell the patient should be questioned about such disorders as hay fever, sinusitis and catarrh and the nasal passageways should be inspected.

The sense of smell should be tested separately in each nostril, the other being occluded by finger pressure. The patient, with the eyes closed, is asked to sniff test substances through each nostril in turn and to name the odours. Irritating, pungent substances such as ammonia or vinegar should be avoided since these stimulate the trigeminal nerve rather than the olfactory nerve. Easily recognised substances such as coffee, cocoa, oil of almonds or vanilla are suitable. If bottles of these are not available, an orange, toothpaste or soap from the patient's bedside locker will serve.

Interpretation

Loss of the sense of smell (anosmia), if due to a neurological lesion, is most commonly the result of trauma. Head injuries, even of minor degree, accelerate the brain differentially from the skull. The olfactory filaments are subjected to shearing strain and are readily torn. Less common causes of anosmia are lesions within the anterior cranial fossa. Tumours may arise from the frontal lobe or in the olfactory groove itself and may cause bilateral anosmia at an early stage. Chronic basal meningitis of tuberculous, syphilitic or neoplastic origin may also involve the olfactory pathways.

Increased olfactory acuity is rarely due to organic disease though it is occasionally a premonitory feature of migraine. Perversion of smell (parosmia) is sometimes of psychological origin but may occur from the partial recovery of traumatic anosmia, a severe nasal infection or the ingestion of drugs (e.g. phenytoin).

Olfactory hallucinations, usually of an unpleasant nature, are characteristic of epilepsy arising in the uncinate gyrus of the temporal lobe and then are often accompanied by smacking gustatory movements of the lips.

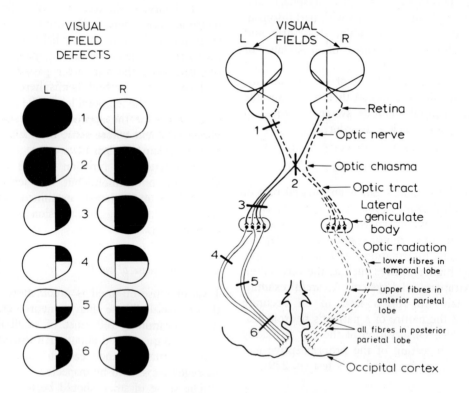

Fig. 8.2 Visual field defects. (1) Total loss of vision in one eye due to a lesion of the optic nerve. (2) Bitemporal hemianopia due to compression of the optic chiasma. The upper quadrants are usually first affected. (3) Right homonymous hemianopia from a lesion of the optic tract.
(4) Upper right quadrantic hemianopia from a lesion of the lower fibres of the optic radiation in the temporal lobe. (5) Less commonly a lower quadrantic hemianopia occurs from a lesion of the upper fibres of the optic radiation in the anterior part of the parietal lobe. (6) Right homonymous hemianopia with sparing of the macula from a lesion of the optic radiation in the posterior part of the parietal lobe.

The optic (second cranial) nerve

The basic anatomy of the visual pathways is shown in Figure 8.2. The examination consists of inspecting the optic nerve head and fundus by ophthalmoscopy as described in Chapter 11, and the testing of visual acuity, the visual fields, pupillary responses and colour vision.

Examination of visual acuity

Visual acuity should be measured for both near and distant vision. The latter should be estimated by the ability of the patient, with each eye in turn, to read standard Snellen types at a distance of six metres. The results are recorded as 6/6, 6/18, etc., the latter meaning that at 6 m, the patient can just read what should be read at 18m. Near vision is tested by using standard reading charts such as the Jaeger card. Each of the patient's eyes is covered in turn and spectacles can be worn if required. Patients should be asked, with each eye, to read the smallest print possible. The result is recorded by noting the chart number of the passage read. If a refractive error is suspected (e.g. because of disparity between near and distance acuity) having the patient look through a pin-hole increases depth of field for focus and partially corrects the defect.

Examination of visual fields

The defects in the visual fields resulting from lesions of the visual pathways are shown in Figure 8.2.

At the bedside it is possible to obtain a rough assessment of the visual fields by the technique of *confrontation*. The patient and the examiner look into each others eyes from a distance of about one metre. After an initial assessment made with both eyes open, the examiner shuts one eye and the patient covers the opposite so that the left visual field will correspond to the examiner's right and vice versa (Fig. 8.3). If the patient looks away from the examiner's eye the test is invalidated. The clinician then proceeds to test the outer limits by bringing a target into the field of vision from the periphery at several points on the circumference. The direction of approach should be distributed over upper and lower quadrants and

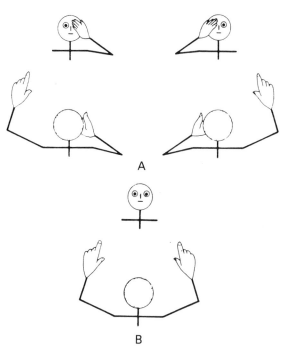

Fig. 8.3 Testing the visual fields. (A) Testing the temporal field in each eye separately. (B) Testing both eyes simultaneously for inattention hemianopia.

nasal and temporal aspects of the visual fields. A satisfactory way to test each of the four quadrants is to advance the target towards the centre of gaze along lines at 45° to the vertical and horizontal axes of the field. The test object should be moved on a plane midway between the patient and the examiner so that a direct comparison can be made between the examiner's visual field and that of the patient. However, a normal patient who is looking straight ahead can see a moving object directly to one side, and also to the side and downward (infero-temporally) even when the object is at right angles from the line of vision. In order to test peripheral vision in these areas, it is necessary to place the test object somewhat behind the patient, and well within the examiner's own field of vision. A finger is a satisfactory target but a more accurate assessment may be made by using a pin with a large head (e.g. a hat pin). This has the advantage of enabling an estimate to be made of the extent of the visual fields to different coloured objects by using pins with white, red and green heads. The visual fields for coloured objects are concentric with, but smaller than, those for white objects.

When using a pin the distraction caused by movement of the examiner's hand is minimised if the pin is stuck into the end of a pencil. A pin can also be used to plot gaps in the central areas of the fields (scotomas) and to assess the size of the physiological blind spot.

If the patient is unable to cooperate by fixing on the examiner's eye, other techniques may be used roughly to map out hemianopic or quadrantic field defects. The patient may be asked to look at the examiner's nose with both eyes open. The examiner then stretches out both arms and moves the fingers asking the patient to point to the moving hand. When the patient, as the result of disturbed consciousness or because of a dysphasic defect is unable to cooperate at all, it may be possible to demonstrate gross defects in the visual fields by rapidly moving one hand towards the patient's face from the side. This menacing stimulus will usually evoke reflex blinking but the patient will not blink when menaced from a hemianopic side.

A patient suffering from a lesion in a parietal lobe may see the test object perfectly well when presented in isolation in each visual half field but will consistently fail to perceive an object in one half of the visual field when stimuli are presented simultaneously and bilaterally (Fig. 8.3). This is called an inattention hemianopia and is an example of perceptual rivalry (p. 231).

In most cases confrontation will map out visual defects with sufficient precision for clinical purposes but the method does not define the full extent of the lateral aspects of the normal visual fields. When minor defects are present or when the shape of the visual defect is important in localisation, the visual fields should be mapped out more accurately by using a tangent (Bjerrum) screen and a perimeter.

Colour vision

Although tests of colour vision are not carried out routinely, they may reveal subtle defects of the retina or optic nerve. The most commonly used method is to present, to each of the patient's eyes separately, plates made up of coloured dots containing numerical shapes (Ishihara plates). The patient is asked to discern the numbers shown in each pattern.

The oculomotor, trochlear and abducent (third, fourth and sixth cranial) nerves

During the close inspection of the eyes and their movements which examination of the third, fourth and sixth cranial nerves requires there should be concurrent observation of local abnormalities of the eye (pp. 58–61). The examination of the functions of these three nerves requires knowledge of the anatomy and physiology of the nerves and of the muscles they supply. There are interconnections between the nuclei of the three nerves and pathways to them from higher centres of control.

Ocular muscles. The principal voluntary muscle of the upper eyelid is the levator palpebrae superioris. Fibres of the orbicularis oculi and involuntary (tarsal) muscles are also found in the network of muscle fibres in the eyelids.

The involuntary muscle fibres in the iris subserve two functions. Concentric fibres form the sphincter pupillae which constricts the pupil; radial fibres within the iris dilate the pupil. The ciliary muscle, when contracted, causes an increase in convexity of the lens.

Six external ocular muscles supply and move the eyeball. Whenever movement of the eye occurs, all the external ocular muscles participate to a greater or lesser extent but individual muscles are particularly responsible for individual movements.

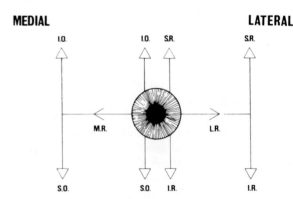

MEDIAL   **LATERAL**

Fig. 8.4 Testing of ocular movements. Medial and lateral rectus (MR and LR) move the eyes medially and laterally respectively. With the eyes in the mid position inferior oblique (IO) and superior rectus (SR) elevate the eye and superior oblique (SO) and inferior rectus (IR) depress the eye. When the eye is turned medially inferior oblique moves the eye upwards and superior oblique moves it downwards. When the eye is turned laterally superior rectus elevates the eye and inferior rectus depresses it.

It can be seen from Figure 8.4 that the lateral rectus is almost solely responsible for turning the eye outwards (abduction) and the medial rectus for adduction of the eyeball. When the eye lies in the mid position the movement of the eye in the vertical plane is a function of four muscles. The inferior oblique and superior rectus are responsible for upward movement, the superior oblique and inferior rectus for downward movement. Upward and downward movements of the eyes in the mid position do not separate the actions of these muscles. The actions of the four muscles are easily elucidated if Figure 8.5 is studied. It can be seen that when the eye is adducted the superior oblique is a pure depressor of the eye and the inferior oblique is almost solely responsible for elevation of the eye. When the eye is turned outwards, or abducted, the superior rectus bears the main responsibility for upward movement and the inferior rectus for downward movement.

Nerve supply. The *oculomotor* or *third cranial nerve* originates in a series of nuclei in the midbrain whence fibres run anteriorly in close relationship to the red nucleus, the substantia nigra and the pyramidal pathways in the cerebral peduncle (Fig. 8.58, p. 249). After leaving the midbrain the third nerve enters the cavernous sinus on its lateral wall, there lying lateral to the internal carotid artery. It then enters the orbit through the

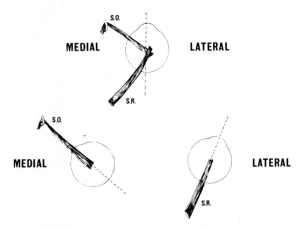

Fig. 8.5 Testing of ocular movements. To show the actions of the superior oblique (SO) and superior rectus (SR) muscles. The dotted line represents the optical axis. It will be seen that when the eye is turned medially, superior oblique is a depressor of the eye. When the eye is turned laterally superior rectus elevates the eye. The actions of inferior oblique and inferior rectus are similar.

superior orbital fissure and separates into branches which supply the levator palpebrae superioris, the superior, medial and inferior recti and the inferior oblique muscles.

The *trochlear* or *fourth cranial nerve* arises from its nucleus anterior to the aqueduct of Sylvius in the mid-brain just below the third nerve nuclei. The fourth nerve passes posteriorly and the fibres from the right and left trochlear nuclei decussate on the dorsum of the mid-brain, They pass through the cavernous sinus, lying immediately below the third nerve and enter the orbit through the superior orbital fissure. The fourth cranial nerve supplies only the superior oblique muscle. Because of the decussation on leaving the brain stem, the left trochlear nucleus sends fibres to the right orbit and vice versa.

The *abducent* or *sixth cranial nerve* arises in the lower pons anterior to the fourth ventricle (Fig. 8.59, p. 250). The fibres of the seventh cranial nerve loop around the abducent nucleus. The sixth nerve fibres leave the brain stem at the junction between pons and medulla and then run a very long intracranial course. As it passes forward and laterally the nerve lies over the petrous part of the temporal bone. It then pierces the dura near the dorsum sellae to enter the cavernous sinus, passing along the lateral aspect of the sinus to enter the orbit through the superior orbital fissure and supply the lateral rectus muscle.

Parasympathetic fibres take origin from cells within the nuclear complex of the third nerve. Preganglionic fibres pass with the fibres of the third nerve. Most run to the ciliary ganglion whence postganglionic fibres arise to supply the ciliary muscle and sphincter of the pupil. A smaller number of parasympathetic fibres bypass the ciliary ganglion to end in episcleral ganglia. It is thought that these latter fibres are responsible for the reaction of accommodation.

Sympathetic fibres arise in centres in the hypothalamus and run through the mid-brain, pons, medulla and cervical cord and emerge through the ventral roots of the first two or three segments of the thoracic spinal cord. These fibres then ascend through the sympathetic chain to the superior cervical ganglion. From here postganglionic fibres arise and ascend in the carotid plexus and enter the orbit with the oph-

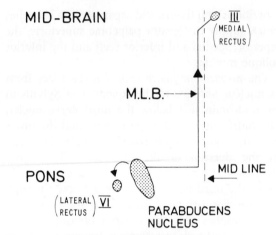

MID-BRAIN

III
(MEDIAL RECTUS)

M.L.B.→

PONS

(LATERAL RECTUS) VI

MID LINE

PARABDUCENS NUCLEUS

Fig. 8.6 Coordination of lateral gaze. Fibres from the parabducens nucleus (pontine center for conjugate lateral gaze) run to the immediately adjacent sixth nerve nucleus. Other fibres run in the medial longitudinal bundle (MLB) to that part of the third nerve nucleus on the opposite side which activates the medial rectus. Thus the lateral movements of the abducting eye and medial movements of the abducting eye can be synchronised.

thalmic artery to terminate on the radial (dilator) muscle of the iris. Sympathetic fibres also supply the tarsal muscles and the orbital muscle, the latter tending to hold the eye forward in the orbit.

Internuclear connections. The medial longitudinal bundle (fasciculus) coordinates the activity of the motor nerves to the eye. It connects the nuclei of the three ocular nerves to each other and to other nuclear masses, particularly the vestibular nuclei. A diagram of this system is shown in Figure 8.6. Near to the sixth nerve nucleus in the pons is a centre, the parabducens nucleus, which co-ordinates conjugate lateral movements of the eyes. Fibres from this centre run to the sixth nerve nucleus on the same side. Other fibres cross the mid line and run in the medial longitudinal bundle to that part of the contralateral third nerve nucleus which supplies the medial rectus. This provides a mechanism which ensures that the optical axes remain parallel when the eyes are turned conjugately to the side.

Supranuclear connections. There lies in the cortex of the frontal lobe at the posterior end of the second frontal convolution an area which when stimulated causes conjugate deviation of the eyes away from the stimulated side (frontal eye field).

Fibres from this area probably run through the anterior part of the internal capsule, through the basal ganglia to terminate in the pontine centres coordinating lateral gaze. Damage to these frontal centres, paralysing or weakening their function leads to impairment of voluntary conjugate deviation of the eyes away from the side of the lesion.

There are also centres in the occipital cortex concerned with conjugate eye movements but these are less well defined than are those in the frontal area; it is likely that they are important for maintaining visual fixation on a moving target (pursuit movements).

Examination

Inspection. The examination should be prefaced by a detailed inspection of the eyes commencing with the *eyelids*. The size of the palpebral fissures and any asymmetry between the two should be noted. Any ptosis (drooping of an eyelid) or any widening of the palpebral fissures should be observed. Involuntary movements of the eyelid, particularly spasms which also usually involve the orbicularis oculi, may be seen. The rate of blinking should be estimated. The patient should be asked fully to open and forcibly to close the eyes.

The *pupils* should be inspected. Pupils normally are round, regular in outline and equal in size. The size of the pupils varies with the amount of ambient lighting but is usually between 3 and 5 mm in diameter, being greater in childhood and smaller in old age. Pupils which are less than 3 mm in diameter in average conditions of illumination are called miotic and dilation of the pupils above 5 mm is referred to as mydriasis. The size of the pupils on the two sides should be compared.

Pupillary reflexes. If a light is shone on the retina, the pupil on the same side, as well as that on the opposite side, constricts. The reaction of the pupil on the side stimulated is called the *direct light reflex* and the constriction of the other pupil is the *consensual light reflex*. The speed and extent of constriction should be assessed in each eye separately, shielding the other from the light while doing so in order to test both direct and consensual reflexes. The light should approach from the side in order to avoid an accommodation response. Occasionally an initial constriction is followed rapidly by alternating dilation and constriction. This is called hippus and is a normal variation.

The *reaction of accommodation* refers to the constriction of the pupils which accompanies convergence of the eyes when the patient looks at a near object. The patient should be asked to relax accommodation by gazing into the distance at, say the ceiling and then asked to shift the gaze to fix on the observer's finger, held near the patient's nose. Alternatively the patient may be asked to keep the gaze fixed on the clinician's finger which at first is held several feet away and is then brought nearer and nearer to the patient's face. The significance of abnormal pupillary reflexes is discussed on page 199.

Constriction of the pupils. Miosis may be due either to paralysis of the sympathetic system or to stimulation of the parasympathetic system. Some drugs such as neostigmine, by inhibiting the action of cholinesterase, cause constriction of the pupil. Constriction of a pupil may be due to a lesion of the cervical sympathetic nerves when it will usually be accompanied by a degree of ptosis and with enophthalmos and impaired sweating on the same side, comprising *Horner's syndrome* (Fig. 8.7). A reduction in pupillary size is a normal manifestation of ageing sometimes called senile miosis.

Dilatation of the pupils. Mydriasis is often a manifestation of anxiety. It can also result from stimulation of the sympathetic system or paralysis of parasympathetic nerves. Drugs such as atropine and homatropine paralyse cholinergic nerves and therefore give rise to mydriasis whilst amphetamine and similar drugs dilate the pupil by sympathetic stimulation. Enlargement of the pupil may result from blindness due to damage to the optic nerve.

Abnormal pupillary reflexes. Impairment or absence of the pupillary reaction to light may be due to interruption of afferent or efferent sides of the reflex arc. Since both pupils constrict in response to light shone into one eye afferent lesions can easily be distinguished from damage to efferent pathways. If a pupil constricts when light is shone into the opposite eye, (i.e. the consensual light reflex is preserved), the motor pathway for constriction to that eye is intact and the damage

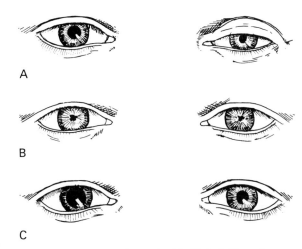

A

B

C

Fig. 8.7 Pupils as a diagnostic aid. (A) Left Horner's syndrome. There is ptosis, the pupil is small and regular. Sweating on the affected side of face is frequently diminished. (B) Argyll Robertson pupils. The pupils are small and irregular. They react to accommodation but not to light. (C) Right Holmes-Adie syndrome (tonic pupillary reaction). Reaction to light appears absent but to accommodation is preserved with delayed relaxation.

must lie on the sensory side of the reflex arc. Lesions of the optic nerve such as acute retrobulbar neuritis, damage the afferent side of the arc. In such cases there will be no direct light reaction but the consensual light reaction will be observed. This is the '*amblyopic light reaction*'. The afferent side of the reflex arc is impaired also in the *Argyll Robertson pupil* where the affected pupils tend to be small and characteristically the two pupils are unequal and irregular. Here there is loss of the light reaction but preservation of the reaction to accommodation (Fig. 8.7). A lesion in the pretectal area explains most of the phenomena of the Argyll Robertson pupil (Fig. 8.8). Isolated loss of reaction to accommodation with preservation of the light reflex is uncommon but may occasionally occur in some cases of brain stem encephalitis involving parasympathetic fibres (p. 197). Loss of reaction to both light and accommodation may be due to structural damage to the iris itself, occasioned by trauma or by inflammatory lesions, which prevent the pupil from changing size. The motor pathway serving pupillary reflexes may be damaged by a complete third nerve palsy when reactions both to light and to accommodation will be lost.

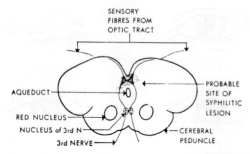

Fig. 8.8 The light reflex pathway in the midbrain and the probable site of the lesion in the Argyll Robertson pupil. The pupillary reflex to accommodation involves a different pathway through the lateral geniculate body and the occipital cortex.

A relatively common abnormality of pupillary reflexes, usually seen in adult women, is the *tonic pupillary reaction (Holmes-Adie syndrome)*. In this condition the reaction to light appears absent and the reaction to accommodation is delayed and sustained in a tonic fashion after convergence ceases. In some instances the light reaction is present but is delayed and sustained (Fig. 8.7). This is a benign condition due to a lesion in the ciliary ganglion, but it needs to be differentiated from the Argyll Robertson pupil. Absence of ankle jerks and other tendon reflexes may accompany these tonic pupillary reactions.

Ocular movements. During inspection of the eyes the direction of any deviation of the optical axes of the eyes from parallel should be noted. The patient should be instructed to report if they see double at any time and then asked to look upwards, downwards, to the left and to the right, and then to look upwards and downwards while gazing to the left and then to repeat this looking to the right. The patient should then be asked to follow with the eyes a target held by the examiner who moves it in the directions listed. The target should be held at least 60 cm — about an arm's length — from the patient's eyes, so that the nose does not interfere with fixation. After testing with both eyes open it may be necessary to test each eye separately, the other being covered by the examiner's hand. If double vision is present, they should be asked in what direction of gaze the objects seem to be most widely separated. In the position of maximal separation of the images the more

peripheral of the two images is the false image. By covering the eyes alternately and asking the patient to say when the outer image disappears it is possible to establish which eye is at fault. The weakened muscle is that which normally moves the affected eye in the direction in which maximal double vision occurs. If diplopia has been present for more than a few months it may be difficult to obtain clear cut answers about the direction of gaze in which maximal separation of images occurs because the patient has learned to suppress the false image. Occasionally double vision is absent despite obvious ocular paresis; this is particularly common when *strabismus* (squint) has been present for many years. The differentiation of paralytic squint from the non-paralytic (concomitant) squint, common in children, is described on page 312.

Nystagmus. Whilst ocular movements are being tested the presence of nystagmus, i.e. involuntary oscillations of the eyes, should be observed. Nystagmus is described as 'pendular' when the oscillations about a central point are equal in rate and amplitude like the swing of a pendulum. Nystagmus is said to be 'jerking' (phasic) when there are quick and slow phases of unequal duration. The quicker phase is arbitrarily used to define the direction of nystagmus. Thus 'nystagmus to the right' refers not to the direction of gaze in which nystagmus occurs but to the direction of the quick phase. Jerking nystagmus may be graded:

1. First degree — only present on lateral deviation of the eyes.
2. Second degree — present on looking straight ahead.
3. Third degree — present on looking in the direction opposite to that of the fast phase.

Note should be made of the directions of gaze which evoke nystagmus, whether nystagmus occurs on vertical movement or on lateral movement, whether it is equal in amplitude and rate in all directions of gaze, or whether rate and amplitude vary with direction of eye movements. Nystagmus usually comprises a to and fro oscillating movement but sometimes there is a rotary component; the eyes turn around their axes. This too should be noted. Normal people may occasionally exhibit jerking movements of the eyes at the extremes of gaze and particularly so when the test object is held close to the subject's eyes.

Interpretation

Ptosis. This may be due to a lesion of the levator palpebrae muscle itself, of its neuromuscular junction, of the third nerve or of the cervical sympathetic pathways. Damage to the sympathetic supply rarely causes more than slight drooping of the eyelid and sympathetic involvement can easily be differentiated from weakness of the levator palpebrae superioris by asking the patient to elevate the eye voluntarily. If the levator muscle is weak the patient will be unable to elevate the lid completely, but will be able to do so if the cervical sympathetic is involved since this results only in weakness of the superior tarsal muscle. Ptosis due to a lesion of the ocular sympathetic fibres is usually accompanied by other features of Horner's syndrome (see below).

Ptosis may accompany some myopathies and is commonly present, often bilaterally but unequally and usually variably in myasthenia gravis (Fig. 10.4). If this is suspected the patient should be asked to look upward at an object whilst keeping the head still. This causes continued elevation of the eyelids and after a period the ptosis will become more marked in patients with myasthenic weakness.

When ptosis is an accompaniment of a third nerve palsy there will usually also be dilatation of the pupil and a pattern of defective ocular movements attributable to a third nerve lesion (p. 198).

Spasmodic closure of the lids is often a psychogenic phenomenon but may occasionally occur in parkinsonism. In the latter condition blinking is infrequent.

Widening of the palpebral fissure or fissures may occur because of lid retraction in thyrotoxicosis. Unilateral widening may be mistaken for ptosis affecting the other eye; it may indicate a paresis of the orbicularis oculi on that side caused by a seventh nerve lesion.

Disorders of ocular movements. Disordered ocular movements may result from lesions of ocular muscles (myopathies), neuromuscular junctions, ocular nerves and their nuclei, or from interruption of internuclear and supranuclear con-

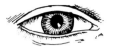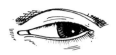

Fig. 8.9 Lesion affecting the third cranial nerve; there is ptosis, pupillar dilatation and lateral deviation looking straight ahead.

nections. Analysis of the defects in ocular movements will help to decide whether they fit a pattern of muscular or neural involvement, and if neural, which nerves are implicated. *Myopathies* tend in the early stages to affect all the muscles equally and partially, presenting a generalised restriction of eye movements. Ptosis accompanies this general impairment in the rare condition of ocular myopathy and a similar picture may be manifest in myotonic dystrophy.

Myasthenia gravis usually effects ocular muscles variably. Characteristically the ocular paresis associated with myasthenia gravis is associated with ptosis but there are no pupillary abnormalities.

Lesions of the third cranial nerve, if complete, cause ptosis, weakness of superior, medial and inferior recti and inferior oblique muscles, as well as pupillary dilatation and absent pupillary reflexes (Fig. 8.9). Third nerve lesions may be incomplete and the pupillary reflex abnormalities and ptosis may be absent. Bilateral third nerve palsies are usually incomplete and most commonly arise from lesions within the mid-brain where the two third nerve nuclei lie very close together (Fig. 8.58, p. 249). Mid-brain lesions affecting the third nerve are often associated with upper motor neurone signs on the side opposite the lesion (Fig. 8.58). Third nerve damage within the cavernous sinus is almost always accompanied by lesions of the fourth and sixth nerves and impaired sensation over the distribution of the ophthalmic division of the fifth nerve (p. 203).

Lesions of the fourth cranial nerve (Fig. 8.10) are rare in isolation but affection of the superior oblique muscle commonly results from trauma to the orbit causing dislocation of the trochlea through which the tendon of the superior oblique muscle runs. The fourth nerve may be involved, together with the third and sixth nerves in diffuse lesions of the brain stem such as multiple sclerosis and acute vitamin B_1 deficiency (Wernicke's encephalopathy). The fourth nerve is also involved with

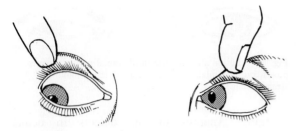

Fig. 8.10 Lesion affecting left fourth cranial nerve. Looking downwards and to the right the eye turns inwards but not downwards.

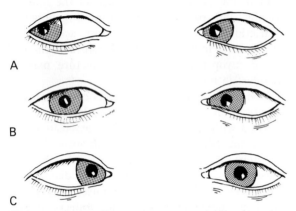

A

B

C

Fig. 8.11 Lesion affecting the left sixth cranial nerve. (A) Looking to the right. (B) Looking straight ahead. (C) Looking to the left.

the third and sixth nerves in lesions within the cavernous sinus.

Lesions of the sixth cranial nerve. Paralysis of the lateral rectus may be due to a lesion affecting the muscle itself, its neuromuscular junction or the sixth nerve, the last being a common accompaniment of raised intracranial pressure whatever the cause (Fig. 8.11). In such instances the sixth nerve palsy constitutes a false localising sign. If the sixth nerve is involved in the brain stem it is usually associated with a seventh nerve palsy on the same side and upper motor neurone signs on the other.

Internuclear disturbances. A lesion of the medial longitudinal bundle (Fig. 8.6) anywhere along its course between the pons and mid-brain will cause a weakness of adduction on attempted lateral conjugate gaze and this is the characteristic clinical phenomenon of internuclear ophthalmoplegia. Such lesions may be unilateral or bilateral. If the medial longitudinal bundle is damaged in the mid-brain, impaired convergence will accompany the

defect of lateral conjugate gaze (anterior internuclear ophthalmoplegia, Fig. 8.58 p. 249). When a lesion lies in the lower part of this tract, in the pons, fibres to the adjacent sixth nerve may also be interrupted so there will be defective abduction as well as restricted adduction on lateral deviation. The weakness of abduction may be reflected by nystagmus in the abducting eye (posterior internuclear ophthalmoplegia, Fig. 8.59, p. 250). This type of nystagmus confined to, or more marked in the abducting eye on attempted lateral gaze, is known as ataxic nystagmus and denotes a pontine lesion. The disconjugation of eye movements caused by internuclear lesions is seen best when the patient makes rapid lateral changes of gaze.

Supranuclear disturbances. Irritative lesions of the frontal lobe, such as occur when an epileptic discharge arises there, cause conjugate deviation of the eyes away from the side of the lesion. An infarct in this area may not only cause hemiplegia but in the early stages also function as an irritative lesion. Thus, immediately after a stroke it may be observed that the patient's head and eyes are turned towards the paralysed limbs. Later there is often a paralysis of function and the patient will find difficulty in conjugate deviation of the eyes towards the paralysed side.

Nystagmus. This may be caused by visual disturbances, or by lesions of the labyrinth, the central vestibular connections, the cerebellum, brain stem or cervical cord. Pendular nystagmus is usually due to a loss of macular vision but is occasionally seen in diffuse brain stem lesions. Jerking nystagmus which is of constant direction regardless of the direction of the gaze suggests a labyrinthine lesion or a cerebellar disturbance. Nystagmus which changes direction with the direction of gaze suggests a widespread central involvement of the vestibular nuclei. Jerking nystagmus absent with the eyes in the mid position but which develops only on lateral gaze and whose fast component is in the direction of gaze indicates a lesion of the brain stem or cerebellum. Nystagmus which is confined to one eye suggests a peripheral lesion of the nerve or muscle responsible for movement in the appropriate direction or it may be due to a lesion of the medial longitudinal bundle. Nystagmus which is restricted to the abducting eye on lateral gaze, ataxic nystagmus, is due to a lesion of the medial longitudinal bundle between the pons and mid-brain as in multiple sclerosis. Nystagmus which occurs on upward gaze, with the fast component upwards, (upbeat nystagmus) may be due to a lesion in the mid brain at the level of the superior colliculi, but is often a component of internuclear ophthalmoplegia from a lesion of the medial longitudinal bundle. Downbeat nystagmus (fast phase downwards) suggests a lesion in the lower part of the medulla.

The trigeminal (fifth cranial) nerve

The trigeminal nerve carries both motor and sensory fibres. The motor nucleus is situated near the floor of the fourth ventricle in the lateral part of the pons from whence the motor root emerges near to the sensory root and passes below the trigeminal (Gasserian) ganglion to leave the skull through the foramen ovale. After joining the mandibular division of the sensory nerve it supplies the muscles of mastication, the masseters, temporals and pterygoids. The masseters elevate the jaw as, to a lesser extent, does the temporalis muscle. The pterygoid muscles depress and protrude the jaw when acting together and when one acts alone it causes the jaw to move laterally away from the side of the contracting muscle.

The sensory part of the trigeminal nerve carries exteroceptive sensation from the face, the anterior part of the head and inside the mouth (Fig. 8.12).

The ophthalmic division supplies the skin of the forehead, the root of the nose and the scalp as far back as a line joining the ears. It also supplies the cornea, conjunctiva and the intraocular structures as well as the mucosae of the frontal, sphenoidal and ethmoidal sinuses and of the upper part of the nasal cavity. It lies on the lateral wall of the cavernous sinus as it passes from the orbit to join the trigeminal ganglion.

The maxillary division supplies the skin of the nose, cheek and upper lip, the mucosae of the maxillary sinus, posterior part of the nasal septum and the lower part of the nasal cavity. The upper teeth and gums, the hard and soft palate receive sensory fibres from this division.

The mandibular division supplies the skin of most of the jaw, other than its angle, the mucosae of

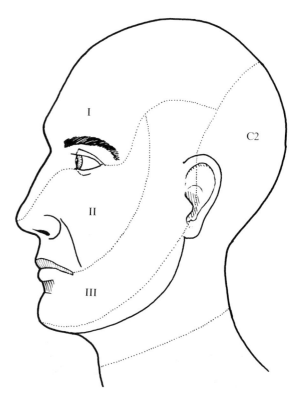

Fig. 8.12 Cutaneous distribution of the trigeminal nerve. (I) Ophthalmic division. (II) Maxillary division. (III) Mandibular division. (C2) Second cervical root. (C3) Third cervical root.

the cheek, jaw, floor of the mouth and the tongue. It also supplies the lower teeth and gums.

The cells of origin of the sensory part of the nerve lie in the trigeminal ganglion.

Tactile impulses conveyed in the central processes of these cells pass into the pons to terminate in the principal sensory nucleus of the fifth nerve. After synapsing here fibres carrying tactile sensation proceed to the thalamus in the ascending tract of the fifth nerve which lies near the medial lemniscus. Impulses concerned with pain, temperature and some concerned with tactile sensation terminate in the nucleus of the spinal tract which extends downwards from the principal sensory nucleus, through the pons and medulla into the spinal cord where it reaches the third cervical segment. Nerve fibres from different parts of the face are grouped in the following manner. The area around the mouth is supplied by fibres which synapse with second order neurones lying in the

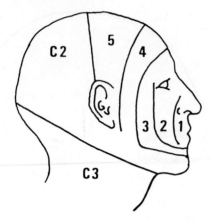

Fig. 8.13 Pain fibres to the head. Areas marked 1 to 5 indicate the central distribution within the spinal tract of the fifth cranial nerve. 1 is represented in the pons, 2 the pontomedullary region, 3 the lower medulla, 4 and 5 the upper cervical cord. The areas labelled C2 and C3 derive from the spinal segments directly.

highest part of the spinal tract. Concentric areas spreading outwards from the mouth are supplied by fibres which synapse at progressively lower levels in the spinal tract. The outermost segment of the face is represented by fibres which descend to the lowest part of the tract. These arrangements give rise to the so-called 'onion-skin' distribution of facial sensory representation (Fig. 8.13). The fibres arising from the neurones in the spinal tract, cross to the opposite side and pass upwards to the thalamus and thence with those from the body, to the sensory cortex.

Examination

Sensory functions. Light touch and pain sensation is tested in the territory of the three sensory divisions using cotton wool and pin prick respectively. Temperature sense can also be tested. The methods of examination conform to those for sensory testing in general (p. 228). The two sides of the forehead, of the cheeks, and of the jaw should be compared.

Sensory deficits occasionally may involve the periphery of the face whilst sparing the central area, or the converse may occur. In addition to testing sensation in the major divisions some comparison should be made between the sensation in the 'snout' area around the nose and mouth and the sensitivity at the periphery of the cheek.

Motor functions. This starts with inspection of the muscles of mastication. Muscle wasting may be revealed by a flattening of the face above and below the zygoma. In some instances fasciculation may be seen in the masseters and temporal muscles. If there is bilateral weakness of the muscles of mastication the jaw may hang loosely open.

The patient should be asked to open and close the jaw against resistance. As the patient clenches the teeth hard the masseters should be palpated and an estimate made of their bulk and symmetry. When the patient opens the jaw against resistance, the jaw will deviate towards the weakened muscle if there is unilateral weakness of the pterygoids. If this is suspected patients should be asked to move the jaw laterally against resistance; it may then be found that the jaw can be moved towards the affected muscle but cannot be deviated towards the normal side. Facial asymmetry, resulting from a seventh nerve palsy, may give rise to a misapprehension that the jaw is deviated.

Reflexes. The *corneal reflex* comprises a brisk contraction of the orbicularis oculi evoked by touching the cornea. The afferent part of the reflex arc is the first division of the trigeminal nerve; the motor limb lies in the facial nerve. Each fifth nerve communicates with both seventh nerves and therefore both eyes close when either cornea is stimulated.

The corneal reflex is elicited by touching the cornea, not the conjunctiva, with a wisp of cotton wool. The cornea is extremely sensitive and is vulnerable to injury, so that the touch must be light. The wool should approach the eye from the side (Fig. 8.14) as an object jabbed at the patient from

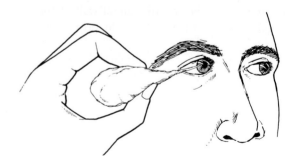

Fig. 8.14 Testing the corneal reflex.

directly in front will elicit a reflex closure of the eyes which is a response to menace and is not dependent on fifth nerve stimulation. The contraction on both sides should be observed. This will enable lesions of the fifth cranial nerve to be differentiated from damage to the efferent pathway of the reflex. If there is a seventh nerve palsy on the side stimulated there will be no direct response of the orbicularis oculi on that side but the patient will feel the touch on the cornea and there will be a brisk closure of the other eye. The briskness of the direct response on each side should be compared. Impairment of the corneal reflex may be the earliest sign of a lesion affecting the ophthalmic division of the trigeminal nerve and may be observable before cutaneous sensation is demonstrably impaired. Pontine lesions affecting the fifth and seventh nerve nuclei or their interconnections will also cause impairment of the corneal reflex. Acute pyramidal tract damage (e.g. in a cerebral hemisphere stroke) may also cause transient loss of the corneal reflex contralateral to the lesion.

The *jaw jerk* is analogous to the tendon reflexes in the limbs. The afferent and efferent pathways are subserved by the fifth cranial nerve. The effective stimulus is a brisk downward stretch of the masseter muscles which is best evoked by placing

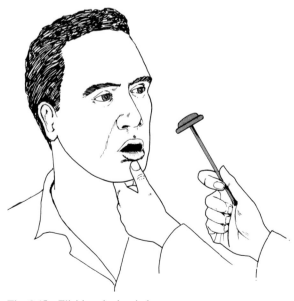

Fig. 8.15 Eliciting the jaw jerk.

the thumb or forefinger over the tip of the patient's mandible and then tapping the examiner's finger downwards with a tendon hammer (Fig. 8.15). This manoeuvre should be performed with the patient's jaw hanging open. The reflex response comprises a brisk closure of the jaw. Measured by electrophysiological methods the jaw jerk is always present. It is often not visible in young people unless they are anxious but is commonly seen above the age of 50; the decision as to whether a jaw jerk is merely present or is pathologically exaggerated is sometimes difficult.

Interpretation

Peripheral lesions. Facial pain may be difficult to localise and frequently arises from the structures supplied by the fifth nerve such as dental abscesses or caries, inflammation of the sinuses and abnormalities of the temporomandibular joints. Trigeminal neuralgia gives rise to no signs. If sensory changes are present, it is likely that there is a structural lesion of the fifth nerve. Multiple sclerosis in young people, or tumours invading the fifth nerve may give rise to episodic trigeminal pain which mimics trigeminal neuralgia.

Peripheral divisions of the fifth cranial nerve may be damaged by trauma, or may be involved in neoplastic processes at the base of the skull. Nasopharyngeal tumours may also cause pain and diminished sensation if they erode the base of the skull.

Herpes zoster (p. 76) often affects the ophthalmic division of the fifth cranial nerve and in elderly people is liable to cause persistent burning pain in the distribution of the nerve. Post-herpetic neuralgia is usually accompanied by scars and by slight impairment of sensation over the forehead in the distribution of the affected ophthalmic division.

Central lesions. When the fifth cranial nerve is affected more proximally it is often associated with other cranial nerve signs which indicate the site of the lesion. The first division of the trigeminal nerve may be implicated in lesions within the cavernous sinus, in company with the third, fourth and sixth nerves. Tumours lying in the cerebellopontine angle often impinge on the trigeminal sensory nerve root, giving rise to paraesthesiae and numbness affecting almost all the face of the appropriate side. Lesions here are frequently associated with deafness, cerebellar signs and seventh nerve signs and this combination suggests the site.

Motor lesions of the trigeminal nerve are much less common. Bilateral involvement of the masticatory muscles may occur in myasthenia gravis and as part of a bulbar palsy in motor neurone disease, when wasting and fasciculation may be observed. In bilateral lesions of the upper motor neurones above the level of the pons the jaw jerk is abnormally brisk.

The facial (seventh cranial) nerve

The facial nerve consist of two parts. The larger motor component supplies all muscles of facial expression. The smaller part (nervus intermedius) comprises sensory and parasympathetic constituents which carry taste fibres from the anterior two thirds of the tongue and visceral efferent fibres to the lacrimal, submaxillary and sublingual

glands. There are a few somatic sensory fibres which carry cutaneous sensation from a small area of the external ear.

The motor nucleus of the facial nerve is found in the pons medial to the descending nucleus of the fifth nerve. Efferent fibres loop round the nucleus of the sixth cranial nerve before leaving the pons on its lateral aspect (Fig. 8.59 p. 250). It is there joined by the nervus intermedius in the cerebello-pontine angle near the sixth and eighth nerves. Motor fibres and the nervus intermedius then enter the facial canal. The afferent fibres of the nervus intermedius have their cells of origin in the geniculate ganglion and terminate in the upper medulla. From the geniculate ganglion secretory fibres pass via the petrosal nerves to the lacrimal glands. The facial nerve then runs through the facial canal, gives off two branches and leaves the skull at the stylomastoid foramen. The first branch is the nerve which supplies the stapedius muscle, which limits the movement of the ear drum and ossicles in response to loud noise. The more distal branch is the chorda tympani (Fig. 8.16) which

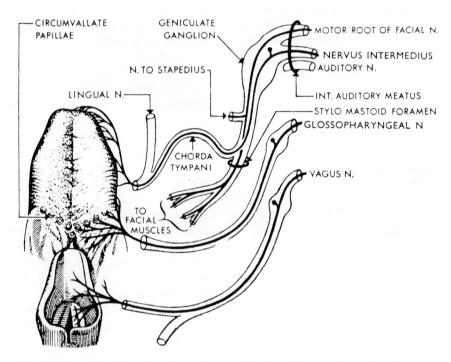

Fig. 8.16 Seventh, ninth and tenth cranial nerves. To show (1) taste pathways from the tongue in the facial and glossopharyngeal nerves, (2) the essential components of the facial nerve as it passes through the skull and (3) the vagus nerve and the larynx.

joins the lingual nerve (a branch of the mandibular nerve) and carries taste fibres from the anterior two-thirds of the tongue as well as parasympathetic fibres to the submandibular and sublingual salivary glands.

After leaving the stylomastoid foramen the facial nerve passes anteriorly through the substance of the parotid gland and is then distributed via a number of branches to all the musculature of the face. Among the more important muscles of facial expression are the frontalis which raises the eyebrows, the orbicularis oculi which causes closure of the eyes and the corrugator which draws the eyebrows downwards to produce a frown. The nares may be constricted or dilated by muscles supplied by the seventh nerve. The orbicularis oris closes and purses the mouth whose angles are raised by the levator anguli oris. The platysma draws down the lower lip and depresses the chin.

Examination

Motor functions. Any involuntary movements should be noted. These may take the form of tics or habit spasms (p. 218) which are stereotyped but may comprise very complex movements in certain individuals. Isolated twitches and more prolonged spasms may affect one side of the facial musculature (hemifacial spasm).

The two sides of the face should be compared. Signs of facial palsy may be obvious on inspection; there may be a widened palpebral fissure on the affected side with absence of wrinkling on that side of the face causing drooping of the corner of the mouth with dribbling of saliva and flattening of the nasolabial fold. Bilateral weakness of the facial muscles may be manifest in pouting of the lips and a transverse smile. Movements of the upper part of the face should be compared with activity in the lower face.

Voluntary contractions of facial muscles should be examined. The patient should be asked to frown, raise the eyebrows, wrinkle the forehead and to close the eyes as strongly as possible. The examiner should attempt to open the eyes when the patient is forcibly closing them. The patient should be asked to show the teeth, to blow out the cheeks, to purse the mouth and to whistle. The

response to an emotional expression, such as smiling, should be noted (p. 208).

Sensory functions. The sensory examination involves testing of taste over the anterior two thirds of the tongue. The primary tastes, sweet, salt, bitter and sour, should be tested using sugar or saccharin, salt, quinine and vinegar respectively. The examiner should hold the protruded tongue gently with a swab. The test substances are placed on each side in turn and the patient, whose eyes should be closed, is asked to identify the tastes by opening the eyes and pointing to the apposite word written on a card. The patient should be instructed not speak, because this will cause the tongue to be retracted into the mouth and saliva will flow over the tongue carrying taste to both sides, and to the posterior third, of the tongue.

Secretory functions. These are usually not tested. If lacrimation is excessive, it will be observed during the taking of the history; it is often due to obstruction of a tear duct. The patient will complain if there is increase or decrease of salivation.

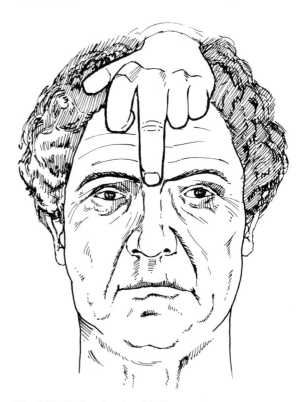

Fig. 8.17 Performing the glabellar tap.

Reflexes. The *glabella* or *nasopalpebral reflex* is elicited by percussion with the finger over the root of the nose (Fig. 8.17). It is important that the tap is light and that the patient is not visually menaced by a direct stab of the fingers from in front. The reflex response to a tap over the glabella is a brisk bilateral closure of the eyes. In most normal people repeated percussion evokes three or four contractions and then the response ceases. Exaggeration and prolongation of the glabellar tap response is seen in disorders of the extrapyramidal system, most commonly in some patients with parkinsonism.

Snout reflex. Tapping the upper lip or stroking it with the edge of a wooden tongue depressor normally produces no visible response except during infancy. In bilateral upper motor neurone lesions it may give rise to puckering and protrusion of the lips.

Interpretation

Impaired facial movements may be due to disturbance of supranuclear motor pathways which influence the activity of the facial nerves, to affections of the seventh cranial nerve itself or to lesions within the facial muscles. The first stage of interpretation involves the assessment and differentiation of lesions at these various levels.

The paucity of spontaneous facial movements and of emotional expressiveness in *parkinsonism* may at first suggest bilateral weakness of the facial musculature. But the parkinsonian patient will exhibit no weakness when performing voluntary facial movements on request. A sustained glabellar reflex may help to support the diagnosis of parkinsonism, but some anxious, normal people continue blinking as long as the tapping is repeated.

Upper motor neurone. *Unilateral lesions* (above the level of the pons) characteristically weaken movements of the lower part of the face more than those of the upper face. This discrepant affection is due to innervation of the upper facial structures from both hemispheres whilst lower facial movements are represented largely in the contralateral motor cortex. This pattern of weakness is the rule in upper motor neurone lesions but there are occasional exceptions. A patient who has recently and suddenly sustained a hemiplegia may initially suffer from paresis equally affecting both upper and lower face.

Patients with *bilateral upper motor neurone lesions* may exhibit an obvious snout reflex. Such patients may also show a lability of emotional expression and a dissociation between emotional and voluntary movements may be observed. For example some patients with a marked voluntary weakness may yet move the paralysed side normally when they smile. The reason for this dissociation is not known but presumably there are alternative pathways subserving emotional movement.

Lower motor neurone. The facial nerves may be affected anywhere along their pathways from the pons to peripheral branches to give a lower motor neurone palsy.

Unilateral affection of a seventh nerve is a common clinical presentation, most frequently arising without known cause in the condition called *Bell's palsy*. It is often possible to localise the site of damage. Interruption of the facial nerve after its emergence from the stylomastoid foramen may be due to trauma or to lesions of the parotid gland. Characteristically these distal lesions involve only some of the muscles of facial expression on the appropriate side. Involvement of the facial nerve proximal to its exit from the facial canal causes a paresis of all the muscles. Facial asymmetry will be apparent on inspection with widening of the palpebral fissure and flattening of the facial groove. However where a facial palsy has been present for some time the muscles undergo shortening and contracture and the nasolabial fold and other facial markings may be more deeply etched than on the normal side. Therefore, the diagnosis of facial nerve palsy should not be made without asking the patient to move the facial muscles.

One diagnostically useful sign is an exaggeration of a normal reflex; when the patient attempts to close the eye on the affected side there will be restricted movement of the orbicularis oculi but there is a brisk upward movement of the eyeball, often to such an extent that the pupil becomes completely hidden under the eyelid. This (Bell's phenomenon) occurs only in lesions of the seventh nerve and is not a feature of upper motor neurone facial weakness.

The site of lesions within the facial canal can be

assessed (Fig. 8.16). Lesions below the chorda tympani will only cause facial palsy. In lesions above the chorda tympani there will be additional loss of taste over the anterior two thirds of the tongue and diminished salivation. Proximal to the nerve to stapedius, hyperacusis in the ear on the same side is added to the other features; such is the picture presented by lesions of the geniculate ganglion. Affection of the geniculate ganglion is rare and in nearly all cases is due to herpes zoster. Damage to the facial nerve in the most proximal part of the facial canal is uncommon. When it occurs defective lacrimation is added to the manifestations of more distal lesions.

Within the *cerebello-pontine angle* lesions of the seventh nerve, together with the nervus intermedius, are often accompanied by signs of damage to some or all of the eighth, fifth and sixth nerves as well as by cerebellar disturbance. *Pontine lesions* of the seventh nerve affect only its motor component and usually cause a concurrent sixth nerve palsy on the same side together with contralateral upper motor neurone signs (Fig. 8.59 p. 250), due to involvement of the pyramidal tract.

Bilateral facial weakness due to neural lesions is uncommon. Both motor nuclei may be implicated in motor neurone disease causing a bulbar palsy and a few generalised polyneuropathies may extend to involved both seventh nerves. Guillain-Barré syndrome, an immunologically-precipitated, demyelinating polyneuropathy, has a predilection for the facial nerves.

Facial muscles. Mysathenia gravis tends to affect facial muscles variably with facial weakness and the attendant dysarthria becoming more apparent as the patient uses the facial muscles and as the day wears on. *Myopathic weakness* of the face is bilateral and symmetrical; pouting of the lips, a transverse smile, and flattening of the facial creases on both sides present a characteristic picture. In almost all instances muscles other than the facial muscles will also be affected.

The vestibulocochlear (eighth cranial) nerve

The eighth cranial nerve comprises two components — auditory fibres which arise from the cochlea and vestibular fibres which arise from the otolith organs (saccule and utricle) and semi-circular canals. The functions of these two distinct elements are considered separately.

The cochlear (auditory) division. Sound waves are normally conducted by air to the ear but they may also be transmitted through bone if a vibrating object is in contact with the skull. Central processes from the cochlea within the inner ear enter the skull through the internal auditory meatus near to the facial nerve, pass through the cerebello-pontine angle to enter the brain stem, eventually to synapse in the cochlear nuclei in the lower pons. Second order fibres ascend in the lateral lemnisci of both sides. There are side connections to cell groups such as the superior olive but most fibres pass to the medial geniculate body. Thence the final sensory relay is conveyed in the auditory radiations to the anterior transverse temporal gyrus which is the auditory receptive area; each receptive area receives impulses from both ears.

The vestibular division. The end organs of the vestibular nerves are situated in the semicircular canals and in the utricle and saccule. Fibres are thence carried to the cells of origin in the vestibular ganglia in the internal auditory meatus whose central processes form the vestibular nerve. This passes through the internal auditory meatus in company with the cochlear nerve to enter the upper medulla. The vestibular fibres terminate on the vestibular nuclei whence a new relay of fibres runs to the medial longitudinal bundles of both sides, establishing communications with the third, fourth and sixth nerve nuclei. There is a major connection from the vestibular nuclei to the vermis of the cerebellum. Some fibres pass from the nuclei downwards into the spinal cord to form the vestibulospinal pathway. The vestibular system coordinates the motor reflexes which maintain equilibrium and make the postural adjustments occasioned by movements of the eyes, head and body. Some vestibular information also makes its way to the posterior temporal lobes where it contributes to the awareness of body position and movement.

Examination

The cochlear component. The findings on auriscopic examination of the external ear passages and of the drums (p. 61) are relevant to the assessment of hearing. This should be tested in each ear in turn by whispering to the patient whose eyes are closed and whose other ear is occluded by finger pressure on the tragus. Normally a whisper can be heard at a distance of three metres. A wristwatch or rubbing of the forefinger and thumb together beside the patient's ear provide alternative stimuli.

If there is some impairment of hearing the next step is to determine whether this results from a lesion within the external auditory meatus or middle ear, i.e. conduction deafness, or whether it is due to a defect of the cochlea or its nerve, i.e. perceptive or nerve deafness. Normally air conduction of sound is more efficient than bone conduction, but when there is conduction deafness, the reverse is the case. A *tuning fork* may be used to make the differentiation (*Rinne's test*). A vibrating fork (256 or 512 cycles per second) is held close to the external auditory meatus. Its base is then pressed against the mastoid bone (Fig. 8.18). The patient is asked which of these two stimuli seems to be the louder.

Weber's lateralising test provides supplementary information (Fig. 8.19). The vibrating tuning fork

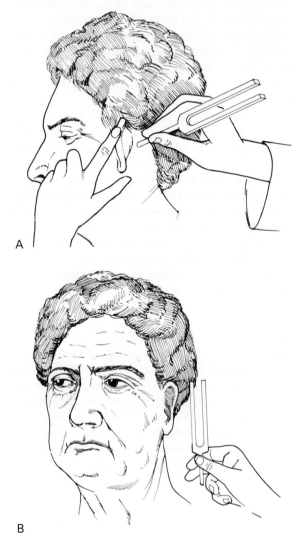

Fig. 8.18   Rinne's test. (A) Bone conduction. (B) Air conduction.

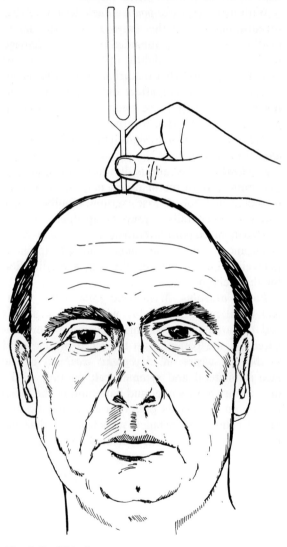

Fig. 8.19   Weber's test.

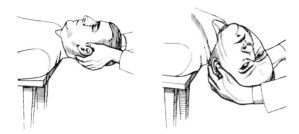

Fig. 8.20 Testing for positional nystagmus.

is applied to the midline of the forehead and the patient is asked whether the sound is heard in the midline or whether it seems to come from one or other ear. Normally the sound appears to arise in the midline. If there is damage to the cochlea or its neural connections the sound will be perceived less well on the affected side and will appear to arise on the healthy side. If there is a lesion in the middle ear or blockage of the meatus, the sound is referred to the affected ear.

Audiometry. Patients with defective hearing should be assessed by audiometry which measures the degree of hearing loss at different sound frequencies. Pure tone audiometry combined with speech discrimination audiometry will differentiate neural deafness from conductive deafness.

Vestibular function. This cannot effectively be evaluated at the bedside, but *positional nystagmus* may be sought. The patient is asked to lie on the back, with the shoulders at the end of the couch (Fig. 8.20). The head, projecting beyond the couch, is supported by the examiner's hands; the head is then fully extended and turned to one side. The patient's eyes should remain open. Nystagmus is not seen in normal people. When present, it may develop immediately or up to ten seconds after the head has been positioned and may persist or disappear spontaneously after about a minute. Nystagmus which appears and then subsides spontaneously indicates a lesion of the otolith organs in the ear which lies inferiorly. Positional nystagmus of this 'peripheral' type is usually accompanied by marked vertigo. Nystagmus which persists usually indicates a lesion affecting the brain stem or cerebellum. After a short interval the test should be repeated with the head extended and rotated to the other side.

Interpretation

Damage to the cochlear part of the eighth nerve results in diminished hearing and tinnitus. *Tinnitus* is a subjective awareness of noise, such as a hissing. The noise may be high or low pitched and often seems to be originating in the affected ear. Lesions of the vestibular pathways give rise to an abnormal sensation of movement — vertigo. In many instances both components of the eighth nerve are affected together, as in Ménière's syndrome characterised by a combination of tinnitus, deafness and vertigo associated with a progressive dilatation and oedema of the cochlea and the vestibular parts of the labyrinth.

Deafness. Conduction deafness most frequently results from chronic otitis media or from blockage of the external meatus by wax. Perceptive deafness most often has its origin in the cochlea as a result of aging processes, damage from measles, from antibiotics such as gentamicin, or from trauma. A blow, blast injury or noise of high intensity may cause deafness particularly for high frequency sounds.

Vertigo. This may result from a large number of conditions of which the vast majority affect the labyrinth itself or the most peripheral part of the vestibular nerve. In almost all cases these peripheral lesions also involve the cochlea or its nerve; a notable exception to this rule is vestibular neuronitis in which a viral infection causes intense vertigo without deafness or tinnitus.

Vertigo may be due to lesions of the cerebellum and is then usually not associated with auditory loss or with tinnitus. In general, bouts of vertigo, separated by periods of normality, are due to labyrinthine lesions. If paroxysms of vertigo are accompanied by persistent ataxia the lesion probably lies centrally, in the brain stem or cerebellum. In labyrinthine lesions nystagmus is often prominent only during attacks of vertigo and in general the degree of nystagmus is proportional to the vertiginous disturbance. In central lesions affecting the brain stem or cerebellum there is often persistent nystagmus with relatively slight vertigo.

Peripheral lesions. Assessment of lesions of the cochlear and vestibular divisions of the eighth nerve in its peripheral path requires specialised knowledge and apparatus and includes audiometry, caloric testing with nystagmography, electrocochleography and evoked potential audiometry (p. 242).

Central lesions. In the cerebello-pontine angle the commonest lesion is a neuroma of the eighth nerve itself causing tinnitus followed by deafness and occasionally vertigo. Neoplasms of the fifth nerve, meningiomas and tumours arising from the cerebellum may also affect structures in the cerebello-pontine angle where space occupying lesions are often accompanied by cerebellar ataxia, facial palsy, or sensory disturbances of the fifth nerve and, later, raised intracranial pressure.

Perceptive deafness on the same side as the lesion may result from damage to the brain stem by such conditions as infarcts of the pons or plaques of multiple sclerosis. In most instances intrinsic lesions of the brain stem will be accompanied by other cranial nerve disturbances as well as by long tract signs.

Since auditory impulses are relayed to both temporal lobes unilateral damage to the cortical auditory receptive area usually produces only very transient impairment of hearing. However, vertigo is a relatively common symptom in temporal lobe epilepsy.

The glossopharyngeal (ninth cranial) nerve

The motor part of this nerve arises in the nucleus ambiguus in the medulla and in company with the tenth and eleventh cranial nerves leaves the skull through the jugular foramen. The ninth nerve supplies the stylopharyngeus muscle which elevates the upper pharynx, in combination with the palatopharyngeal muscle which is supplied by the tenth nerve.

The glossopharyngeal nerve contains a large sensory component which transmits common sensation from part of the lining of the tympanic cavity and the Eustachian tube. It also carries pain fibres from the pharynx and the tonsillar region and general afferent sensation from the posterior third of the tongue, the soft palate and the uvula. These sensory fibres run back through the medulla; those subserving touch terminate in the solitary nucleus in the medulla and pain fibres end in the nuclei of the fifth nerve. The glossopharyngeal nerve conveys taste from the posterior third of the tongue and these fibres terminate in the solitary nucleus. The ninth nerve also transmits impulses from chemoreceptors and baroreceptors in the carotid body and sinus. It conveys parasympathetic fibres to the parotid gland and partially supplies the submaxillary and sublingual salivary glands.

Examination

Sensory functions. Many of the functions of the glossopharyngeal nerve are intermingled with those of the tenth cranial nerve. Taste on the posterior third of the tongue can be tested in isolation but only with great difficulty. Taste in this area is most conveniently, though rarely, tested by applying a weak electric current to the back of the tongue. This normally evokes an acid taste if sensation is intact.

The sensory supply to the posterior third of the tongue and the pharynx can be tested by touching these areas with the point of a long pin or a wooden stick. The procedure is unpleasant and should be performed only when it is important to define ninth function exactly.

Reflexes. Touching the posterior wall of the pharynx evokes its constriction and elevation. This is the 'gag' reflex whose afferent arm is the glossopharyngeal nerve and whose efferent path is the vagus nerve. It may occasionally be absent in normal people. When there is no reflex response the patient should be asked if the pharyngeal stimulus is felt, in order to differentiate interruptions of the afferent or efferent limb of the reflex arc. A similar reflex arc supplies the *palatal reflex*. When the soft palate is touched it moves upwards. When testing these reflexes the stimulus should be applied to each side in turn.

Motor functions. These cannot be tested satisfactorily since paralysis of the stylopharyngeus muscle is not manifest clinically if tenth nerve function is intact.

Interpretation

Lesions of the ninth nerve are extremely rare in isolation. It may be implicated by lesions at the base of the skull such as fractures or invasive tumours but usually other cranial nerves will be involved. Glossopharyngeal neuralgia is the most important condition solely affecting the ninth nerve. This is felt in the back of the throat and resembles trigeminal neuralgia in its lancinating character, in its episodic occurrence and in the absence of any detectable disturbance of ninth nerve function.

The vagus (tenth cranial) nerve

The motor part of the vagus nerve originates in the nucleus ambiguus of the medulla which it leaves in a series of rootlets adjacent to the glossopharyngeal nerve. It passes through the jugular foramen to the neck, chest and abdomen, supplying motor fibres to the soft palate, the pharynx and, via its recurrent laryngeal branch, to all the intrinsic muscles of the larynx.

The tenth nerve conveys sensory impulses from the dura mater of the floor of the posterior cranial fossa and from part of the external auditory meatus. These sensory fibres, after they enter the medulla, pass to the fifth nerve nucleus. Tactile impulses from the pharynx are also conveyed in the vagus to the fifth nerve nucleus. The vagus has extensive afferent and efferent connections with the heart, lungs and gut.

Examination

Clinical examination of the tenth cranial nerves includes close attention to the patient's *speech*. Lesions of the vagus nerve or its recurrent laryngeal branch may give rise to dysphonia (p. 192); interruption of its motor fibres, by paralysing the palate, will give a nasal quality to the voice.

The *soft palate* should be inspected. In bilateral lesions of the tenth nerves the whole soft palate droops; in a unilateral palsy there will be drooping of one side of the soft palate, the uvula being deviated to the normal side (Fig. 8.21). The patient should be asked to sustain phonation by uttering a prolonged 'Ah' and palatal movements should be observed whilst doing so. In bilateral palsies the palate will not elevate and in unilateral lesions one side of the palate remains immobile, and the uvula moves towards the normal side. Movement of the posterior pharyngeal wall should

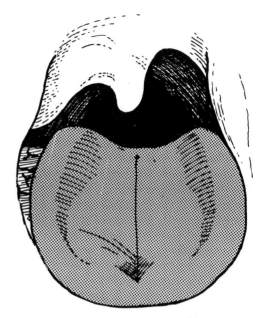

Fig. 8.21 Right tenth nerve palsy.

be observed during phonation. If one side is paralysed it tends to move laterally, like a curtain, towards the normal side. The palatal and pharyngeal reflexes should be examined (p. 212).

In the presence of dysphonia or whenever a lesion of the tenth nerve is suspected, the *vocal cords* should be inspected (p. 135).

Interpretation

Unilateral lesions of the tenth cranial nerve occur at the base of the skull as a result of fractures, tumours or chronic basal meningitis, and the adjacent ninth and eleventh nerves are usually also implicated. Isolated lesions of the vagus nerve are uncommon but its *laryngeal branch* may be damaged in the neck by trauma or by malignant tumours. Inoperable bronchial carcinoma is the most common cause of a left recurrent laryngeal palsy. Abductor vocal cord palsy is often the earliest sign of recurrent laryngeal nerve palsy. Later the adductors are also affected and the cord lies in the midway position between abduction and adduction. In a unilateral palsy the voice is usually hoarse but the degree of dysphonia is variable since compensatory movements by the unaffected cord across the midline mitigate the disability. If the palsy is bilateral and partial the cords do not abduct on inspiration so giving rise to inspiratory stridor. When there is complete interruption of both recurrent laryngeal nerves, the cords rest in the cadaveric position and cannot abduct or adduct. Phonation is thus impossible; if asked to cough, the patient cannot build up intrathoracic pressure by closing the cords and thus produces a 'bovine' cough which is a prolonged, low-pitched noise, without the explosive quality of a normal cough. Isolated paralysis of the adductors of the cords is usually bilateral and of hysterical origin. The patient loses voice volume but can talk in a whisper. There is no respiratory disturbance and the cough has its normal explosive quality, indicating that the adductors can in fact function normally.

Bilateral tenth nerve lesions are seen as part of true bulbar palsy and bilateral supranuclear affection of the structures innervated by the tenth nerve contribute to the picture of supranuclear bulbar palsy (p. 215).

The spinal accessory (eleventh cranial) nerve

The major part of the eleventh cranial nerve derives from the anterior horn cells of the first to the fourth cervical segments. Fibres leave the lateral aspect of the cord and ascend, uniting as they course upwards with fibres from higher cervical segments. Eventually the spinal part of the nerve enters the skull through the foramen magnum. Within the skull the nerve is joined by its smaller cranial component which arises in the medulla. The two constituents separate as they leave the skull through the jugular foramen. The spinal accessory nerve again descends into the neck where it supplies the sternomastoid and the upper half of the trapezius muscles. The lower half of trapezius obtains its nerve supply directly from the third and fourth cervical segments.

Examination

The eleventh cranial nerve is tested by examining the bulk and power of *the sternomastoid and trapezius muscles*. When testing the former both sides can be examined together by asking the patient to press the chin downwards against the

resistance of the examiner's hand. In normal circumstances, both sternomastoids will stand out and can be inspected and palpated. Differences in bulk can quickly be recognised. Each sternomastoid should afterwards be tested by asking the patient to turn the chin against resistance to each side; there will be weakness on turning the head away from the side of a muscle whose strength is impaired.

When examining the upper fibres of the trapezius the patient, standing upright, should be inspected from behind. Wasting of the upper trapezius will produce a flattening of the affected muscle. The vertebral border of the scapula will be displaced away from the spine in its upper part and towards the spine at its lower end. The whole arm droops and hence the finger tips on the involved side reach nearer the ground than do those on the normal side. The power of the trapezius should then be tested by asking the patient to shrug the shoulders against resistance.

Interpretation

Involuntary movements frequently implicate the sternomastoid muscles. Turning movements of the head due to contraction of one sternomastoid may occur as part of the picture of chorea or dystonia. Spasm of the sternomastoid may be a feature of spasmodic torticollis (p. 218) but usually other nearby muscles are also involved.

Upper motor neurone lesions produce only slight weakness of the sternomastoid muscles and cause little disability. However when sternomastoid weakness is found in an upper motor neurone lesion, the muscle ipsilateral to the lesion is affected. This is because the motor programmes represented in the cerebral cortex activate patterns of movement rather than individual muscles. Since the left sternomastoid turns the head to the right side, it is this muscle which is weakened by a left hemisphere lesion. Upper motor neurone weakness of trapezius may be seen as a delay in shoulder elevation when the patient is asked to shrug.

Bilateral lower motor neurone affections of the spinal accessory nerves may occur as part of the picture of true bulbar palsy. Marked weakness on the two sides is manifest by the head falling backwards. Bilateral wasting of the sternomastoid muscles is more often due to a myopathy rather than a neural lesion but the former is itself rare. Myasthenia may cause intermittent weakness of both sternomastoids.

Unilateral lower motor neurone lesions of the eleventh nerve are uncommon and, in isolation, are rare. Lesions of the nerve at the jugular foramen by fractures of the skull, basal meningitis or tumours usually also implicate the ninth, tenth and twelfth nerves. Within the neck, trauma, particularly missile wounds, may damage the nerve.

The hypoglossal (twelfth cranial) nerve

The hypoglossal nerve arises from its nucleus in the medulla which it leaves medial to the ninth, tenth and eleventh nerves. It then passes through the hypoglossal canal into the neck and on via the angle of the mandible to supply all the muscles of the tongue. Each twelfth nerve nucleus receives an upper motor neurone supply from the precentral gyri of both cerebral hemispheres.

Examination

Inspection is the most important aspect of the examination of the tongue which should first be scrutinised as it lies on the floor of the widely opened mouth; it should then be protruded and again carefully inspected. Atrophy is usually easily recognised since the tongue becomes wrinkled and thinner. Spontaneous contractions (fasciculation) of the muscles may be apparent (p. 217). They persist when the tongue is at rest and may also be seen on its underside. Tremors usually are prominent when the tongue is protruded and are much less evident when the tongue is in the mouth.

If there is unilateral weakness of the tongue, it deviates, on protrusion, towards the paralysed side, because of the action of the normal genioglossus (see Fig. 8.22). The patient should be asked to move the tongue in and out and from side to side, slowly and rapidly in turn and then should press the tongue against the cheek whilst the examiner's finger resists the movement by pressure on the outside of the cheek. If there is unilateral paresis there will be an impairment of the ability to move the tongue towards the normal side.

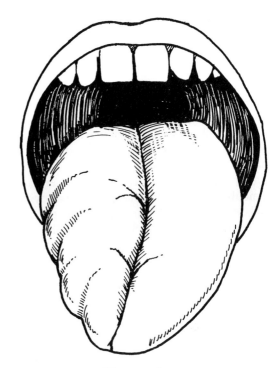

Fig. 8.22 Right twelfth nerve palsy.

Interpretation

Involuntary movements of the tongue may occur. Rapid protrusion and retraction, called a 'trombone' tremor may be seen in parkinsonism. Choreiform movements of the tongue may be a feature of Sydenham's or Huntington's chorea. Irregular and continual rotatory movements of the tongue may be induced by drugs, such as levodopa and the phenothiazines. This possibility should be considered in any patient with oro-facial dyskinesia.

Bilateral upper motor neurone lesions cause the tongue to assume a more conical form and its voluntary movements are sluggish. Bilateral supranuclear lesions are sometimes due to vascular lesions in both internal capsules and they may also result from the generalised degeneration of motor neurone disease. Such supranuclear lesions invariably affect others of the lower cranial nerves and usually also implicate the fifth nerves. This produces the picture of *supranuclear or pseudobulbar palsy*, where dysarthria, dysphonia and dysphagia are accompanied by a spastic, immobile tongue and an abnormally brisk jaw jerk and gag reflex.

Unilateral upper motor neurone lesions above the medulla cause the protruded tongue to be deviated slightly towards the paralysed side. There is no accompanying weakness or fasciculation nor does the slight weakness produce any significant disability. The abnormality is more striking after an acute lesion (e.g. hemisphere stroke) and tends to diminish after a few days.

Bilateral lower motor neurone lesions are most commonly part of a *true bulbar palsy* and will be found in association with weakness of the other motor cranial nerves. Severe disability with dysarthria, dysphagia and dysphonia results. Bilateral wasting of the tongue accompanied by fasciculation is often observed in motor neurone disease and much less frequently may result from poliomyelitis, from tumours or vascular lesions in the medulla, or from syphilis.

Unilateral lower motor neurone lesions of the twelfth nerve are uncommon but may arise occasionally from vascular disease in the medulla or from lesions at the base of the brain such as chronic syphilitic or tuberculous basal meningitis. Tumours arising in the post-nasal space may erode the skull base and implicate the twelfth nerve. Trauma may also damage the nerve and is particularly liable to do so after its exit from the hypoglossal canal. When the twelfth nerve is unilaterally involved by these processes there are usually attendant lesions of ninth, tenth and eleventh cranial nerves.

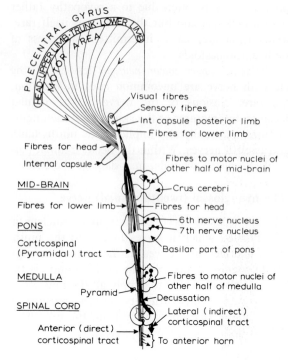

Fig. 8.23   The motor pathways.

THE MOTOR SYSTEM

It is convenient to consider motor and sensory functions separately but precise movements require an intact sensory system as well as a properly functioning motor apparatus. Normal motor activity may be disturbed by:

1. A loss of learned movement patterns. The organised sequences of motor activation which underlie voluntary actions may be impaired in the absence of paralysis. This is called dyspraxia or apraxia.
2. Paralysis or weakness.
3. Impairment of coordination.

4. Changes in tone.
5. Involuntary movements.
6. Hypokinesis.

The motor pathways are shown in Figure 8.23. Assessment of motor function includes detailed inspection, and examination of tone, power, coordination and fine movements. In some cases more specialised tests designed to reveal dyspraxia may also be employed.

Inspection

Careful inspection is an important aspect of the examination of the motor system which may reveal the nature of the patient's disability.

Posture. The posture of the patient should be noted. The distinctive hemiplegic picture resulting from intracranial lesions of the pyramidal pathways is the posture of unilateral *decorticate rigidity*; the affected arm is flexed and adducted across the chest with the leg on the same side stiffly extended (Fig. 9.3). The features of *decerebrate rigidity* are extension of the neck, back and legs; the arms are internally rotated, adducted and extended except at the wrist where they are flexed. Such a posture immediately suggests the presence of a lesion of the motor pathways in the mid-brain. Flexion at neck, hip, knee and elbow presents a posture characteristic of parkinsonism. A patient suffering from this disease may, when lying, hold the head above the pillow for long periods.

Muscle wasting. Differences in bulk between corresponding muscle on the two sides of the body may provide valuable clues to the presence of wasting or atrophy but the dominant arm and hand in manual workers often show disproportionate muscle hypertrophy. This is illustrated by the marked increase in size of muscles in the racket arms of professional tennis players. The assessment of wasting should include comparisons of the relative affection of proximal and distal parts of limbs. In most instances muscle wasting is more easily and more certainly detected by inspection than with a tape measure.

Fasciculation. In wasting muscles it is often possible to see fasciculation. This is produced by the spontaneous contractions of large groups of muscle fibres or of whole motor units. The contractions commonly occur sporadically and successively involve different parts of the muscle. The movements are usually of fine amplitude. Fasciculation suggests a lower motor neurone lesion lying proximally near the anterior horn cells as in motor neurone disease. It is not always present when there is denervation.

Sometimes fasciculations are seen in normal people. In such instances the movements are not associated with muscle wasting and are usually rather coarser and tend to affect the same area of muscle in the thighs or the thenar eminences after unwonted exercise. A similar phenomenon

(myokymia) may cause spasmodic contractions of the orbicularis oculi, levator palpebrae superioris or other facial muscles. This is a benign condition commonly produced by fatigue and anxiety. Benign fasciculation and myokymia are liable to arouse fears in medical students and doctors who may interpret them as having sinister significance.

Voluntary movements. Clumsy movements of the hands may imply incoordination or dyspraxia. Delay in initiation of movements and reduction in their amplitude once initiated will suggest extrapyramidal hypokinesis. The complete lack of use of one limb or of one side of the body may indicate the presence of a monoplegia or a hemiplegia.

Involuntary movements. There should be a careful inspection and analysis of any involuntary movements, of which tremors are the commonest.

Tremors are defined as rhythmic movements resulting from alternating contraction and relaxation of groups of muscles. In the limbs, where they are usually seen, tremors produce oscillations about a joint or group of joints. When a tremor is observed its rate and amplitude should be estimated and the directions of movements analysed. The tremor most frequently seen is rapid and fine in amplitude and is an exaggeration of normal physiological tremor. All apparently smooth movements are underlain by a tremor whose rate is 10 per second in adults. This oscillation can be demonstrated by amplication; if a large sheet of paper is laid over the outstretched hand of a healthy subject it will be seen that the edges of the paper are in continuous fine movement. If normal physiological tremor is increased in amplitude it becomes visible to the naked eye. This is often seen in anxious patients, in hyperthyroidism, in alcoholics and in those who over-indulge in tea,

Table 8.1 Types of tremor

Name	Frequency	Examples	Rest	Posture	Movement
Action (or postural)	10 Hz	Hyperthyroidism Anxiety and fatigue	−	+	+
Intention	5 Hz	Cerebellar		+	+ +
Resting	5 Hz	Parkinsonism	+ +	±	±

coffee, tobacco and other drugs (Table 8.1). A slow, coarse tremor is a cardinal feature of parkinsonism and characteristically involves a beating of the thumb towards the index finger. In its fully developed form it is of 'pill-rolling' type when the thumb runs across the tips of all the fingers. Parkinsonian tremor is reduced during a voluntary movement. Intention tremor is described on page 222 and flapping tremor on page 47.

Myoclonus is a term used to describe sudden shock-like contractions which involve one or more muscles or a whole limb. Myoclonic jerks may occur singly or repetitively. They may occur in a normal person. They are common in generalised epilepsy and when falling asleep but also are an uncommon manifestation of some degenerative diseases of the brain.

Choreiform movements are irregular, jerky, semi-purposive and ill-sustained. They tend to move from one part of the musculature to another in quick succession. This distinguishes choreiform movements from the much commoner *tic* or *habit spasm*. The tic of an individual is a repetitive, stereotyped movement. The same movement, even if complex, is repeated over and over again. Facial grimaces are frequently encountered.

Hemiballismus is similar to choreiform movement but is more proximal and much greater in amplitude and more forceful. There are violent flail-like, throwing movements of the limbs which, as the name implies, are usually unilateral. These tend to occur acutely as the result of vascular damage to the sub-thalamic nucleus.

Athetoid spasms are slow writhing movements principally affecting the distal parts of limbs. Many extrapyramidal diseases lead to involuntary movements which are both choreiform and athetoid in type.

Dystonic movements (sometimes called *torsion spasms*) are similar to athetoid movements but tend to affect the proximal part of the limb or the trunk so that turning, twisting movements of the trunk or limbs occur.

Spasmodic torticollis is a common type of involuntary movement, representing a segmental form of dystonia and usually comprises repetitive, rotatory movements of the head and neck to one side, sometimes accompanied by extension of the neck.

Palpation

Palpation of muscles may sometimes give information of value. Muscles may be tender in inflammatory conditions (myositis). Palpation of the apparently large muscles in the Duchenne type of dystrophy reveals the doughy consistency of fatty infiltration (pseudo-hypertrophy) rather than the elastic feel of normal muscle tissue. In some forms of acute muscle necrosis (e.g. alcoholic rhabdomyolysis) the muscles may have a firm 'woody' consistency. Palpation of the bulk of a fully contracted muscle is sometimes useful in confirming minor degrees of wasting suspected on inspection.

Examination of tone

Tone, for clinical purposes, may be defined as the resistance felt when a joint is moved passively. In normal people who are relaxed the manipulation of a joint evokes a slight, elastic resistance from the adjacent muscles. The degree of this normal tension can be gauged only by repeated examination and abnormalities in tone are often difficult to evalue.

The patient should lie supine with the head and neck resting in the neutral position, comfortably upon a pillow. Time must be spent, if necessary, in achieving the cooperation and relaxation of the patient. It may help to ask the patient to 'go floppy'. The elbow joint and the wrist, hip, knee and ankle should then be put through a full range of passive movements. The knee, for instance, should always be put into a position of full extension and then flexed (Fig. 8.24A). Each of these joints should first be manipulated rapidly and then more slowly. It is a useful preliminary, having got the patient relaxed, to grasp the forearm and shake the upper limb gently. The resulting passive movements at the wrist joints can then be observed. This is a valuable way of checking that the patient is relaxed as well as providing information about the muscle tone around the wrist. A similar manoeuvre can be employed in the legs. The patient's leg, supported on the bed, should be grasped below the knee and the leg gently rocked from side to side. The evoked passive movements of the ankle are observed (Fig. 8.24B). Any local

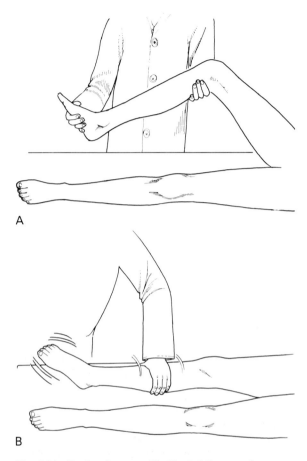

Fig. 8.24 Testing for tone. (A) Check full range of movement at the knee. (B) Rock the relaxed leg to and fro.

lesion such as arthritis should be excluded before ascribing neurological significance to increased resistance to joint movements. Tone may be increased (hypertonia) or decreased (hypotonia).

Hypertonia. There are two distinct types, spasticity and rigidity. Spasticity accompanies upper motor neurones lesions. It is characterised by a rapid build-up in resistance during the first few degrees of passive movement and then, as the movement continues, there is a sudden lessening of resistance. This phenomenon is likened to the sensations encountered when opening a clasp knife and is called 'clasp-knife spasticity'. It is much more commonly and more easily detected in passive movements of the knee joint than it is in the upper limbs. Spasticity is generally more marked on passive extension (as opposed to flexion) of the elbow.

Rigidity is the term used to describe sustained resistance to passive movement. This phenomenon occurs in diseases of the basal ganglia and is similar to the sensation produced by bending a lead-pipe. It is variously referred to as lead-pipe, plastic or extrapyramidal rigidity. When tremor is superimposed on rigidity the resistance to passive movement is jerkily increased. This is called cogwheel rigidity and is commonly felt in parkinsonism. Extrapyramidal and cogwheel rigidity are most easily detected at the wrist when relatively slow manipulation is employed.

Hypotonia. This is usually hard to assess. Decreased resistance is difficult to distinguish from good relaxation. A more useful sign of hypotonia in the arms is a change in posture. When a patient suffering from rheumatic chorea (which is attended by hypotonia) is asked to stretch out the hands and spread the fingers it will be found that the wrists are flexed and the metacarpophalangeal joints are hyperextended giving rise to the so-called 'dinner fork' deformity.

Associated features. Alterations in tone may only achieve clinical significance because there are associated features such as clonus and increased tendon reflexes.

Clonus. This is the term applied to a rhythmic series of involuntary muscular contractions evoked by a sudden stretch of muscle. A few beats of clonus are commonly elicited in nervous patients, especially in the calf, and may not be significant. Sustained clonus, i.e. contractions which continue as long as stretch is applied, reflects exaggerated tendon reflexes as a result of damage to the upper motor neurones and is a 'hard' neurological sign. Clonus is most commonly evoked at the knee and ankle joints. Patellar clonus is elicited by sharply pushing the patella towards the foot whilst the patient lies supine and relaxed with his knee ex-

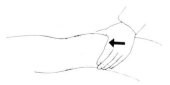

Fig. 8.25 Testing for knee clonus.

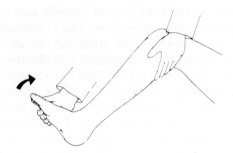

Fig. 8.26   Testing for ankle clonus.

tended and supported by the bed as illustrated in Figure 8.25. Clonus at the ankle is produced by a firm dorsiflexion of the foot with the leg in the position shown in Figure 8.26.

Testing of power

There are two methods by which muscle power can be tested. *Isometric testing* involves asking the patient to contract a group of muscles as powerfully as possible, and then to maintain that position whilst the examiner tries to restore the part to its original position. Alternatively the patient may be asked to put a joint through a full range of movement using maximal power whilst the examiner opposes the movement. This is *isotonic testing*. Both methods are effective; many clinicians employ either technique at will. To detect minor degrees of weakness isotonic testing is more sensitive than the isometric method. Any variability and undue fatiguability of muscle power should be noted.

The testing of power should not degenerate into an unseemly trial of strength between the patient and the examiner. Assessment of muscle power relies on the patient's co-operation, and is therefore partly subjective. Sudden changes in power should alert the examiner to variable effort by the patient, and suggest a non-organic explanation.

Major movements. In most instances it is necessary only to test the power of movements of major joints. It is recommended that a regular routine be followed. One satisfactory sequence is first to test the power of flexion and extension of

the neck; then abduction and adduction, flexion and extension of the shoulders should be examined. Flexion and extension at the elbow, flexion and extension of the wrist, pronation and supination of the forearm, abduction and adduction of the fingers, the power of opposition of thumb and little finger and the power of the hand grip should be assessed.

Trunk muscles should be tested by examining the power of flexion and extension and of lateral flexion of the trunk against gravity and against resistance. The muscles of the anterior abdominal wall may best be examined by asking the supine patient to raise the head from the pillow against resistance. Whilst the patient performs this manoeuvre the abdominal muscles should be observed and palpated. If upper or lower segments of the rectus abdominis are weak, the umbilicus will be drawn away from the weakened muscles.

In the lower limbs, flexion, extension, abduction and adduction of the hips, flexion and extension of the knees, dorsiflexion and plantar flexion, inversion and eversion of the ankles and flexion and extension of the toes should be tested.

Individual muscles. If there is localised weakness or wasting a more detailed examination of appropriate individual muscles should be made. The evaluation of muscle power should be recorded quantitatively using the grading recommended by the Medical Research Council, viz:

0 — No active contraction
1 — Visible or palpaple contraction without active movement
2 — Movement which is possible with gravity eliminated
3 — Movement which is possible against gravity
4 — Movement which is possible against gravity plus resistance but which is weaker than normal
5 — Normal power

Sensitivity can be improved by sub-dividing grade 4 into 4+, 4, and 4–.

The methods by which the actions of individual muscles are tested, details of motor nerve distribution and the segmental derivation of nerves need to be known. These details are described in *Aids to the examination of the peripheral nervous system*

(Ballière Tindall). Examples of the testing of individual muscles are given on page 267.

Significance of loss of power. Weakness may result from generalised loss of muscle tissue associated with some systemic or metabolic disease. Myopathic weakness is often most evident in the proximal limb musculature. Myasthenia gravis produces loss of power which fluctuates in severity and which can be improved transiently by the intravenous injection of edrophonium. Weakness due to lower motor neurone lesions is attended by wasting of muscles. The pattern of weakness produced by lower motor neurone lesions may conform to the distribution of one or more peripheral nerves or of motor roots. Systematised affection of lower motor neurones as in motor neurone disease tends to produce weakness which is often distal and is usually symmetrical.

Damage to upper motor neurones causes weakness of movements not of individual muscles and tends to affect whole limbs. Paresis of one limb (monoplegia) usually results from a lesion near the motor cortex (Fig. 8.23). A hemiplegia is commonly caused by interruption of the upper motor neurones in the opposite internal capsule where the fibres are closely packed together and all are damaged by quite a small lesion. Pyramidal tract damage at this site or more caudally causes more profound weakness in shoulder abduction, elbow and finger extension and intrinsic hand muscles than in adductors and flexors. In the leg, it is hip and knee flexion and dorsiflexion and eversion of the foot which are most prominent in this 'pyramidal distribution'. Paraparesis, weakness of both legs, is usually caused by lesions in the lower spinal cord. Tetraplegia refers to paralysis of all four limbs and is produced by high spinal cord lesions.

The examination of motor power should assess the presence and severity of weakness and define its distribution to determine the site of the causative lesion.

Coordination

The smooth and accurate performance of purposeful movements requires intact sensory and motor functions as well as efficient control by higher centres. Any lesion which causes weakness may be accompanied by clumsiness but incoordination is particularly prominent in sensory and cerebellar ataxia.

Sensory ataxia. This results from defective proprioception and can to some extent be mitigated by visual control of movements. It is, therefore, exacerbated when the eyes are closed.

Cerebellar ataxia. The posterior lobe of the cerebellum functions as a feed-back centre. The progress of a limb in motion is monitored by proprioceptive information fed to the cerebellum. Through its connections with the motor cortex the cerebellum causes adjustments to be made in patterns of motor activation so that the limb's movements are accurately and smoothly aimed. When this guidance system is disturbed the incoordination thus produced, cerebellar ataxia, is not susceptible to visual compensation.

Testing coordination. A most useful test of coordination in the arm is the *finger-nose test*. The patient is asked to hold an arm outstretched and then to touch the tip of the nose with the tip of the index finger (Fig. 8.27). A variation on this test which renders it more sensitive requires patients to touch first the tip of their own nose and then the end of the examiner's index finger held at arm's length away from the patient. The sensitivity of this test may still further be increased if the examiner moves the index finger from place to place whilst the patient's finger is en route to it. An alternative manoeuvre is the *finger-to-finger test* in which the patient is asked to extend and abduct the arms fully and then to bring the tips of the index fingers through a wide circle to the midline until they are separated by about a quarter of an inch. The smoothness and accuracy of movements

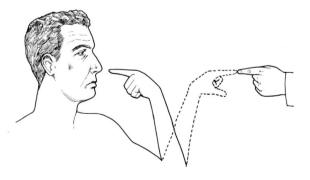

Fig. 8.27 The finger-nose test.

are observed. The patient with sensory ataxia may perform smoothly when the eyes are open but performance will markedly deteriorate when the eyes are closed due to loss of awareness of the position of the limbs in space. In cerebellar ataxia movements are clumsy and jerky (dyssynergia). The patient may overshoot the target (dysmetria). If a movement is attempted with the eyes closed, the finger overshoots towards the side of the cerebellar lesion (past pointing). *Intention tremor* is most characteristic of damage to the posterior lobe of the cerebellum. Here the patient's hand is steady at rest but develops a tremor of increasing amplitude as it approaches its target.

In the lower limb the patient is asked to perform the *heel-shin test* by placing one heel on the opposite knee and then sliding the heel accurately down the front of the shin to the ankle and back again (Fig. 8.28). This test too can be made more sensitive by first making the patient raise a leg to touch the examiner's index finger with the great toe before proceeding to perform the heel-shin test.

Rapid alternating movements are rendered irregular in force and rhythm by cerebellar disorders. They may be tested by asking the patient quickly to pronate and supinate the

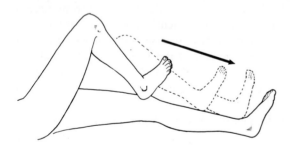

Fig. 8.28 The heel-shin test.

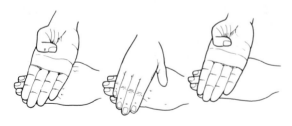

Fig. 8.29 Testing for dysdiadochokinesis.

forearms or quickly and repeatedly to slap one hand alternatively with the front and back of the other hand (Fig. 8.29). Impairment of rapid alternating movements is called *dysdiadochokinesis*. Patients vary widely in their abilities to perform such movements. Most people perform the tests more precisely with the dominant hand and some are very clumsy when using the other hand.

Assessment of fine movements

The examination of the motor system should assess the patient's capacity to carry out small, precise, coordinated finger movements. Such movements are usually the earliest to be affected by lesions of upper motor neurones and may be the last to recover. The hypokinesis associated with diseases of the basal ganglia is often most easily and earliest detected by slowing and poverty of fine finger movements; one of the signs of cerebellar defect is the inability to make rapid movements of the hands.

The most useful and the simplest of the various tests of fine movements is to ask patients, as rapidly as possible, with each hand in turn to make 'piano-playing' individual finger movements. A supplementary test consists of rapidly touching the tips of the little, ring, middle and index fingers successively with the tip of the thumb of the same hand.

The patient should also be observed carrying out those everyday activities which demand precise coordination of finger movements, such as fastening buttons, tying ties and shoe laces.

Testing for dyspraxia and apraxia

Difficulty in the performance of fine movements may have been noted in the absence of incoordination, weakness or sensory defect. This would suggest that the patient has difficulty in formulating and synthesising movement patterns, i.e. suffers from dyspraxia. This can be assessed by asking the patient to pick up small objects from a table, to wind a watch, and to simulate throwing a ball, combing the hair and putting on spectacles. Cutting paper with scissors, tying a knot in a piece of string and folding paper and placing it in an envelope are other examples. These simple tests may be supplemented by constructional tasks such as asking the patient to draw geometrical figures such as a square or a triangle and to make similar figures from matchsticks.

The patient's writing should be examined. Dyspractic patients write slowly and with difficulty. The formation of letters may be incomplete and their size variable; what is written rarely keeps to the horizontal.

Suspected dyspraxia may sometimes be confirmed as patients dress for they may attempt to put their coat on back to front or in extreme instances try to put their trousers on their arms. Bilateral dyspraxia may arise from a lesion in the parietal lobe of the dominant hemisphere. A lesion in the non-dominant parietal lobe may give rise to dressing and constructional dyspraxia or to motor dyspraxia confined to the non-dominant arm and hand. Often the localising of a lesion causing dyspraxia will be facilitated by the presence of other signs of cortical disturbance such as dysphasia (p. 190) or agnosia — loss of the ability to recognise a previously familiar object such as a pen or key. The bizarre nature of dyspractic disturbances may sometimes lead the unwary to make a diagnosis of hysteria.

Summary of examination of the motor system

The examiner should develop an approach which will enable the information outlined above to be elicited with economy of effort and the minimum of duplication of tests. A useful preliminary to the examination of the motor system is to ask the patient to hold the arms out straight with the fingers spread, first with the eyes open and then maintain this position with the eyes closed. Observation of this very simple manoeuvre will often give information which will direct the emphasis of the rest of the examination. Involuntary movements of the arms will be apparent. Abnormal postures may be seen. If one arm tends slowly to drift downwards this will be an indication of paresis of that arm. Intention tremor revealed during the initial examination of the arms may indicate the need to examine other cerebellar functions with care.

In general the scheme for examination of motor function will be applied first to the upper limbs and then repeated in the lower limbs.

1. *Inspection* should take note of posture, of wasting and its distribution, of the presence or absence of fasciculation and of voluntary and involuntary movements.
2. *Tone* should be assessed by passive movement of all joints of the relaxed patient. Attempts should be made to elicit clonus at knee and ankle.
3. *Power* in muscle groups should be tested and if necessary it should be evaluated in individual muscles.
4. *Coordination* and fine movements should be examined and in appropriate instances the patient should be set specialised tests to explore the possibility of dyspraxia.
5. Reflexes should be elicited and compared.

Interpretation of abnormalities of motor function

Examination of motor functions will determine which of the six modes of disturbance considered on page 216 are operative. The next stage in analysis is to decide where the lesion is situated. Motor function may be disrupted at any of seven levels, viz.:

1. **The highest level.** Parts of the cortex of the frontal and parietal lobes are especially concerned with the formulation and storage of patterns of movement. Derangement causes apraxia or dyspraxia.

2. **The level of the upper motor neurone.** This comprises a motor system which originates in cortical neurones whose axonal prolongations run downwards to establish connections with the contralateral motor cranial nerves and through the pyramidal tracts with the lower motor neurones on the opposite side of the spinal cord (Fig. 8.23). Interruption of this system anywhere along its extensive course causes paralysis of movement often in the 'pyramidal distribution' (p. 221), and an increase of tone accompanied by clonus. Attendant reflex changes are discussed on pages 233 to 237.

3. **The level of the lower motor neurone.** This provides a link between the higher motor path-

ways and the final effector apparatus where axons of the anterior horn cells terminate as part of the neuromuscular junctions. Dissolution at this level causes weakness and wasting of those muscles innervated by the damaged lower motor neurones. If there is widespread wasting of muscles in a limb or around a joint then tone may be decreased.

4. *The level of the neuromuscular junction.* This constitutes a communication between the neural motor pathway and the muscle. The electrical impulses carried along the lower motor neurone evoke the release from the neural termination of a transmitting substance, acetylcholine, which causes depolarisation of the muscle membrane. Interference with the chemical transmitter's role causes a variable weakness of muscles, usually unaccompanied by wasting.

5. *The muscular level.* This is the terminal and effector part of the motor pathway. Depolarisation of muscle, biochemically initiated, spreads electrically and causes the muscle fibres to shorten or contract. Impairment of this process leads to weakness which is usually attended by loss and atrophy of fibres.

6. *The cerebellar level.* The cerebellum takes part in a feedback system, processing information about the state of motor activity and by modifying cortical activity adjusts the rate and direction of movements and provides a stable postural base for movements. Disruption at the cerebellar level does not lead to weakness but to incoordinate, imprecise movements including those affecting ocular movements and speech, thereby producing nystagmus and dysarthria. These features sometimes are associated with hypotonia and hyporeflexia.

7. *The extrapyramidal level.* This comprises a complex lattice work of fibres and interspersed nuclear masses running from the cortex to the brain stem whence descending motor fibres pass downwards into the cord to influence lower motor neurone activity. Impairment at this level causes a delay in initiation and a poverty of movement, attended by involuntary movements and alterations in tone.

To localise the level of motor dysfunction supplementary evidence about reflex functions may be required and the process of final synthesis occurs when the whole examination of the nervous system is completed (p. 248).

THE SENSORY SYSTEM

For clinical purposes sensation is divided into:

1. *Exteroception* — Superficial modalities comprising touch, pain and temperature.
2. *Proprioception* — Deep sensations concerned with muscle and joint (or position) sense.
3. *Enteroception* — Visceral sensations largely served by the autonomic nervous system.
4. *Distance reception* — Senses of smell, sound, sight and taste providing information about the distant environment.

Information from all the active sensory pathways is integrated and interpreted in the cerebral cortex.

There is still a divergence of opinion as to whether the different modalities of sensation are subserved by specialised end organs or by end organs which are flexible and which respond to different types of energy. Touch end organs are distributed in a punctate manner over the skin and are activated by pressure which distorts or deforms them. Pain may arise superficially in the skin, from deep structures such as muscles or tendons or from viscera. Pain endings have the capacity to respond to high intensity stimuli of any nature, such as extremes of heat and cold which are potentially damaging to the tissues. Deep pressure and deep pain are probably subserved by end organs similar to those of pain in the skin.

Clinically it is customary to refer to temperature sensation but it seems clear that there are discrete receptors distributed in a punctate manner over the skin, some of which respond to heat and others which respond to a fall in temperature.

Proprioceptive function comprises two components. The first concerns the appreciation of passive movement, and the second an awareness of the position of body parts after movement.

Vibration sense is not a specific sensory modality. Rather, the term refers to discernment of repeated patterns of pressure mediated by end organs in the skin as well as in deeper structures. Vibration sense is analogous to the appreciation of flicker by the visual system. Vibration is felt particularly well through bone which probably serves merely to amplify the stimulus.

Sensations of touch, pressure and position are

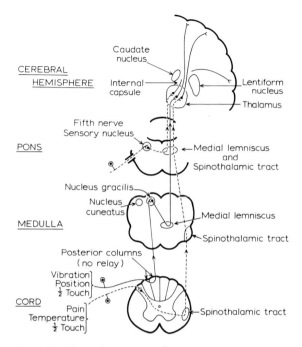

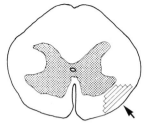
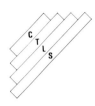

Fig. 8.31 Spinothalamic tract. To show layering of the spinothalamic tract in the cervical region: C represents fibres from cervical segments which lie centrally; fibres from thoracic lumbar and sacral segments (labelled T, L and S respectively) lie progressively more laterally.

Fig. 8.30 The main sensory pathways.

carried in the peripheral nerve in relatively large, fast-conducting afferent fibres. Both pain and temperature modalities are served principally by smaller, slower conducting fibres.

Sensory pathways. The cells of origin of peripheral sensory fibres lie in the dorsal root ganglia whence proximal processes enter the spinal cord via the posterior spinal nerve roots. On entering the cord the fibres separate into two groups which then travel in the spinal cord by two distinct pathways (Fig. 8.30). Some of the fibres which subserve the sensations of touch and light pressure and all of those subserving joint position sense and perhaps all concerned with vibration sense, ascend in the posterior columns to the gracile and cuneate nuclei at the lower end of the medulla. Here second order neurones arise; their fibres decussate and pass upwards through the medial lemniscus to the ventral nucleus of the thalamus.

Fibres which transmit pain and temperature sensation and some of those subserving touch, synapse in the posterior horn, in the cord, near to their point of entry. Thence fibres from second order neurones, cross to the opposite side and ascend in the lateral spinothalamic tract. This tract preserves its laminated structure in its passage up-

wards through the cord. Those fibres from the lowest segments lie outermost in the tract whilst those arising from more proximal segments lie nearer the centre of the cord (Fig. 8.31). Those fibres concerned with touch which cross within the cord lie anteriorly in the anterior spinothalamic tract. The spinothalamic pathways run to the ventral nucleus of the thalamus. From the thalamus third order neurones, transmitting all forms of sensation, pass to the sensory cortex.

Symptoms. The most frequent sensory symptoms are pain, numbness and altered sensation or paraesthesiae. Pain due to neural lesions is often described as burning or stabbing. Lesions of dorsal spinal roots or the dorsal columns may cause sensations of 'tightness' or band-like constrictions in the limbs or trunk. Patients usually describe impairment or loss of sensation as numbness. Paraesthesiae may also be referred to as numbness or as 'pins and needles' by the patient but sometimes the altered or perverted sensation may be more imaginatively interpreted for instance, as a feeling of wet sand on the limbs or of hot water running down the skin.

Patients usually are aware of any significant reduction of temperature sensation. They may know that they can grasp hot objects without discomfort or realise that they burn themselves, or scald themselves in their baths without being alerted by a painful warning.

In many instances patients will be able to delineate the distribution of their sensory symptoms fairly precisely and hence guide the examiner to the areas which need careful examination.

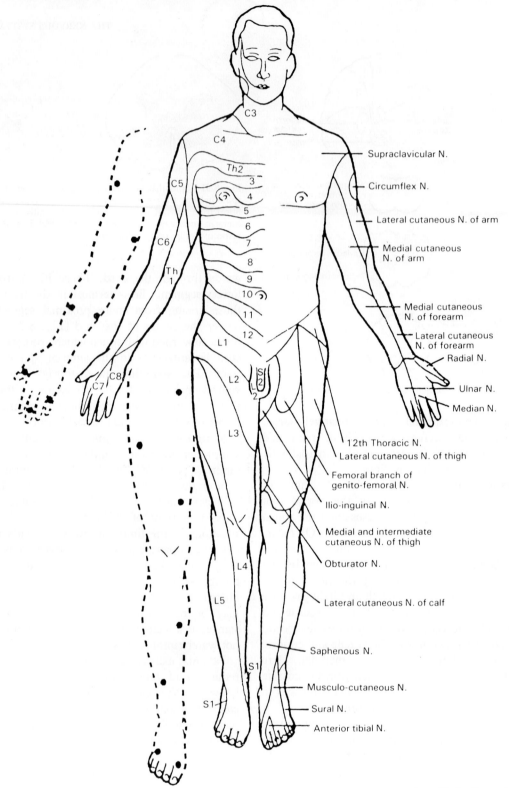

Supraclavicular N.

Circumflex N.

Lateral cutaneous N. of arm

Medial cutaneous
N. of arm

Medial cutaneous
N. of forearm

Lateral cutaneous
N. of forearm

Radial N.

Ulnar N.

Median N.

12th Thoracic N.

Lateral cutaneous N. of thigh

Femoral branch of
genito-femoral N.

Ilio-inguinal N.

Medial and intermediate
cutaneous N. of thigh

Obturator N.

Lateral cutaneous N. of calf

Saphenous N.

Musculo-cutaneous N.

Sural N.

Anterior tibial N.

Fig. 8.32 Segmental and peripheral nerve innervation and points for testing anterior cutaneous sensation of limbs. By applying stimuli at the points marked within the dotted outline both the dermatomal and main peripheral nerve distribution are tested simultaneously.

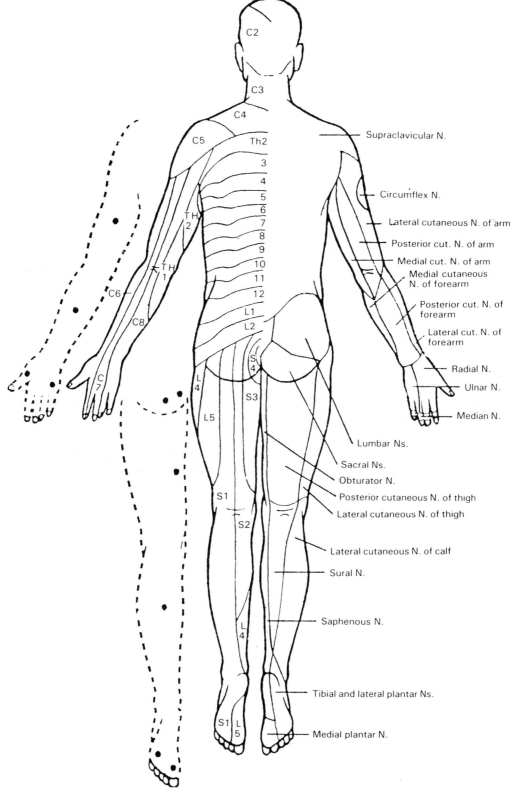

Fig. 8.33 Segmental and peripheral nerve innervation and points for testing posterior cutaneous sensation of limbs. By applying stimuli at the points marked within the dotted outline, both the dermatomal and main peripheral nerve distribution are tested simultaneously.

Examination of sensation

The object of sensory testing is to delineate the extent of sensory impairment and to determine which modalities are involved. It is important to evolve efficient yet time-saving methods of examination. The first competent examination of a patient's sensory system is the one most likely to provide accurate information. Routine testing of cutaneous sensation is relatively easy if the anatomical distribution of sensory nerves is used to determine those points which must be surveyed in order to cover the territories of peripheral nerves as well as posterior nerve roots. These are indicated in Figures 8.32 and 8.33. On the trunk the effects of root lesions are easily identified by the orderly arrangement of dermatomes.

Touch. This is usually tested using a small point of cotton wool which should be laid directly on the skin and not moved over it since moving the wool produces a tickling sensation which is mediated by the pathways for pain rather than those for touch. A light camel hair brush, or a piece of paper can also be used to test touch. The borders of any area of altered sensation should be mapped out. This depends on the patient's responses and it is easier for a patient to detect enhancement of a sensation rather than its diminution. The stimulus should, therefore, be moved from a region of diminished sensation towards normally sensitive areas. In the less common circumstance when sensation in an affected area is abnormally heightened, the stimulus should be moved from the normal into the hypersensitive area. Light touch testing is more reliable if the patient's eyes are closed during the assessment. The patient is asked to report when he feels the cotton wool. The examiner should avoid making touches regularly in time, since the patient may anticipate the stimulus and report it even if it is not felt.

Pain and temperature sensations. These are tested respectively by pin prick and by hot and cold water contained in tubes. The pin should be used gently. Transmission of infection, notably of type B hepatitis and HIV, is a danger if the same pin is used to test sensation in different patients. Disposable, sterile, hypodermic needles, discarded after one examination, obviate this danger but

their sharp edges easily penetrate and lacerate the skin. It is best to use a new, cheap, steel, dressmaker's pin for the sensory testing of each patient.

The patient should be asked, with the eyes closed, to distinguish between stimulation with the point and the head of the pin answering respectively 'sharp' or 'blunt'. The territory of each dermatome, or sensory nerve must be tested with sharp as well as blunt sensation. Patients should also be asked to comment on any heightening or lessening of pain felt as the pin is moved along the trunk or along the limb at the points indicated in Figures 8.32 and 8.33. Temperature sensation is tested only in special circumstances as, for example, if there is reason to suspect dissociated anaesthesia (p. 232). Then hot and cold tubes should be applied in random sequence to the skin; the patient with the eyes closed attempts to distinguish between them. A cruder but readily available bedside test is to assess cold perception using the metal of a tuning fork or similar object.

Deep pain. This is tested by firm squeezing over the muscles and tendons. The patient is asked to indicate when the pressure becomes painful and the examiner gauges whether the force applied would be painful in normal people.

Position sense. The distal part of the limbs are almost always first affected. In the lower limbs it is customary to test position sense first at the terminal interphalangeal joint of the great toe. The proximal phalanx is fixed by grasping it firmly in the finger and thumb of the examiner's left hand. The thumb and forefinger of the right hand grip the terminal phalanx on its lateral borders. Avoiding contact with the second toe because this could indicate the direction of movement (Fig. 8.34). The patient is asked to close the eyes and to indicate when the toe is flexed or extended passively. If the sensation of passive movement is only moderately impaired, the patient may be aware that movement has taken place but will be unable correctly to assess the direction of movement. Many patients will guess and answer 'up' or 'down'. The test, therefore, should be meticulously appraised. When there is gross diminution the movement itself may be undetected. Only if there is impairment of joint position sense peripherally is it necessary to employ additional

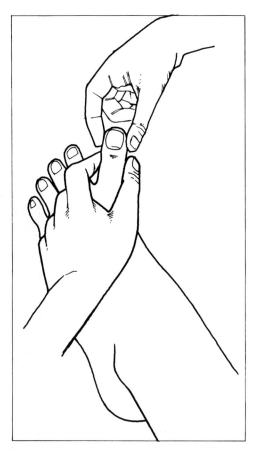

Fig. 8.34 Testing for position sense.

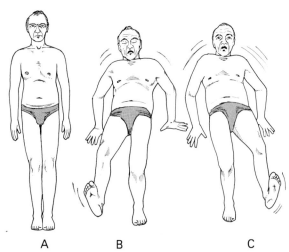

A   B   C

Fig. 8.35 Romberg's test for position sense. The patient can stand with feet together and eyes open (A), but falls with eyes closed (B). In contrast the patient with a cerebellar lesion cannot stand with feet together and eyes open (C).

tests at the ankle and knee. A similar process of testing may be adopted in the upper limbs. The terminal interphalangeal joint of the index finger is first examined and if indicated the proximal joints are studied. It is rare for gross impairment of position sense to be manifest at the hip or shoulder joints.

Concomitant signs of diminished position sense should be assessed. A deterioration in the performance of the finger-nose test (p. 221) when the patient's eyes are closed indicates impaired postural sensibility in the arms. When position sense in an arm is markedly impaired involuntary movements occur in the limb when the patient holds it outstretched with the eyes closed (pseudo-athetosis). These are abolished by visual control of the arm's posture when the eyes are open.

Rombergism may be observed. To demonstrate this phenomenon the patient stands upright with the feet together and eyes closed. If there is loss of postural sensation the patient rocks and sways (Fig. 8.35). Sometimes symptoms suggestive of rombergism are volunteered by patients. They may state that when they close their eyes whilst washing the face they pitch forward against the washbasin or that they are very unsteady when walking in the dark. Such symptoms strongly suggest marked diminution of position sense. Vestibular impairment may cause rombergism in the absence of defective joint position sense. Unsteadiness due to cerebellar deficit will persist when the eyes are open.

Vibration sense. This also is first impaired at the periphery of limbs. The base of a vibrating tuning fork, ideally a weighty one, with a frequency of 128 cycles per second, is placed on the dorsum of the terminal phalanx (Fig. 8.36). The patient is asked to describe the sensation. The test is positive only if the patient is aware of vibration. If there is any doubt it may be necessary to apply the tuning fork sometimes vibrating, sometimes still to the toe. The reliability of the patient's responses can thus be gauged. Minor degrees of impairment may be detected if the examiner's own appreciation of the fork's vibration is used as a yardstick against which to measure the patient's response but vibration sensation is normally

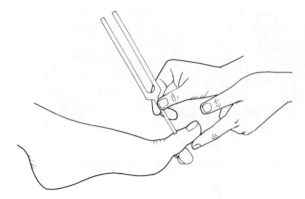

Fig. 8.36 Testing for vibration sensation.

diminished by age. Should vibration sense be lost or impaired distally then the tuning fork should be moved proximally in order to establish the level at which it is appreciated. It is customary to apply the fork to bony prominences; after the dorsum of the terminal phalanx it is placed successively over lateral malleolus, the upper part of the tibia, the iliac crests and if necessary over the costal margin. Similarly in the arm one may proceed from the terminal parts of the fingers to the wrist and the elbow.

Barber's chair sign. A distinctive sensory sign may sometimes be provoked by neck flexion. The patient should be asked to touch the chest with the chin rapidly and to relate any sensations thus evoked. Patients may describe an intense tingling, commonly likened to an electric shock, radiating down the arms, along the spine or down the legs when the head is bent forward. This phenomenon may be volunteered by the patient in the history. It is caused by disruption of the sensory pathways in the mid-cervical region of the spinal cord. The barber's chair sign most commonly occurs in sufferers from multiple sclerosis but it is sometimes a feature of cervical spondylosis, syringomyelia or vitamin B_{12} deficiency or indeed of any lesion in the cervical cord.

Examination of cortical sensory functions

Lesions of the sensory cortex impair the discriminative aspects of sensation. Accurate localisation of stimuli, and the assessment of shape, weight, size and texture of objects are the functions of this highest sensory level. The cortex receives information transmitted by the afferent pathways and then interprets them in the light of previous experience. If there is peripheral disruption of the conducting pathways the tests of the highest sensory level are invalidated. Patients must be able to understand what is required of them during testing and be able to communicate their responses. Intact basic sensations and adequate intellectual and language functions are essential prerequisites for the study of cortical sensory performance. The following tests are employed:

Two point discrimination. This tests the ability to distinguish the contact of two separate points applied simultaneously to the skin. The object is to determine the minimum distance of separation at which two points are identified as two distinct stimuli. Over the finger pulps two points separated by only 3–5 mm are normally so recognised. In the legs a separation of 50–100 mm is required before two discrete stimuli are appreciated and the test is seldom employed there. One or both points of an opened paper clip or preferably of a pair of special dividers, calibrated to show the amount of separation of their blunted points should be applied randomly over the skin of the fingers. The patient, whose eyes are closed, is asked to say if one or two pricks is felt after each stimulation. It is abnormal if the two points need to be separated by more than 5 mm before they are distinguished over the finger pulps, or 40 mm on the soles.

Point localisation. This tests the ability of the patient to localise accurately the point touched with the head of a pin or orange stick when the eyes are closed. The eyes are then opened and a finger placed on the stimulated site. Localisation is more precise at the periphery of limbs than proximally.

Stereognosis. This tests the ability to identify objects by palpation and requires not only intact peripheral sensation but the evocation in the cortex of the constellation of ideas and memories necessary for recognition. Suitable common objects such as a coin, a key, a pen, or a wallet are placed in the patient's hand whilst the eyes are closed. After careful palpation the patient is asked to identify the object.

Identification of textures. This depends on the same mechanism as does stereognosis. A piece of paper, cloth, wood or metal is placed in the hand of the patient who is then asked to identify the nature of the substance from its feel.

Graphaesthesia. This tests the ability to recognise numbers traced by a blunt object on the palm of the hand and, although normally accurate to a surprising degree, is impaired or lost in lesions of the sensory cortex. This test can also be performed on the legs.

Sensory extinction. This tests perception of stimuli at corresponding sites on both sides of the body. It is first necessary to demonstrate that a stimulus, either touch or pin prick, is felt when separately applied to an appropriate point on each side. If like stimuli are delivered, bilaterally and simultaneously, the stimulus may be perceived by the patient only on one side. The test should be repeated several times, the patient's eyes being closed throughout, in order to confirm that the responses are consistent. The stimulus is extinguished, or suppressed on the side opposite that of a lesion in the sensory cortex. This phenomenon is also known as *perceptual rivalry* and it is a feature of parietal lobe dysfunction. It must be re-emphasised that this test is applicable only if cutaneous sensations are preserved on both sides of the body.

Summary of examination of the sensory system

Tests of sensory modalities

Light touch	— cotton wool
Superficial pain	— pin prick
Deep pain	— tendon pressure
Temperature	— warm/cold
Proprioception	— joint position
Vibration	— tuning fork
Cortical localisation	— 2-point discrimination
	— stereognosis
	— graphaesthesia

Interpretation of sensory abnormalities

It may be difficult to decide whether there is significant sensory loss. The intensity of successive stimuli such as pinprick will vary slightly since they are applied by the examiner who cannot deliver identical pressures repeatedly. Some patients will detect and report such minimal variations. Superficial sensation tends to be blunted over the thickened, hard skin of the hands of manual workers, and may appear to be heightened over the face or trunk. Some patients can easily be conditioned to recognise altered sensation in various areas.

Diminution of vibration sense at and below the ankles is a frequent finding in normal elderly people. The perception of deep pain sensation depends partly on the pressure applied to deep tissues by the examiner and partly on the readiness of the patient to interpret the feelings as painful. It follows that an apparent diminution or heightening of deep pain sensation should not be given undue significance. Marked diminution or absence of deep pain, as in tabes dorsalis, can usually be recognised. Excessively tender calf muscles in vitamin B_1 deficiency can also usually be validated by comparison with the patient's responses to similar degrees of pressure applied over the thighs or upper arms.

In general, organic alterations of sensation are consistent and reproducible in their nature, degree and extent. This will help to distinguish between significant and spurious sensory signs. The history is also important. Patients of normal intelligence who have considerable alteration of superficial sensation will volunteer sensory symptoms. The finding of extensive or severe sensory loss in the absense of such symptoms should cause the examiner to review the signs sceptically. Close observation of patients' reactions will often help to confirm their spoken interpretations. When the pricking of a pin crosses the boundary between a cutaneous area wherein pain is diminished to one of normal pain appreciation the transition is usually accompanied by a facial grimace or a withdrawal movement of a limb. Such involuntary responses are strong evidence of organic sensory affection.

Once the extent and nature of sensory loss has been determined the localisation of lesions is comparatively simple.

Peripheral nerves. Lesions of individual peripheral nerves or sensory nerve roots commonly give rise to subjective feelings of numbness and to diminution of all sensory modalities in their areas of distribution (Figs. 8.32 and 8.33). Less commonly, partial lesions of peripheral nerves give rise to pain of a burning, exquisitely unpleasant quality. It is thought that this type of pain is mediated through the slower conducting, smaller pain fibres (p. 225). It is called 'delayed' or 'second' pain to distinguish it from the 'normal', 'first' or 'bright' pain which is conducted at faster rates in the larger pain fibres. This peculiarly unpleasant pain (causalgia) is liable to occur when nerves have been damaged, but not completely disrupted, by trauma. The median and sciatic nerves are vulnerable to this type of reaction. Causalgia is accompanied by diminished sensation in the cutaneous area of the nerve involved and the skin itself may become thin, red and hairless.

Generalised polyneuropathies uncommonly give rise to similarly unpleasant pain in those few instances when smaller pain fibres are relatively spared in the 'burning feet syndrome' sometimes caused by prolonged vitamin B deficiencies. Much more commonly generalised polyneuropathies cause numbness or paraesthesiae. The subjective and objective sensory features then affect the distal parts of limbs and usually involve the legs before the arms. Superficial sensory loss in a polyneuropathy is found over the distal parts of the extremities and extends along the limbs to a level which is uniform around their whole circumference. This is the 'stocking' and 'glove' type of sensory disturbance. Deep sensation, such as proprioception and vibration may be affected in polyneuropathy. If they are significantly impaired in association with glove and stocking anaesthesia it suggests that there is involvement of large sensory fibres, the dorsal root ganglia, or that there is a concurrent affection of the dorsal columns.

Spinal cord. Sensation may be disturbed in several ways by lesions involving the spinal cord. Tumours which compress the cord may also impinge on an adjacent sensory root and hence give rise to diminution of all modalities in the corresponding dermatome. Sensory fibres may be damaged in the dorsal root entry zone, and lesions here also cause sensory loss in segmental dermatomes. The spinal sensory tracts may be interrupted and the level reflected in a loss of sensation at and below the segmental level of the lesion in the cord.

When the spinothalamic pathway is disrupted

there will be a diminution of pain and temperature sensation below the level of the lesion on the opposite side of the body. The upper border of this impairment will not necessarily correspond to the segmental level of the lesion because of the laminated structure of the tract. Such considerations help in the clinical differentiation between intramedullary tumours, which are rarely removable, and extramedullary tumours which may be curable with surgery.

Spinal cord lesions may cause loss of one modality of sensation in an area wherein other modalities are preserved. This is called 'dissociated' sensory loss. Most commonly pain and temperature sensations are lost whilst touch, vibration and position senses are intact. This pattern results from lesions which interrupt the lateral spinothalamic system but do not impinge on the dorsal columns. Dissociated anaesthesia is found in cases of syringomyelia (Fig. 8.56) but may also result from other processes, such as a tumour, damaging the central or lateral parts of the spinal cord.

Intracranial lesions. Within the *lower brain stem* lesions may give rise to impairment of pain and temperature on the ipsilateral side of the face and on the contralateral side of the body (sometimes called alternating analgesia).

Above the pontine level the spinothalamic tract and the medial lemniscus lie close together and are often damaged together. Lesions here which cause sensory impairment affect all modalities on the face, as well as on the body, on the side opposite the lesion. A hemianaesthesia involving the face and body is often due to interruption of the closely-packed sensory radiations in the contralateral *internal capsule*.

Lesions of the *thalamus* may give rise to spontaneous, intense, burning pain on the contralateral side, associated with diminution to touch over the same area. Pain can be provoked on the affected side of the body only by a painful stimulus of greater than normal intensity, i.e. the threshold of painful stimuli is raised. Pain, when thus evoked, has an ill-localised, particularly unpleasant quality.

Damage to the *sensory cortex* does not impair perception of pain, temperature and touch but causes a loss of discriminatory and correlative sensory appreciation.

EXAMINATION OF THE REFLEXES

A neurological reflex depends on an arc which consists of an afferent pathway triggered by stimulating a receptor, an efferent system which activates an effector organ and a communication between these two components. Since a reflex response to an appropriate stimulus is involuntary, disturbances of reflexes afford objective signs of neural malfunction. Some of the reflexes subserved by cranial nerves such as the corneal reflex and jaw jerk are described on page 204. The routine neurological examination should include elicitation of tendon (deep) reflexes in the limbs and of some superficial (cutaneous) reflexes, including the plantar responses.

Tendon reflexes

The tendon reflexes are phasic stretch reflexes, which involve only two neurones, one afferent and one efferent with one synapse between them. Tendon reflexes depend on a sudden brief stretch of muscle spindles which evokes from them a synchronous afferent discharge. A volley of sensory impulses is conducted to the spinal cord wherein they activate motor neurones whose axons run back to the stretched muscles causing them to contract. Each reflex is subserved by its own spinal cord segments. During routine clinical examination the biceps jerk, the jerk from brachio-radialis (earlier called the supinator longus and hence referred to as the supinator jerk) and the triceps jerk are tested in each upper limb; the knee and ankle jerks in the lower limbs. The segmental innervation of these reflexes is illustrated in Figures 8.37–8.42. There are suprasegmental influences which modify the function of the tendon reflex arc.

Elicitation of tendon reflexes

These reflexes are most efficiently evoked by a tap from a tendon hammer. The instrument should have a firm but flexible shaft and should contain most of its weight in its head which should preferably be made of metal and well padded with soft rubber. The tendon, not the muscle, should be struck by the hammer as mechanical stimu-

lation of a muscle belly produces a contraction of the muscle which is not dependent on the reflex arc.

The patient should be placed in a comfortable, relaxed position which allows the examiner easily to reach the limbs. The muscle being tested should be visible. One tendon jerk should immediately be compared with its fellow on the opposite side. Convenient positions and methods are illustrated in Figures 8.37–8.42.

Interpretation of tendon reflexes

A tendon reflex results in a sudden displacement of part of a limb which then rapidly returns to its original position. The normal amplitude of such movements may be increased or decreased or there may be no movement.

Increased tendon reflexes. Many patients are anxious. This is reflected in slight contractions of their muscles which facilitate tendon reflexes which become brisker than usual. A decision about whether reflexes are abnormally brisk is not always easy and may depend upon other evidence such as asymmetry or the plantar responses. When assessing a reflex response other muscles in the limb, as well as the one stimulated, should be observed. When tendon reflexes are pathologically exaggerated there is often a spread of the evoked contractions beyond the muscle stimulated, as, for example, the finger flexion which often accompanies biceps and supinator jerks when they are pathologically exaggerated.

The finger flexion jerk (C.7, 8 and T1) may help to confirm the presence of significant hyperreflexia. The tips of the examiner's middle and index fingers are placed across the palmar surfaces of the proximal phalanges of the patient's relaxed fingers; the examiner's own fingers are then tapped lightly. A slight flexion of the patient's fingers often occurs normally but a brisk contraction suggests hyperreflexia.

Hoffman's sign is another manifestation of hyperreflexia in the flexor muscles of the fingers. It is elicited by first flexing the distal interphalangeal joint of the patient's middle finger and then flicking it down farther so that it springs back to normal Figure 8.43. When tendon reflexes are hyperactive the thumb quickly flexes in response to

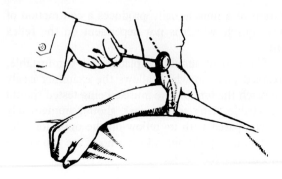

Fig. 8.37   Eliciting the biceps jerk, C.5 (C.6)

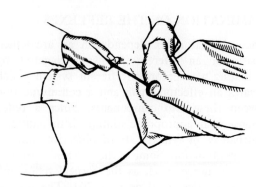

Fig. 8.38   Eliciting the triceps jerk, C.6, C.7.

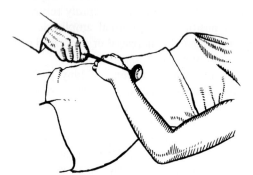

Fig. 8.39   Eliciting the supinator jerk, (C.5), C.6.

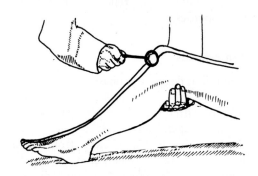

Fig. 8.40   Eliciting the knee jerk (note, the legs must not be in contact with each other), L.3, L.4.

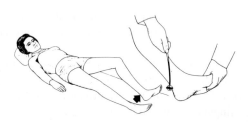

Fig. 8.41   Eliciting the ankle jerk of recumbent patient, L.5, S.1.

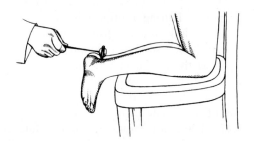

Fig. 8.42   Eliciting the ankle jerk of kneeling patient, L.5, S.1.

this manoeuvre. Minimal flexion of the thumb may sometimes be evoked in normal people, particularly if they are apprehensive. If Hoffman's sign is unilaterally positive, it is a very strong indication of a significant increase in finger flexion reflexes on that side.

Diminished or absent tendon reflexes. A few normal people have tendon reflexes which are dif-

ficult to obtain or, rarely, are absent. Some patients who regularly take hypnotic or anticonvulsant drugs show a generalised reduction in the amplitude of their tendon reflexes. The significance of depressed tendon reflexes needs to be appraised by a comparison between the responses obtained on the two sides and between the amplitude of the jerks in the arms and those in the

THE NERVOUS SYSTEM 235

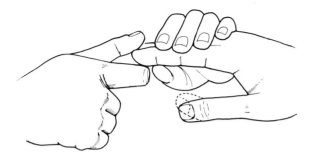

Fig. 8.43 Hoffman's sign.

legs. If normally brisk contractions are seen in the arms and very poor responses are evoked at knee and ankles then it is probable that the latter findings are pathological.

Usually absence of one or more tendon jerks denotes a neural lesion. When no response is obtained the absence of the reflex should be confirmed by 'reinforcing' the jerk. Tendon reflexes are increased in amplitude (i.e. potentiated or reinforced) by forcible contraction of muscles remote from those being tested. To reinforce the knee and ankle jerks the patient may be asked forcibly to clench the hands or to hook the fingers of the hands together and then forcibly to attempt to pull one away from the other without disengaging the fingers (Fig. 8.44). Reinforcement of the reflexes in the upper limbs may be obtained by asking the patient to clench the jaws or to push the knees hard together. It is important to remember that the phenomenon of reinforcement lasts for less than a second. The patient should, therefore, be told to perform the appropriate manoeuvre (previously demonstrated) almost synchronously with the examiner's tap of the tendon. The patient should also be told to relax after the tendon has been struck.

Site of lesion. Lesions of muscle, neuromuscular junction, peripheral nerve or spinal cord may cause loss or reduction of reflexes. Tendon reflexes disappear very late in the course of diseases which primarily affect muscle (i.e. myopathies). Whilst the neural arc remains intact surviving muscle fibres continue to contract even when there is marked muscle wasting and weakness. By contrast lesions which damage peripheral nerves cause very early loss of tendon reflexes. This is because even

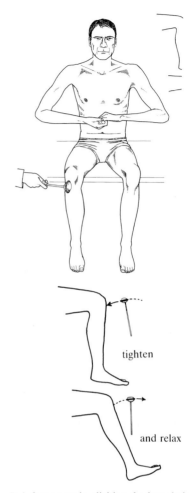

Fig. 8.44 Reinforcement in eliciting the knee jerk.

minor dysfunctions of peripheral nerves cause either or both afferent or efferent impulses to become asynchronous and the tendon reflex is consequently lost.

Myasthenic disturbance at the neuromuscular junction usually causes no change in tendon reflexes though they may occasionally be temporarily diminished during periods of profound myasthenic weakness.

Lesions within the spinal canal may interrupt the connections between the sensory and motor limbs of the reflex arc and cause loss of reflexes. Absent tendon reflexes, caused for instance by the compression of a tumour, are valuable indications of the segmental level of a lesion involving the spinal cord. An uncommon reflex change, but one which is of precise localising significance, is the phenomenon of *inversion*. The transmission of a tendon tap stimulates muscles other than that directly stretched. In normal circumstances the slight contractions thus evoked are submerged by the major response mediated through the monosynaptic reflex arc. If, however, the arc is interrupted and the direct response is lost, the contractions in other muscles may become clinically apparent. This sometimes occurs after stretch of the biceps or brachioradialis tendons; no response is seen in the stretched muscle but the fingers flex. This is called inversion of the biceps or supinator jerk (usually both are involved together) and it is due to a lesion involving the neural structures arising from the fifth cervical segment of the cord. Less common is inversion of the triceps jerk. When this occurs, due to a lesion of the C.7 spinal segmental structures, tapping the tendon of triceps produces no contraction therein but causes a contraction of the biceps.

Other abnormalities of tendon reflexes. In uncomplicated and isolated cerebellar lesions the tendon reflexes are described as pendular; the limb oscillates several times after the initial jerk, before settling again to its original position. This phenomenon is most easily detected in the knee jerk when the patient is seated on the edge of a bed with the feet swinging freely off the ground. It occurs rarely and is not of great clinical value.

On occasions a fairly brisk contraction of a muscle in response to a tendon tap may be followed by very slow relaxation. This delayed relaxation, most often seen at the ankle, is a reliable sign of hypothyroidism.

Superficial reflexes

These consist of muscular contractions evoked by cutaneous stimulation. The plantar response is the best known and most important. Others are the abdominal and cremasteric reflexes.

The plantar response. In normal people stimulation of the lateral border of the sole of the foot causes a 'flexor' response with plantar flexion of the great toe and usually of the other toes. The stimulus should not cause injury but it should be of noxious character since this is a nociceptive reflex. A blunted point such as the end of a car

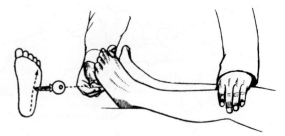

Fig. 8.45 Eliciting the plantar reflex. An extensor response is shown.

key, or an orange stick produces an appropriate stimulus. Some clinicians prefer to use their thumb nail. The patient should lie supine with the legs extended. The stimulating point is drawn slowly along the lateral border of the foot from the heel towards the little toe until a response is elicited (Fig. 8.45). In pathological circumstances, this produces an extensor response with dorsiflexion of the great toe at the metatarsophalangeal joint often accompanied by other phenomena, such as a sluggish spreading or 'fanning' of the other four toes. Sometimes an extensor plantar response is attended by simultaneous reflex contraction of the flexor muscles of the hip, knee and ankle. This is called the withdrawal response of which dorsiflexion of the great toe is a fragmentary manifestation.

Interpretation. There has for many years been extensive investigation into this reflex which is generally accepted as the most significant clinical neurological sign. For practical purposes an extensor plantar response indicates a lesion of the upper motor neurone system. It has been averred that in some instances damage to the pyramidal pathway does not result in an extensor plantar response, and that occasionally an extensor plantar response is observed in the absence of damage to this system. However, such instances are rare and there is no reason to abandon the clinical interpretation which regards the extensor plantar response as pathognomonic of a lesion of the upper motor neurone. The plantar response is normally extensor during the first year of life when the pyramidal tracts are still unmyelinated.

The plantar reflex is normally evoked by stimulation of the sole in the area supplied by the first sacral sensory root. In cases wherein there are widespread and severe lesions of the corticospinal pathways the reflexogenic zone may be greatly enlarged. An extensor plantar response may then be produced by a number of techniques. Rubbing over the crest of the tibia, squeezing the achilles tendon or a tap over the lateral malleolus may each induce dorsiflexion of the great toe. These signs have eponyms but are of little clinical importance. One accessory sign of damage to the pyramidal pathways may sometimes be helpful when an extensor plantar response cannot be obtained because of a concurrent lesion causing paralysis of extensor hallucis longus. *Rossolimo's sign* depends upon plantar flexion of the big toe. The distal phalanges of the toes are flicked into extension by the examiner's fingers and then allowed to fall back into their normal position. A brisk plantar flexion of the great toe is a sign of pathological hyperreflexia. It is the counterpart in the lower limbs of Hoffman's sign.

Occasionally no response is obtained to a nociceptive stimulus applied over the lateral border of the foot. Most commonly this is due to coldness of the feet and the test should be repeated after warming the patient. If no reflex movement is elicited despite warming there may be an impairment of cutaneous sensibility over the S.1 distribution or there may be paralysis of the long flexors or extensors of the great toe. The plantar response may be absent immediately after a complete transection of the spinal cord during the phase of spinal shock.

The abdominal reflexes. Normally a contraction of the muscles of the anterior abdominal wall is provoked when the skin of the abdomen is stroked or scratched. These responses are polysynaptic nociceptive reflexes. The patient should lie warm and relaxed in a supine position with a low pillow supporting the head. The cutaneous nerves derive from the eighth to twelfth thoracic spinal segments. The upper and lower abdominal quadrants on each side are stimulated by drawing an orange stick towards the midline, parallel respectively with the costal margins and with the inguinal ligaments (Fig. 8.46). The stick is best drawn lightly and quickly at an acute angle to the skin, since the reflexes are served by cutaneous touch receptors and are not dependent on muscle stretch or painful stimulation.

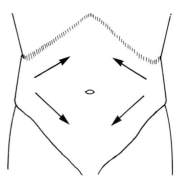

Fig. 8.46 Abdominal reflexes. Site of stimuli for their elicitation.

Interpretation. In most people the muscles underlying the area stimulated will contract briskly. However the reflexes may be absent when the abdominal wall is lax in parous women and in obese patients. Occasionally they may be lost because of impaired pain sensation in the skin or because of lower motor neurone lesions affecting the abdominal musculature, sometimes the legacy of abdominal surgery. In most instances absence of responses in a young relaxed patient with good abdominal muscles strongly suggests an upper motor neurone lesion. The reflexes may be lost on one or both sides, reflecting unilateral or bilateral upper motor neurone involvement. While absence of abdominal reflexes is by no means invariable in upper motor neurone lesions, their loss is often an early manifestation in multiple sclerosis. In upper motor neurone lesions due to motor neurone disease the abdominal reflexes are usually preserved. Loss of abdominal cutaneous reflexes probably results only if other pathways, as well as the upper motor neurones, are interrupted and such widespread lesions are liable to occur in multiple sclerosis.

The cremasteric reflexes. Stroking or scratching the inner aspect of the upper part of the thigh in male patients normally provokes an elevation of the testis on the same side. This reflex response may be lost as a result of an upper motor neurone lesion, or when the genitofemoral nerve or its roots (L. 1 and 2) are damaged.

MISCELLANEOUS TESTS

A number of tests which are not carried out

routinely may yield most important information in appropriate circumstances.

Signs of meningeal irritation

Inflammation of the meninges due to infection or blood in the subarachnoid space evokes reflex spasm in the paravertebral muscles. In the cervical region this manifests itself by *neck rigidity* which impedes passive flexion of the neck. This should be looked for in any patient in whom meningitis or subarachnoid haemorrhage is a possibility (Fig. 8.47). The neck initially should be slowly flexed but in the early stages of a meningeal reaction spasm may be more easily demonstrated if the neck is flexed abruptly. Normally the chin can be made to touch the chest without causing discomfort. Neck rigidity may not be present in patients early in the evolution of a subarachnoid haemorrhage, or in those who are deeply comatose for whatever reason.

Meningeal irritation causing spasm in the lumbar region can be demonstrated by passive movements of the lower limbs (*Kernig's sign*). The patient lies supine with one leg extended; the leg to be tested is flexed at the hip and knee. Whilst the hip joint remains flexed the knee is extended as shown in Figure 8.48. When there is meningeal irritation involving the posterior roots in the lumbar area it will be impossible fully to extend the knee because of spasm in the hamstring muscles.

Signs of nerve root irritation

When lumbar and sacral nerve roots are pressed upon by a prolapsed intervertebral disc, stretching of the sciatic nerve or the femoral nerve may give rise to pain. These nerve stretching tests are described on page 276.

Signs of tetany

In tetany a low plasma ionised calcium concentration causes an increased excitability of nerves. Sensations of pins and needles in the hands, feet and round the mouth often precede painful muscle cramps. *Carpopedal spasm* is the characteristic finding. The hands spontaneously take up the position known as the *main d'accoucheur*, in which there is opposition of the thumb, extension of the interphalangeal and flexion of the metacar-

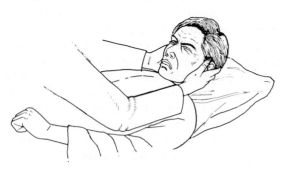

Fig. 8.47   Testing for meningeal irritation (neck rigidity).

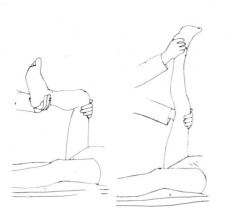

Fig. 8.48   Testing for meningeal irrritation (Kernig's test).

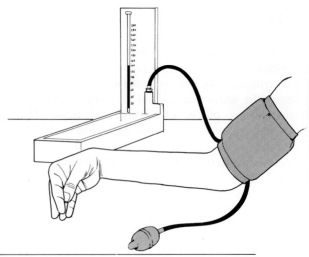

Fig. 8.49   Testing for latent tetany (Trousseau's sign).

pophalangeal joints. In latent tetany the same position can be induced within four minutes by inflation of the sphygmomanometer cuff to a level above the systolic blood pressure — *Trousseau's sign* (Fig. 8.49). An alternative test (Chvostek's sign) is to tap over the facial nerve in front of the ear. When positive this provokes a brisk momentary contraction of the facial muscles, pulling the mouth to that side in latent tetany, but also in some normal subjects.

Signs elicited by palpation, percussion and auscultation

Palpation of the skull and of the spinous processes occasionally reveals local destructive lesions due to tumours or irregularities due to trauma. Percussion may elicit localised tenderness in the spinous processes overlying an epidural abscess.

Auscultation for bruits. As part of the neurological examination, the patient's neck, head and eyes should be auscultated. Bruits due to subclavian or vertebral artery stenosis are heard best at the supraclavicular fossa, whereas stenosis at the origin of the internal carotid artery causes a bruit maximal in the anterior neck just below the angle of the mandible (see Fig. 8.50). Bruits due to tur-

bulent blood flow in intracranial vascular malformations may be heard over the cranium, but are often better detected by listening over the eye. Best results are obtained by placing the stethoscope bell over a gently closed eyelid; muscle noise can be reduced by asking the patient to open the other eye. The precordium should always be auscultated to ensure that cardiac murmurs are not being transmitted to the cranial vessels.

SUMMARY OF EXAMINATION OF THE NERVOUS SYSTEM

This is given in the form of the case recording on page 358.

FURTHER INVESTIGATION

The clinical examination of the nervous system is an integral part of the general medical examination. Similarly, neurological investigations cannot be considered in isolation. In some instances a blood count which reveals a macrocytic anaemia may implicate vitamin B_{12} deficiency as the cause of spinal cord lesions. A leucaemic blood picture or glycosuria may suggest the aetiology of various neurological pictures. These examples emphasis the frequent need to utilise non-neurological tests when evaluating patients with neurological problems.

The intelligent selection of appropriate investigations is based on the clinical picture and should always take account of the discomforts and dangers attendant upon the investigative techniques. In a few cases extreme clinical urgency will demand that the definitive test, even if painful, be performed immediately. In most instances it is wise to instigate those investigations which are least disturbing and only later to proceed to uncomfortable, hazardous or invasive tests.

Radiological examination

Plain radiographs are important preliminary investigations in many neurological problems. A chest radiograph may reveal a bronchial carcinoma and hence explain a wide variety of metastatic and non-metastatic neural complications. Plain radiographs of the skull may show displacement of

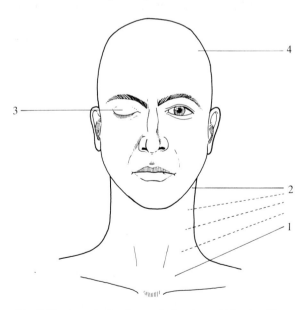

Fig. 8.50 Auscultation for cervical and cranial bruits. (1) Supraclavicular fossa. (2) Carotid bifurcation. (3) Over passively closed eyelid. (4) Over cranium.

a calcified pineal gland, erosions caused by tumours or thickening of the vault of the skull provoked by a subjacent meningioma. Lesions such as gliomas, tuberculomas and arteriovenous malformations may be delineated by abnormal calcification but the definitive investigation of an intracranial lesion often requires CT scanning. Radiographs of the spine should be performed whenever a lesion of the cord or nerve roots is suspected. The vertebral bodies, the pedicles and the disc spaces may display abnormalities which would localise the site and suggest the cause of compression of the spinal cord.

More complex radiological investigation is discussed on pages 244 to 246.

The cerebrospinal fluid

An examination of cerebrospinal fluid (CSF) used to be a common procedure in the investigation of neurological disorders. It still often provides information of value, but with the development of non-invasive methods of investigation the indications for its use are fewer. A lumbar puncture is essential when acute or chronic infection of the brain or meninges is suspected. It should usually be performed in patients in whom the diagnostic possibilities include multiple sclerosis, sarcoidosis, neurosyphilis and the Guillain-Barré syndrome. In suspected subarachnoid haemorrhage, computed tomography is the investigation of choice, but lumbar puncture may confirm the diagnosis if this is negative or unavailable. It is seldom of primary importance in the diagnosis of cerebral tumours or in the investigation of epilepsy.

A lumbar puncture must not be performed if there is suspicion of raised intracranial pressure, irrespective of whether papilloedema is present or not. In these circumstances a CT scan should be preferred first. The danger is of sudden death from 'coning' of the brain through the foramen magnum.

Note should be made of the appearance of the fluid. Normally clear and colourless, the CSF becomes turbid if it contains many cells. If blood-stained, the fluid should be collected in three successive tubes to differentiate between a traumatic puncture in which the later collections will be less contaminated, and a subarachnoid

haemorrhage in which successive tubes will be uniformly red. Blood-stained fluid should also be centrifuged to see whether the supernatant fluid has a yellow tinge (xanthochromia) which develops when blood has been present for several hours. The CSF may also sometimes be yellowish in deeply jaundiced patients or when its protein content is much increased. The CSF pressure can be measured by a simple manometer, and is usually 50–150 mm of CSF.

Laboratory examination of the CSF should include a cell count, estimation of the protein and glucose content and serological examination for syphilis. In appropriate circumstances microbiological studies, bacterial or viral, should be carried out.

Cell count. Normal CSF contains less than five lymphocytes per cubic millimetre. In bacterial meningitis the cell count may rise to many hundreds or several thousands per cubic millimetre with a marked predominance of polymorphs. Lymphocytosis of moderate degree is found in tuberculous meningitis and viral meningitis, though in the initial stages of these conditions there also may be an increase in polymorphs. A slight to moderate rise in the lymphocyte count may be found in viral encephalitis, in active neurosyphilis, multiple sclerosis and sarcoidosis.

Protein. The total protein content in normal CSF lies between 0.2 and 0.5 g/l. A moderate elevation of protein may be found in many intracranial diseases including acute infections, neurosyphilis, vascular lesions and many cases of cerebral tumour. Very high protein contents are found in the Guillain-Barré syndrome and when compression of the spinal cord blocks the CSF flow. A few systemic diseases, notably diabetes and hypothyroidism, may also be accompanied by a rise in CSF protein.

The total protein in most cases of multiple sclerosis is within normal limits, but the IgG level (normally 6 to 12% of the total protein) is significantly raised (greater than 20%) in approximately two-thirds of patients with multiple sclerosis whether or not the disease is active. The IgG is also increased (usually accompanied by a rise in total protein) in neurosyphilis, in sarcoidosis and in some disorders of connective tissue. Local synthesis of IgG within the CNS — a feature of multiple sclerosis — can be inferred with more certainty if the CSF IgG concentration is compared with that in blood, and corrected for the CSF/blood albumin ratio (CSF IgG index). The abnormality most characteristic of multiple sclerosis is the presence of oligoclonal bands in the gammaglobulin region when concentrated CSF is subjected to electrophoresis on a gel with a pH gradient (iso-electric focusing). Similar bands may be seen in other disorders e.g. neurosyphilis.

Glucose. The CSF normally contains between 2.2 and 4.5 mmol of glucose per litre (40 to 80 mg/100 ml). The CSF glucose is normally related to blood glucose being approximately 1.7 mmol per litre below the blood level. A high glucose content, therefore, may be found in diabetes. A marked reduction in CSF glucose is a feature of bacterial meningitis; in severe cases glucose may be absent. A moderate reduction in glucose may be found in tuberculous and carcinomatous meningitis and in neurosarcoidosis. The glucose content is usually normal in viral meningitis and encephalitis.

Serology. Tests for syphilis are still performed routinely. The Wasserman reaction (WR) has largely been replaced by the Venereal Disease Research Laboratories (VDRL) flocculation test, but this may still give false positive and false negative results. The treponema pallidum haemagglutination test (TPHA) and the fluorescent treponema antibody test (FTA) are more specific and more sensitive, but may remain positive for life even after effective treatment. More recently an enzyme-linked sorbent assay (ELISA) for antitreponemal IgG has been introduced. This assay is easier to perform than the older tests, but it is not more specific. A similar ELISA for antitreponemal IgM can be used to detect recent or active infection.

Other serological tests which may be indicated are those for antinuclear factor (ANF) and DNA-binding antibodies which may be positive in connective tissue disorders (e.g. SLE) involving the nervous system. Serum antibodies directed against skeletal muscle acetyl choline receptors are present in more than 80% of patients with myasthenia gravis, and may be valuable in early stages of diagnosis.

Microbiological investigation. Whenever infection is suspected the CSF should be centrifuged and the deposit examined microscopically after Gram staining, and, if tuberculous meningitis is a possibility, after Ziehl-Neelsen staining. Cultures should also be prepared from the CSF in cases of suspected infection and antibiotic sensitivities determined. Occasionally fungi and cryptococci are found in the CSF and the latter is best demonstrated by staining with Indian ink. If the initial bacteriological examination is negative, but the clinical suspicion of meningitis remains high, lumbar puncture should be repeated in an attempt to identify the responsible organism.

In certain instances viruses may be cultured from the CSF, but often the diagnosis of viral infection depends on detecting rising antibody titres in serum or CSF rather than by isolation of the virus in the fluid.

Miscellaneous tests. In certain situations, more specialised and refined examinations of the CSF may be carried out. For example in carcinomatous meningitis examination of a fresh CSF specimen after cyto-centrifugation may reveal malignant cells. In cases of severe meningitis antibiotic levels may be measured in the CSF as a guide to treatment.

INVESTIGATION IN RELATION TO SITE OF LESION

The choice of more sophisticated and specific tests is determined by the site of neurological lesions. Such investigations include clinical neurophysiology (electroencephalography, evoked potentials, and electromyography), radionuclide scanning, computed tomography and other imaging techniques.

Intracranial disease

A wide variety of techniques is available for investigation of intracranial lesions; harmless, non-invasive tests should be employed first.

The electroencephalogram (EEG). This records the electrical potentials of the brain after they are attenuated by passing through the skull and scalp. Potential changes are recorded simultaneously over several areas. Intracranial disease may cause normal electrical rhythms to be suppressed or more commonly, abnormal wave forms may be engendered. Such abnormalities may be generalised or localised. EEG abnormalities are more marked with acute lesions such as cerebral abscess than with slowly progressive or chronic lesions. Lesions within the substance of the brain such as gliomas produce more marked and earlier abnormalities than lesions such as meningiomas or angiomas lying outside the brain tissue. The EEG is more precise in its definition of lesions lying in the cerebal hemispheres than it is in lesions lying within the posterior fossa. The EEG is of prime diagnostic value in functional disorders, especially epilepsy. Generalised or localised paroxysmal activity in the form of spikes or sharp waves may be detected between fits, and may be induced by hyperventilation, photic flicker stimulation, sleep or drugs. It is now possible to record EEGs from ambulant patients for 24 hours or longer, and this may provide diagnostic information in selected cases. A normal EEG does not exclude the diagnosis of epilepsy; likewise, the presence of paroxysmal activity is not in itself diagnostic without an appropriate history. Examples of normal and abnormal EEG records are shown in Figures 8.51 and 8.52.

Evoked potential recording. Over the past decade, the development of digital signal averaging has permitted the measurement of small cerebral and spinal potential changes evoked by visual, auditory and peripheral nerve stimuli. An averaged response, relatively free of muscle and AC interference, is built up by storing responses to 100–1000 sequential stimuli. Visually evoked potentials (VEP) are the most useful clinically, and are recorded with an array of scalp electrodes over the occipital region. Stimulation is usually with a reversing chequer-board pattern which is either projected on to a screen or displayed on a television set. The dominant response from a normal eye is a positive wave with a peak at about 100 milliseconds. Lesions of the retina, optic nerve, chiasma, tract, radiation or occipital cortex may all disrupt or delay the response, but demyelinating lesions of the optic nerve often cause marked delay with relatively good preservation of the wave form. A delayed VEP in a

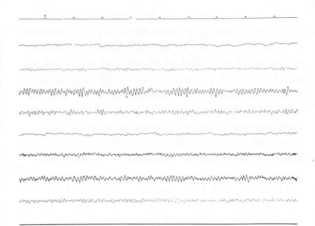

Fig. 8.51 Portion of an 8-channel EEG record taken from a normal adolescent. Four channels running anterior to posterior over the parietal regions are displayed from each side. Top four traces — right side; lower four — left side. Uppermost trace is a 1 second time marker. Note the posteriorly dominant 10/sec waves — the alpha rhythm.

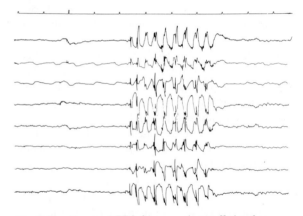

Fig. 8.52 Abnormal EEG from a patient suffering from generalised tonic-clonic seizures. This inter-ictal record shows a paroxysm of generalised spike and slow wave activity lasting about 3 seconds, during which the patient showed no clinical abnormality.

patient with clinically normal vision can therefore be of much diagnostic help in multiple sclerosis.

Somato-sensory evoked potentials (SSEP), recorded from the brachial plexus, cervical spine and contralateral parietal area when the median or ulnar nerve is stimulated electrically, may similarly help detect lesions in the ascending sensory pathways. Similar responses of longer latency can be elicited by tibial or peroneal nerve stimulation in the leg. Auditory evoked potentials (AEP) in response to click stimuli arise largely from the brain stem and may give evidence of cochlear, acoustic nerve or brain stem disorders. Examples of VER and SSEP recording traces are shown in Figures 8.53 and 8.54.

Radionuclide cerebral scanning. This test has largely been superseded by CT scanning. An injected radioisotope (such as technetium) is taken up differentially by diseased intracranial tissue compared to normal brain substance. Differing intensities of radio activities are recorded through the skull and abnormal areas mapped. In this way tumours, particularly meningiomas, can be

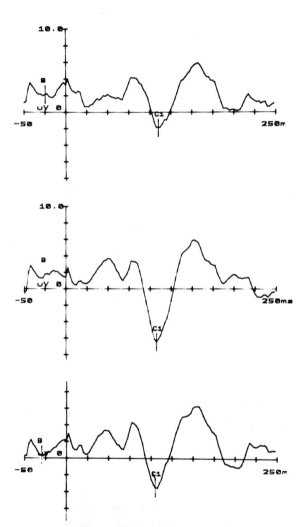

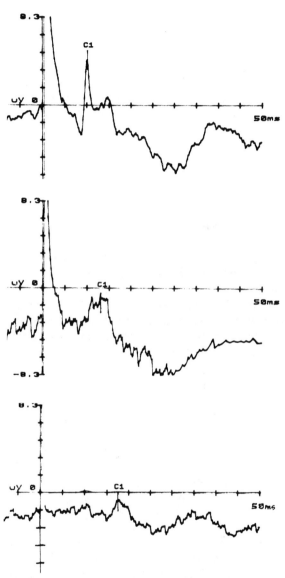

Fig. 8.53 Normal visual evoked responses elicited by reversing chequer-board pattern stimulus to right eye. Top trace — right occipital; middle trace — mid occipital; lower trace — left occipital recording electrode. 100 individual responses are computer averaged to produce these traces. The major positive (downward) deflection occurs about 110 ms after the stimulus (marked C1) and is called the P100 response.

Fig. 8.54 Normal somato-sensory evoked responses elicited by electrical stimulation of the median nerve at the wrist. Each trace is a computer average of 500 responses. Top trace — recorded at supraclavicular fossa, shows a negative (upward) potential at 10 ms. Middle trace — recorded from posterior mid-cervical regional shows at C1 a negative response with a latency of 12–13 ms. Lower trace — recorded from contralateral parietal area shows at C1 a smaller negative response of 17–18 ms latency.

localised and areas of infarction defined in a scintigram.

Computed tomography (CT scan). This radiographic technique detects and displays the differing X-ray densities of cranial structures. Computed absorption coefficients of the cranial structures are translated in analogue form to a cathode ray tube where they are displayed as differing shades of grey. White and grey matter and the fluid filled spaces can be visualised and examined in much the same way as conventional radiographs. The sensitivity of the technique can be increased by the intravenous injection of a water-soluble contrast agent containing iodine which increases the absorption of some intracranial lesions. The technique is atraumatic, takes less than half an hour and the patient is exposed to rather less radiation than that required for a con-

ventional radiograph of the skull. It is an accurate and sensitive tool and, with contrast enhancement, will reveal the vast majority of cerebral tumours, infarcts, haemorrhages, abscesses, arteriovenous malformations and also cerebral atrophy and hydrocephalus (Fig. 8.55). CT scanning has reduced the need for arteriography and markedly reduced the demand for pneumoencephalography. However, it is not infallible; small low-density lesions such as infarcts and some gliomas may be missed. Arteriovenous malformations, small subdural haematomas and intrinsic lesions in the brain stem may also be undetected.

Emission computed tomography. Emission computed axial tomography (ECAT), one form of which is position emission tomography (PET), is a technique of imaging in which radionuclides are injected intravenously and the emitted radiation

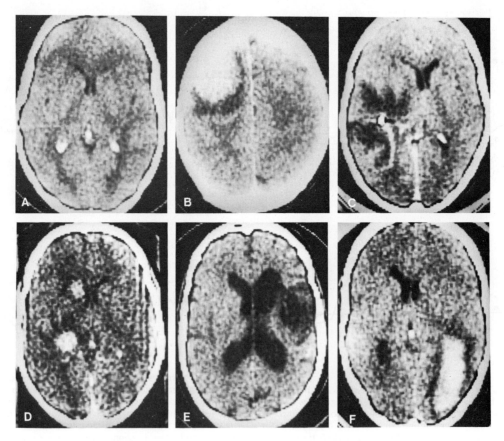

Fig. 8.55   CT scanning as a diagnostic aid. (A) Normal, showing ventricles, choroid plexus and pineal gland. (B) Meningioma. (C) Tumour with metallic body at biopsy site. (D) Metastases. (E) Infarct with dilated ventricles and sulci due to cerebral atrophy. (F) Cerebral haemorrhage. (Courtesy of Dr A A Donaldson.)

from the brain is recorded by scintillation detectors. As with radiation transmission computed tomography (CT scanning), a computer is used in order to construct a two dimensional image of the brain. The technique is highly sensitive and exposes patients to much less radiation than conventional CT scanning. It can reveal morphological abnormalities but with poorer resolution than X-ray CT. However, changes in brain function (e.g. oxygen uptake, glucose metabolism, monoamine storage) may be mapped out by PET scanning. Areas of functional change (e.g. an epileptic focus) can be detected in the absence of structural defects. Since the technique requires a source of short life radioisotopes (a cyclotron), it is limited to major research centres and is unlikely to become a routine clinical investigation.

Magnetic resonance imaging (nuclear magnetic resonance). This procedure utilises the magnetic properties of hydrogen nuclei within the brain. The head is exposed to a magnetic field and the hydrogen nuclei within it are excited by radio frequency radiation and the signals thus produced are detected and computed. The skull is scanned to produce images of brain slices similar to those of conventional CT scanning.

Since grey matter contains much more water (and hydrogen nuclei) than white matter this technique vividly differentiates grey and white matter. It produces imaging of the posterior fossa which is superior to that of conventional CT scanning. As well as revealing space occupying lesions it will demonstrate small lesions within white matter such as those in multiple sclerosis. It is particularly useful in the diagnosis of conditions where demyelination is a feature. Of further value is the facility to construct a midline sagittal image which includes the cerebral cortex, brain stem, cerebellum and upper cervical spinal cord. This provides a very sensitive non-invasive method of looking for lesions at the foramen magnum and upper spinal cord (e.g. syringomyelia, Fig. 8.56). The latest MRI machines are now capable of producing excellent images of the whole spinal cord and subarachnoid space.

Cerebral angiography. With the advent of the CT scan, angiography is rarely the primary investigation in cases of cerebral tumour. However, it still has a place in defining precise anatomy when

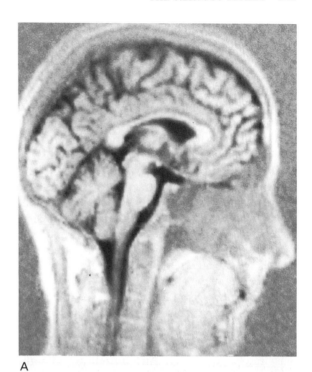

A

B

Fig. 8.56 Magnetic resonance imaging as a diagnostic aid. (A) Normal mid-line sagittal inversion recovery image showing medial aspect of cerebral hemisphere, corpus callosum, brain stem, cerebellum and upper cervical spinal cord. (B) Proton density image of a patient with syringomyelia showing a minor degree of cerebellar tonsillar herniation at the foramen magnum, dilatation of the cervical spinal cord with a syrinx cavity extending down to the centre of the cord. (Courtesy of Professor J J K Best.)

a mass has been demonstrated on the CT scan and operation is contemplated. It is also the appropriate investigation when clinical signs point to a lesion of a blood vessel such as an aneurysm or stenosis. Carotid arteriography and less often vertebral arteriography are performed. These investigations are uncomfortable and potentially hazardous and should be performed only if there are compelling indications.

Digital subtraction angiography employs computer enhancement to subtract soft tissue and bone images from vascular outlines. Using a venous bolus injection of contrast medium, it is possible to obtain reasonable images of the extracranial arteries, but good quality views of intracranial vessels require an arterial injection. With a venous injection it is possible to perform angiographic studies at low risk, but at present the image quality is not usually as good as conventional arteriography.

Pneumoencephalography. This procedure is now rarely performed. Air, introduced into the lumbar subarachnoid space, rises into the basal cisterns and into the ventricles where it can show displacement due to tumour, or dilatation due to hydrocephalus or cerebral atrophy. Pneumoencephalography should not be performed if intracranial pressure is raised. It is frequently followed by severe headache for several days. Although pneumoencephalography is used little in modern practice, a modified limited technique — air CT-meatography — is used to image the internal auditory meatus when an acoustic neuroma is suspected.

Ultrasound scanning. This non-invasive technique has advanced in scope over the last few years. A beam of high frequency sound is transmitted and its echoes detected by a movable probe. Two-dimensional images can be produced to outline different tissue and fluid layers. In infants, the fontanelle can be used as an acoustic window so that some intracranial structures like the cerebral ventricles can be imaged. Neonatal cerebral haemorrhages and hydrocephalus can be demonstrated with ease. In adults, the technique can be used to image the cervical carotid arteries, where even small degrees of atheroma can be detected by an experienced operator. By measuring Doppler frequency shifts, blood velocity and turbulence can be estimated.

Spinal cord

Myelography, or radiculography is often required for the investigation of localised damage to the spinal cord or to outline abnormalities of the nerve roots. A radio-opaque dye is introduced into the subarachnoid space via a lumbar puncture needle. The dye is then manoeuvred along the spinal canal, by tilting the patient. Deformation of the column of dye will reveal compressive lesions and suggest their nature. Various water soluble, non-ionic dyes are used. They give high definition, outline root pockets and are absorbed and excreted.

CT scanning also has a place in the imaging of the spine with or without the addition of contrast. It is a useful adjunct to radiculography, especially in sorting out problems in patients who have had previous disc surgery where it may be important to distinguish between fibrosis and a recurrent disc lesion. MRI is also of use and the ability to produce longitudinal (sagittal) sections is a great advantage.

Muscles and peripheral nerves

The investigation of primary disease of muscle may require extensive biochemical testing. Of general applicability is the estimation of serum enzymes such as aldolase, lactate dehydrogenase and, most specifically, creatine phosphokinase whose concentrations reflect the rate and extent of muscle fibre disintegration.

Peripheral nerve disorders may require a range of investigations to determine the primary cause. These include a chest radiograph, sputum cytology and biochemical tests such as vitamin assays, blood urea, plasma protein electrophoresis, urinary porphobilinogen and glucose tolerance tests.

Electromyography is useful in the investigation of disorders of muscles and peripheral nerves. Muscle and nerve action potentials are detected by skin surface or needle electrodes, and are amplified and displayed on an oscilloscope. Needle electrode study of muscles during voluntary contraction

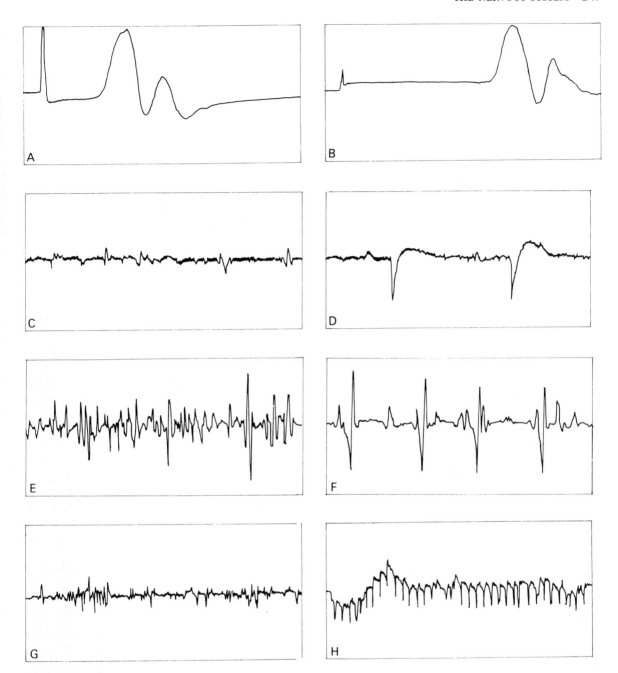

Fig. 8.57 Normal and abnormal electromyographic (EMG) recordings. (A) and (B) show compound muscle action potential responses recorded with surface electrodes on the thenar eminence when the median nerve is stimulated at the wrist (1) and elbow (2). Note the difference in latency; this is used to calculate conduction velocity — usually 50–60 m/sec. 3–8 show EMG recordings made with a concentric needle electrode. (C) shows small short duration fibrillation potentials, and (D) positive sharp waves, both features seen in acute muscle denervation. (E) shows a normal pattern of motor unit recruitment when a subject makes a strong voluntary muscle contraction. Impaired recruitment of enlarged motor units is seen in chronic denervation (F). In myopathy (G) recruitment is full, but the motor units are reduced in amplitude and duration. (H) shows an example of a high frequency burst of muscle activity recorded from a patient with dystrophia myotonica.

helps identify denervation and differentiates it from myopathic disorders. Many peripheral nerves can be stimulated electrically and conduction velocities in motor and sensory fibres be measured separately. Velocity and amplitude measurements help gauge the type and severity in polyneuropathies, and may define the site of localised nerve compression, as in the carpal tunnel syndrome. Disorders of peripheral nerves which are due to demyelination cause marked reduction in conduction velocity, whereas primary axonal degeneration is characterised by reduced amplitude of sensory and motor potentials. Examples of normal and abnormal EMG records are shown in Figure 8.57.

Tests of the autonomic nervous system, dependent on measuring cardiovascular responses to standing, Valsalva manoeuvre, deep breathing and sustained hand grip can be performed in selected cases. Abnormalities are seen particularly in polyneuropathy due to diabetes mellitus, alcoholism and amyloidosis.

THE METHODS IN PRACTICE

Three examples have been chosen. Two of these are general and one is highly specific. The diagnostic process is first discussed and then the examination of the unconscious patient is described. Finally an account is given of the diagnosis of brain death.

1. THE DIAGNOSTIC PROCESS

The completion of the neurological examination is followed by the correlation and interpretation of all the available information in order to reach a diagnosis. The diagnostic formulation should comprise a careful and orderly assessment of the nature of the patient's dysfunction. The neural systems and pathways damaged are then adduced. Next the distribution of lesions is defined. Finally the most likely pathological diagnosis is inferred. In other words what is disturbed, where and why?

a. Disturbance of function

The patient complains of the results of disordered physiological functions whose nature is reflected in the abnormal signs revealed during the examination. The combination of signs attributable to lesions of different parts and paths of the nervous system need to be understood and memorised.

Upper motor neurone (pyramidal tract) lesions. These cause (i) weakness or paralysis of movement; (ii) increase of tone of 'clasp-knife' type; (iii) increased amplitude of tendon reflexes; (iv) diminution of abdominal reflexes; (v) an extensor plantar response.

Lower motor neurone lesions. These give rise to (i) weakness or paralysis of muscles; (ii) wasting of muscles; (iii) there may be fasciculation in the involved muscles; (iv) if many muscles in a limb are wasted, tone will be reduced therein; (v) if affected muscles subserve tendon reflexes, these will be diminished or absent.

Cerebellar lesions. Damage to the posterior lobe of the cerebellum or of its connections with the brain stem are accompanied by (i) ataxia of gait; (ii) intention tremor of limbs; (iii) jerking nystagmus; (iv) dysarthria of staccato or scanning type; (v) dysmetria and past pointing; (vi) impaired alternating movements; (vii) hypotonia and pendular tendon reflexes; (viii) occasionally, smooth movements may be broken up into their constituent parts producing jerking, marionette-like, decomposition of movements.

Generalised polyneuropathies. These often cause (i) diminution of superficial sensation affecting the distal aspect of limbs over 'stocking' and 'glove' distributions; (ii) wasting and weakness of distal limb musculature; (iii) early loss of tendon reflexes.

Spinal or cranial nerve damage. This results in combinations of signs which depend on the area of supply of the individual nerves.

Muscles. Primary affections of muscle fibres lead to wasting and weakness of muscles usually (but not invariably) in the proximal parts of limbs. Fatty infiltration of muscle may cause an apparent increase in size of the affected muscles. Reflexes are preserved until muscle wasting is very marked.

Sensory tracts. Interruption of *dorsal columns* causes (i) ataxia of gait and limb movements aggravated by eye closure; (ii) impaired position sense; (iii) diminished appreciation of vibration. Lesions of the *spinothalamic* system cause impairment of pain and temperature sensation.

These combinations of signs are those of fully developed pictures. Every abnormality is not to be expected in every case and the clinician must be prepared to deduce that a tract has been damaged when incomplete patterns of signs have been demonstrated.

b. Distribution of lesions

The identification of damaged neural structures is followed by the definition of the site or sites of their involvement.

Single lesions. All the observed signs may be due to a localised lesion affecting adjacent structures.

Impairment of specialised functions of the *cerebral cortex* result in dementia, dysphasia, apraxia, astereognosis and other forms of agnosia. Upper motor neurone lesions at the cortical level cause signs similar to those due to interruption of the pyramidal tract at more caudal sites but since the upper motor neurones are spread over a wide area in the cortex, lesions here typically effect only part of the opposite side of the body. A paresis confined to one limb (monoplegia) or to one side of the face is likelier than a hemiplegia. Bilateral upper motor neurone signs result from a solitary cortical site only in the rare instance of a parasagittal lesion, such as a meningioma. This may impinge on both hemispheres on the neurones which lie close together on each side of the sagittal plane and which supply the legs. The demonstration of cortical abnormalities will often enable the extent of a lesion to be mapped out fairly precisely.

Localisation within the *cerebral hemispheres* is helped if a pattern of visual deficit has been elucidated; thus an upper quadrantic homonymous hemianopia points to a lesion in the temporal lobe on the side opposite the field defect (Fig. 8.2).

A profound hemiplegia equally affecting face, arm and leg, associated with loss of sensation of all modalities on the paralysed side suggests a lesion affecting the *internal capsule* where the upper motor neurone and sensory pathways are packed closely together.

Lesions of the *brain stem* are characterised by ipsilateral impairment of one or more cranial nerves with concurrent contralateral affection of one or more long tracts usually the upper motor neurones. Which cranial nerves are implicated will depend on which part of the brain stem is affected. A midbrain lesion is suggested if there is a third nerve palsy on one side and signs of upper motor neurone involvement on the other. Pontine damage is indicated by sixth and seventh nerve signs accompanied by contralateral upper motor neurone signs. Occasionally other tracts such as the spinothalamic pathway are interrupted. Examples of lesions involving the midbrain, pons and medulla are given in Figures 8.58, 8.59 and 8.60.

Spinal cord damage is localised by correlating motor, sensory and reflex changes.

Upper motor neurone signs arising from cord lesions are often, but by no means always, bilateral. The location of the site of upper motor neurone lesions can be made only very roughly on the basis of upper motor neurone signs alone; if they are present in the arms then the lesion must be above the fifth cervical segment; if the abdominal reflexes are all lost then a segment above the eighth thoracic must be implicated; signs in the legs indicate a lesion above the conus medullaris.

The site of upper motor neurone damage is localised much more precisely if the offending lesion also involves the anterior horn cells or motor

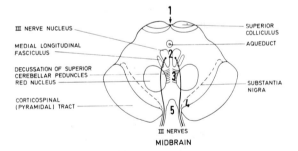

Fig. 8.58 Lesions of midbrain. Lesions at (1), e.g. pressure from a pineal tumour, cause weakness of upward gaze which may first be manifest as nystagmus in a vertical plane. Lesions at (2) produce bilateral, partial lesions of the third nerve and anterior internuclear ophthalmoplegia, (p. 202 damage to medial longitudinal fasciculus). Lesions at (3) cause ipsilateral third nerve palsy and contralateral cerebellar signs (damage to decussating cerebellar peduncles) and/or tremors and athetoid movements (damage to red nucleus). Lesions at (4) cause ipsilateral third nerve signs and contralateral pyramidal involvement. Lesions at (5) cause bilateral third nerve palsy and bilateral pyramidal signs.
Lesions which affect the midbrain immediately below this level also implicate the fourth nerve.

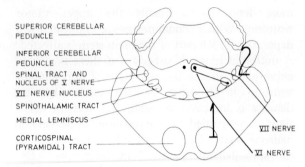

SUPERIOR CEREBELLAR PEDUNCLE

INFERIOR CEREBELLAR PEDUNCLE

SPINAL TRACT AND NUCLEUS OF V NERVE

VII NERVE NUCLEUS

SPINOTHALAMIC TRACT

MEDIAL LEMNISCUS

CORTICOSPINAL (PYRAMIDAL) TRACT

VII NERVE

VI NERVE

Fig. 8.59   Lesions of the pons. Lesions at (1), e.g. haemorrhage, cause ipsilateral sixth and/or seventh nerve palsies and contralateral pyramidal signs. Lesions at (2), e.g. basilar thrombosis, cause ataxia on the side of the lesion (damage to the cerebellar peduncles). There may also be impaired sensation on the ipsilateral side of the face (spinal tract and nucleus of fifth nerve) and on the contralateral side of the body (spinothalamic tract) and occasionally a seventh nerve lesion. Lesions in the pons often cause posterior internuclear ophthalmoplegia (p. 202) and ataxic nystagmus.

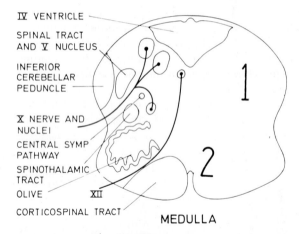

IV VENTRICLE

SPINAL TRACT AND V NUCLEUS

INFERIOR CEREBELLAR PEDUNCLE

X NERVE AND NUCLEI

CENTRAL SYMP PATHWAY

SPINOTHALAMIC TRACT

OLIVE   XII

CORTICOSPINAL TRACT

MEDULLA

Fig. 8.60   Lesions of the medulla. Lesions affecting lateral medulla (1) e.g. thrombosis of posterior inferior cerebellar artery, cause ataxia and intention tremor on ipsilateral side, jerking nystagmus on turning eyes to the side of the lesion (damage to the spinocerebellar tract in the inferior cerebellar peduncle); analgesia on ipsilateral side of face and contralateral limbs (affection of spinal tract of fifth nerve and the lateral sphinothalamic tract); Horner's syndrome (involvement of the central sympathetic pathway); dysphonia, dysphagia and weakness of soft palate and paralysis of vocal cords on the side of the lesion (damage to the tenth nerve).
Lesions affecting the paramedian area (2), e.g. infarction, cause a crossed paralysis — wasting and fasciculation of ipsilateral side of tongue (damage to twelfth nerve) and contralateral pyramidal signs.

roots. Lower motor neurone signs, with wasting in a segmental distribution define the cord lesion accurately. Sensory signs may help to delineate the position of cord lesions; thus impairment of sensation over a segmental dermatome will indicate the level of a lesion on occasion. Interruption of sensory tracts may give rise to a level of sensory loss which sometimes corresponds to the site of the spinal lesion but often extends only to a more caudal level (p. 232). Spinal cord lesions disrupt reflex arcs and loss of tendon reflexes will reflect the segments which have been damaged.

Often the segmental level and the cross sectional areas of a spinal cord lesion may be gauged (Fig. 8.61). Below a hemisection of the cord on the ipsilateral side there will be found (1) upper motor neurone signs, (2) impaired position and vibration senses, (3) signs of vasomotor disturbance. On the contralateral side there will be reduced sensation to pain and temperature. This composite picture is called the *Brown-Séquard syndrome*.

Multiple lesions. The analysis of a patient's signs may show that they cannot be explained on the basis of a single lesion. Two or more separated, *discrete lesions* may be defined, as for instance when lesions in optic nerves are found concurrently with evidence of spinal cord damage in multiple sclerosis.

Lesions may be systematised, i.e. similar types of fibres or cells may be affected in different parts of the nervous system. A symmetrical polyneuropathy is a systematised affection of peripheral nerves. Damage may be confined to groups of upper and lower motor neurones as in motor neurone disease or to dorsal root ganglion

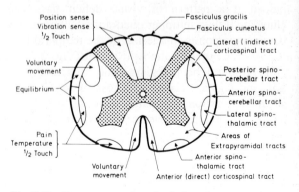

Position sense
Vibration sense
½ Touch

Voluntary movement

Equilibrium

Pain
Temperature
½ Touch

Voluntary movement

Fasciculus gracilis
Fasciculus cuneatus
Lateral (indirect) corticospinal tract
Posterior spino-cerebellar tract
Anterior spino-cerebellar tract
Lateral spino-thalamic tract
Areas of Extrapyramidal tracts
Anterior spino-thalamic tract
Anterior (direct) corticospinal tract

Fig. 8.61   Transverse section of spinal cord.

cells as in one form of carcinomatous neuropathy. Spinal tracts may be selectively damaged, singly or in combination as when dorsal and lateral columns are disrupted by vitamin B_{12} deficiency.

Diffuse damage may be demonstrated when disorders affect wide areas of grey and white matter traversing structural and functional boundaries. Thus alcohol may cause generalised cortical loss, cerebellar degeneration, selective damage to the mid-brain and adjacent structures, as in Wernickes encephalopathy, and peripheral neuropathy. All of these disturbances do not present concurrently but combinations of several such lesions are commonly found in the same patient. Repetitive head injuries also cause randomised, diffuse cerebral affection which results in the dementia, cerebellar ataxia and parkinsonism of the 'punch-drunk' state. The recognition of the patterns of neural lesions provides part of the information needed to make the final aetiological and pathological diagnosis.

c. Pathological diagnosis

In the first instance the development of the illness is reviewed and interpreted in order to estimate the general nature of the neural lesion. More specific clues to aetiology may be contained in the history. The story of an antecedent head injury in an elderly patient with a progressive intracranial lesion may suggest the likelihood of a subdural haematoma. A family history of epilepsy, muscle disease or ataxia may clarify the nature of a patient's illness. Circumstantial evidence from the general medical examination may indicate that the neural lesion is due to the same process which involves other systems. Thus evidence of peripheral vascular disease or of a cardiac arrhythmia might imply that a cerebral lesion was of vascular nature. Clinical evidence of anaemia and a smooth tongue would implicate B_{12} deficiency as the likely cause of a myelopathy. Features of hepatic cirrhosis may suggest an alcohol-related problem.

Finally the nature and distribution of neurological signs might suggest some lesions and help to exclude others. If a patient has signs of intracranial damage together with papilloedema then a space occupying lesion, such as a tumour, is likely. The reflex changes of the Argyll Robertson pupil have been found occasionally in patients with midbrain encephalitis, sarcoidosis or tumours, but their presence, in company with neurological deficit of almost any type, should suggest syphilis as the probable diagnosis. Patients with marked neurological abnormalities, particularly drowsiness and nystagmus, which disappear after a period in hospital may well be suffering from intoxication by either alcohol or drugs.

If the patient with neurological disease is approached in this manner it is often possible to make a firm diagnosis on clinical grounds alone. On those occasions when the information is insufficient the probable causes should be deduced and a rational scheme of investigation designed. Many neurological investigations cause discomfort and some are hazardous; they should be performed only if they are essential in order to define potentially curable lesions. There is no justification for subjecting patients to angiography or lumbar puncture as a substitute for an adequate clinical examination.

2. THE EXAMINATION OF THE COMATOSE PATIENT

The usual orderly and logical approach of history taking, followed by examination and leading to a diagnosis, must be abandoned where the patient's conscious level is impaired. Particular emphasis must be placed on the provision of an adequate airway and ventilatory function together with steps to ensure adequate circulating blood volume and perfusion of vital tissues. Where trauma is suspected, the examination and any movement of the patient with altered consciousness must be performed on the assumption that an unstable spinal injury may be present.

Useful clues to the cause of altered consciousness may be obtained from external examination of the patient to look for needle puncture marks, suggesting an insulin-dependent diabetic or intravenous drug abuser, together with an examination for 'medic alert' bracelets, neck chains or identity cards which list pre-existing medical conditions. Palpation of the scalp for swellings related to local trauma together with careful examination of the head for lacerations must be performed. The ears and nose should be carefully examined to look for blood and/or CSF leakage indicating underlying skull fractures.

History

Wherever possible an account of the circumstances and development of the unconscious state should be obtained from relatives, friends or other witnesses, together with other sources of information, such as ambulance crew or emergency service personnel.

Assessment of conscious state

For clinical purposes, consciousness is defined as the patient's awareness of and response and reaction to the environment. Objective methods of assessing conscious level are important to permit inter-observer communications, together with an ability to assess responses to therapy or deterioration in the primary condition. The most universally applied method of assessment of altered consciousness is by the Glasgow Coma Scale (see Appendix 3 p 356). This was primarily established to assess conscious levels in patients following trauma but also has proved useful in patients with medical causes of coma. Single sets of observations taken on initial examination, are of limited, baseline value only. Repeated clinical examinations are vital. The results of serial examinations should be plotted so that progress can easily be seen. A fall in the numerical value of the Glasgow Coma Scale indicates a decreasing level of consciousness which may represent either a primary neurological deterioration, or impairment of other vital processes, eg respiration and circulation, which are essential to normal neurological function.

General observation

The pattern of respiration should be watched and heard. Deep regular breathing occurs in postictal states. Hyperventilation may be due to metabolic acidosis, e.g. diabetic keto-acidosis or salicylate poisoning. Shallow, slow respiration is commonly seen in opiate overdose. Periodic respiration may result from cardiorespiratory disease, raised intracranial pressure or brain stem lesions. Disorganised, irregular breathing patterns may be seen in severe medullary lesions.

The smell of alcohol on a patient's breath may suggest that this has contributed to an altered state of consciousness. However, patients who have been drinking may have co-existently sustained a head injury or developed any of the other medical causes of altered consciousness. There is a very poor correlation between blood or breath alcohol levels and conscious state and the measurement of these levels is of no immediate additional clinical relevance. Characteristic odours are present in hepatic and severe renal failure and deliberate self poisoning with substances such as bleach and antifreeze. The smell of acetone on the breath may be present in patients with diabetic ketoacidosis. Hypoglycaemia must be excluded in every patient with altered consciousness initially by means of a bedside test on a fingerprick specimen of blood. Where present, hypoglycaemia should be immediately corrected by the administration of intravenous glucagon or dextrose. Where the stix test indicates hypoglycaemia the examining clinician should not wait for the result of a formal blood glucose estimation prior to the administration of glucagon or dextrose.

In patients with altered consciousness with no clearly identifiable cause, the administration of a specific opiate antagonist (Naloxone) is indicated as 'classical' signs of opiate intoxication, i.e. small pupils and a depressed respiratory pattern, are not invariably present.

Examination of the pupillary responses may give a valuable insight into the site of the lesion or lesions leading to altered conscious state. The pupillary pathways are relatively resistant to metabolic insults, therefore the assessment of normal pupillary function may be useful in differentiating structural from metabolic causes of coma. Other pupil signs that may be of value in the unconscious patient are those of unilateral fixed and dilated pupil which may be caused by uncal herniation related to raised intracranial pressure, local ocular trauma or a Holmes Adie pupil. Pinpoint pupils are commonly seen with opiate intoxication and in pontine lesions but may also be present in patients who take miotic eye preparations routinely. Dilated pupils which are reactive to light are a common feature of overdosage with amphetamines and tricyclic anti-depressant drugs.

3. THE DIAGNOSIS OF BRAIN DEATH

It may seem macabre and unnecessary to discuss the diagnosis of death but it has important ethical and legal implications. It has long been accepted that death has occurred when respiration and circulation have ceased. It is now possible to maintain these functions artificially for long periods. It is also generally agreed that permanent cessation of brain function constitutes death and criteria have been established which usually enable this diagnosis to be made with confidence. The need for decision will arise in deeply comatose patients in whom curable causes of coma have been excluded. It is essential to eliminate hypothermia, drug intoxication, hypoglycaemia or other gross metabolic defect before assessing brain stem function. Neuromuscular block can be ruled out either by the presence of tendon reflexes or by direct electrical stimulation of peripheral motor nerves. The following is a checklist for the diagnosis of brain death.

Exclude: hypothermia
drug intoxication
metabolic defect
neuro-muscular block

Test: pupil reflexes
corneal reflexes
vestibulo-ocular reflexes
gag reflex
cough reflex
spontaneous respiration
(and any other cranial nerve response)

Examination

The brain stem reflexes are carefully tested and should be absent. The pupils are unresponsive to bright light, fixed either in wide dilatation or in the mid-position (approximately 5 mm in diameter). The corneal reflex is absent. Twenty ml of ice cold water is slowly injected into each external auditory meatus in turn. If no eye movement occurs the vestibulo-ocular reflexes are absent. The gag and cough reflexes are absent. The patient should show no spontaneous movement nor any reaction to the environment. Spinal reflex activity, though usually absent, may be preserved, but this does not constitute evidence of persisting cerebral function. Usually the patient is hypotonic.

No spontaneous respiration occurs if the patient is removed from a mechanical ventilator long enough to ensure that arterial carbon dioxide rises above the threshold for stimulating respiration. Blood gases should be measured to ensure that this level (6.6 k Pa; 50 mmHg) has been achieved.

Electroencephalography is not an essential prerequisite for the diagnosis of brain death, but if available it can provide supporting evidence thereof. The EEG shows no sign of any electrical activity of cerebral origin in recordings made at high amplification.

It is customary to repeat the testing after an interval, usually a day later. If any doubt still remains then further examinations should be made in succeeding days.

Conclusion

Brain death should be diagnosed only after consultation between two medical practitioners who are experts in the field. One at least should be a consultant and the other a consultant or senior registrar. Each should establish that the preconditions noted above — a deeply comatose patient in whom curable causes of coma have been excluded — have been met before testing is carried out. The length of time before the pre-conditions can be satisfied varies. It is rarely less than twenty-four hours, and may be as long as several days.

The two doctors concerned may carry out the test separately or together. If the tests, on the first occasion, confirm brain death they should nonetheless be repeated. The duration of the interval between tests varies but it should allow adequate time for explanation to be given to relatives and friends of the patient.

FURTHER READING

Cull R E, Simpson J A 1987 Diseases of the nervous
  system. Macleod J, Edwards C, Bouchier I (eds) In:
  Davidson's principles and practice of medicine, 15th edn.
  Churchill Livingstone, Edinburgh
Ross Russell R, Wiles C M (eds) 1985 Integrated clinical
  science: neurology. Heinemann, London

Walton J (ed) 1985 Brain's diseases of the nervous system,
  9th edn. Oxford University Press, Oxford
Walton J et al (eds) 1986 Aids to the examination of the
  peripheral nervous system. Bailliere Tindall, London
Lenman J A R, Ritchie A E 1987 Clinical electromyography,
  4th edn. Churchill Livingstone, Edinburgh

9. The locomotor system

P. J. Abernethy

In the first part of this chapter a simple but comprehensive method of examining the locomotor system is described which can be included with the routine physical examination. This is designed to achieve a rapid assessment of the patient indicating which region, or regions, require more detailed review should any abnormality be found on physical examination or suspected from the history. The second part of the chapter deals with the detailed examination of the various regions. The junior student should initially limit study to Part 1 of the chapter and thereafter refer to the regional examination in Part 2 as specific problems arise.

PART 1
GENERAL EXAMINATION

THE HISTORY: PAIN PATTERNS IN THE LOCOMOTOR DISORDER

Pain is the principal sympton of locomotor pathology and should be analysed as described on page 25. It often has a characteristic pattern in time or in relation to certain activities. This is frequently so clear that the diagnosis can be made from the history alone especially when the clinical signs are few or absent as may occur, for example, in the carpal tunnel syndrome. (p. 55).

The pattern of complaints can often be delineated by taking the patient through a typical day. The following questions cover most activities without suggesting replies.

How do you feel on rising and dressing?
How long can you remain comfortably on your feet?
How far can you walk?
(It is useful to refer to a well-known thoroughfare to estimate distance.)
How long can you sit in comfort?
How do you feel at the end of the day?
How do you sleep?
What makes the pain worse?
What makes the pain better?

This routine also gives an estimate of the patient's abilities which can be compared with findings at a later date. When organic disease is present, a consistent story usually enfolds in contrast to the vague indifference of the hysteric or the aggressive resentment of the malingerer who fears too detailed investigation.

The following notes provide a guide to the characteristic features of pain patterns encountered in specific lesions.

Traumatic lesions

Sprained ligaments. After the initial acute phase when the pain may be severe and constant, pain only occurs with movement which stretches the damaged structure and is relieved when the ligament is relaxed.

Chronic strain of ligaments. In weight-bearing ligaments, in the back or in the foot for example, the patient is most comfortable in the morning. As the day goes on the supporting muscles tire and an aching pain develops which is relieved by rest.

Fracture. There is marked pain with interference of function to a greater or lesser degree. Pain occurs on attempted movement especially when the fracture is not impacted.

Inflammatory lesions

Acute lesion.   The pain steadily increases even at rest. It is throbbing in character and the patient becomes ill and febrile, especially with the formation of pus and the increasing tension within the joint or marrow. Remission of pain and fever occur if pus escapes. When a joint is involved, all movement is inhibited by protective spasm of the controlling muscles. Any attempt at movement whether active or passive causes severe pain. If the patient sleeps deeply the spasm may relax and the patient wakes with a characteristic cry if some movement occurs causing recurrent painful muscle spasm. When there is infection in bone near a joint, movement of the joint may be inhibited by muscle spasm. Gentle examination, however, under these circumstances can often demonstrate that a small range of joint movement is present. In infants localising signs are less easy to discover, but immobility of the affected part is present accompanied by fever, irritability, crying and vomiting.

Chronic lesions.   The features are similar but more prolonged than in acute inflammation. Local and general reactions are less severe. Some movement will still be possible in an early low grade infection of a joint. In rheumatoid arthritis pain and stiffness are characteristically worse in the morning and the patient may take several hours 'to get going'.

Degenerative lesions

Osteoarthritis.   The affected joints are stiff and difficult to move after disuse but move more freely with use. Thus pain and stiffness after prolonged rest relieved by activity but recurring as the patient tires are characteristic of this condition. Night pain may be a disturbing feature.

Prolapsed intervertebral disc.   The history may extend over several years. Prior to any acute episode there is frequently a period of vague aches and pains often accepted by the patient as a normal reaction to activity. An acute episode frequently occurs when bending and lifting or on the day following such activities, but sometimes it can occur for no discernible reason. Pain subsides with rest but may take several weeks to disappear. Thereafter periods of relief are interspersed with major or minor episodes of pain. This characteristically episodic pattern emerges into that of osteoarthrosis.

Ischaemia.   Intermittent claudication is described in Chapter 5.

Spinal stenosis.   Narrowing of the spinal canal and neuroforamina are usually caused by degenerative changes and can result in back pain with radiation to the legs. The pain is often diffuse accompanied by tingling and numbness and by malfunction of the muscles. These symptoms, which the patient finds difficult to describe, increase with standing and walking and are relieved by sitting or lying down. Forward flexion of the spine can also afford relief, sometimes allowing the patient to cycle in comfort despite their limited walking distance.

Instability.   Unstable lesions, such as spondylolisthesis, are associated with increasing pain as the day goes on. After rest the muscles and ligaments are relaxed. As the supporting muscles tire, the related ligaments stretch and pain increases. The pain is aggravated by straightening up and by active, especially bilateral, straight leg raising when supine.

Tumours

With the exception of osteoid osteoma, benign bone tumours do not cause pain unless by pressure on neighbouring structures. Pain is not an invariable feature of malignant tumours but when present it is not related to any special activity, is not relieved by rest and may even be worse at night, disturbing the patient's sleep. Pathological fracture may occur as a result of trivial trauma and causes sudden acute pain.

Secondary gain or 'compensation' pain

There is an astonishing consistency in history and pattern of pain associated with claims for compensation. The patient can recall the accident in minute detail including the date and time, almost to the second, even if it occurred years before. The accident was always some other agent's fault. The pain is constant with dramatic exacerbations always vividly described. It shows no sign of improving and may even be worsening. The patient remains off work and is often accompanied by the spouse or some other supporter who will testify to the worrying amount of analgesics which has to be consumed to relieve the pain.

THE PHYSICAL EXAMINATION

There are three main components, namely the examination of (1) posture, (2) gait and (3) the limbs and spine. The ideal arrangement is that the patient is observed walking into the consulting room allowing an early assessment of posture and gait. Good lighting and adequate space are essential. The examination couch should be accessible from both sides and there must be no obstacle preventing a full range of movement of the patient's limbs.

1. Posture

For adequate assessment the patient should be able to stand and walk. Where this is not possible some idea of the posture can be gained by examination of the patient in the supine and prone positions. Normal posture varies from age to age, passing through a cycle of change as we 'ripe and rot' (Fig. 9.1). In utero and for a short time after birth there is a generalised dorsal convexity of the spine or kyphosis. When the child holds up its head the cervical spine develops a curve convex ventrally — a lordosis. When the child begins to walk a secondary lordosis develops in the lumbar region, often an exaggerated amount, and the legs remain flexed and abducted at the hips and flexed at the knees. Only in the juvenile and the young adult does the typical human erect posture pertain.

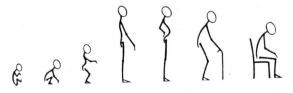

Fig. 9.1 The seven ages of man. Posture change.

Pregnancy or obesity again exaggerate the lumbar lordosis. Thereafter the lumbar discs degenerate and the lumbar lordosis is lost. Flexion of the hips dating from the previous era is unmasked and with sticks a second quadruped stage is reached. The cervical discs degenerate further and finally the general kyphosis of the foetus is reproduced in the wheelchair. In pre-history the cycle was often completed by burial in the womb posture of the foetus.

Thus variations in the curves of the spine are to be expected throughout life. When exaggerated or when angular rather than curved, they become abnormal.

Viewed from the front or behind, the pelvis should be level, the iliac crests being on the same horizontal plane and the spine in a vertical line. Lateral curvature (scoliosis) is always abnormal. In the cervical region it is termed torticollis or wry neck. In the thoraco-lumbar region the scoliosis may be due to faulty posture and be correctable. It may be due to protective spasm where a painful lesion is present or it may be permanent due to an overlying structural change. These can be differentiated by getting the patient to bend forward keeping the legs straight. A postural scoliosis will be corrected. A curve due to a painful condition will be associated with limited flexion to a greater or lesser degree. Scoliosis due to a painless structural lesion will persist even on flexion and a hump will be revealed on the convex side of the curve because the lateral curvature of the spine is accompanied by rotation of the vertebra at the apex of the curve (p. 274). The terms valgus and varus are applied to deviation of the limb away from (valgus) and towards (varus) the midline.

The posture of the limbs varies in the sexes when seen from in front. In the male the arms almost hang straight from the shoulders with the forearm in supination. There is a valgus angulation at the elbow to allow the hand to lie away from the side to permit function in the carrying position. The pelvis in the male is narrow and the femora do not have to converge sharply to allow the tibiae to be parallel and together (Fig. 9.2). The female is pear-shaped. To clear the broad pelvis the forearm is further abducted at the elbow increasing the carrying angle. Because of the width of the female pelvis the femora slope more acutely to the

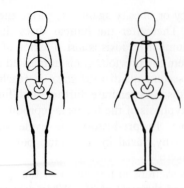

Fig. 9.2   Skeletal differences in male and female.

knee giving a greater valgus angulation of the tibia on the femur. Where this is exaggerated and the tibiae no longer lie parallel it is known as genu valgum or knock knee deformity. The reverse angulation of the tibia adducted on the femur produces the deformity of genu varum, or bow legs.

2. Gait

The normal human gait is a complex phenomenon in which movement occurs in several joints simultaneously in three dimensions. Biped gait would be expected to result in abrupt oscillations of the body up and down and from side to side. It is converted into an even undulation of small amplitude, at least in the male, by movements occurring between the spine and pelvis and at the hip, knee and ankle. Interference with more than one of these components results in an obvious limp. Although there are great variations in normal gait and in the pattern of abnormal gaits, the latter can be divided into two types; those that are painful and those that are not.

Painful gait

The rhythm more than the contour of the gait is disturbed. The patient takes weight off the painful limb as quickly as possible and the timing is dot-dash, painful-normal, painful-normal. When the pain is severe the limb, flexed at hip, knee and ankle, is placed delicately on the ground and the patient hops quickly onto the sound leg. The painful region, if it is within reach, is supported by one hand and the other arm is outstretched to counterbalance. At the other extreme, the only sign may be shortening of the stride on the affected side.

Painless gait

The contour rather than the rhythm of the gait is abnormal. The different varieties can be classified as follows:

Ostoegenic — due to shortening or deformity of the bone
Arthrogenic — due to joint stiffness, laxity or deformity
Myogenic — due to weakness of muscle
Neurogenic — due to organic disorder of the nervous system
Psychogenic — due to psychiatric causes
Prosthetic — due to wearing an artificial limb

   a. Osteogenic gait. With the patient clothed and wearing special footwear there may be little or no evident disturbance of gait, but when stripped for examination no difficulty should be encountered in detecting the cause of the abnormal gait.
   b. Arthrogenic gait. Complete loss of movement due to ankylosis of the hip or ankle often results in suprisingly little disturbance of gait and may pass unnoticed in the clothed patient. When the hip is fixed in a few degrees of flexion and neutral abduction and adduction, the contour of the gait is little disturbed. With the common deformity of more severe fixed flexion of the hip the gluteal region becomes prominent as the leg extends and the gait is awkward. With bilateral hip flexion contracture of this magnitude, the patient adopts a 'Charlie Chaplin' type of gait with both buttocks prominent. If the hip has an abduction deformity, an unsightly gait results as the leg has to swing out and round with each step. The effect of a stiff knee is immediately obvious and the patient has to mount the stairs one at a time with the sound leg leading and descend with the stiff leg leading, (the 'good leg leading up to heaven' and the 'bad leg down to hell').
   A stiff ankle or foot causes little interference with normal gait unless accompanied by deform-

ity. If the foot is plantar flexed in equinus (p. 288) the gait will resemble that of a drop foot (p. 260), but this may not be obvious if high heels are worn.

c. Myogenic gait. The effect of muscle weakness will depend on site and degree. For example, in muscular dystrophy or as a result of the myopathy occurring in severe osteomalacia in the elderly there is a characteristic waddling gait due to involvement of the gluteal muscles.

d. Neurogenic gait. *Spastic paralysis.* The typical spastic gait is seen in patients severely brain damaged from birth. The arms are adducted at the shoulder and flexed at the elbow and wrist. The posture is stooping with legs flexed and adducted at the hip and flexed at the knee and ankle. The patient hitches each knee round and past its neighbour with a jerk, scraping the plantar flexed foot along the ground. In the mildly affected patient, the only noticeable abnormality will be the curious impression that the patient is wearing heavy boots giving rise to difficulty raising the effect off the ground at the beginning of each step. Likewise a patient with a hemiparesis will often exhibit a characteristic gait. The affected leg is stiff and swings forward in a circular fashion rather than being lifted from the ground (Fig. 9.3).

Flaccid paralysis. In contrast to the gaits of an ankylosed hip or foot the corresponding gaits in muscle paralysis are very obvious.

(i) Hip. Normally the abductors of the hip on the weightbearing limb contract to elevate the pelvis on the opposite side to allow that limb to clear the ground on walking. If the abductors are paralysed the pelvis tilts down on the opposite side and to counteract this the patient has to lean towards the affected side (Fig. 9.39). This gives the impression of the patient lurching or dipping towards the paralysed side. A similar gait is seen in congenital dislocation of the hip. When both limbs are involved in this way, a waddling gait results.

(ii) Knee. Paralysis of the muscles controlling the knee may be compensated by the hip and calf muscles and there may be no limp. This occurs as a result of the joint being locked in full extension by the extensors of the hip and the calf. Locking of the knee may be assisted in these circumstances if the foot is in equinus. If the hip extensors are

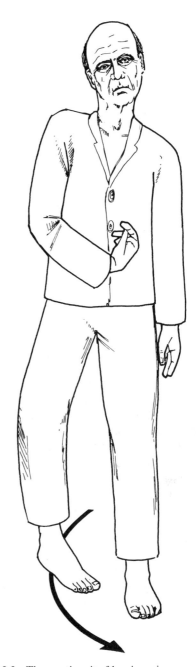

Fig. 9.3 The spastic gait of hemiparesis.

also weak the patient may push back with the hand on the thigh at each step in an attempt to lock the knee in extension. If, in addition, the calf muscles are weak, the patient will be unable to walk without a supporting caliper.

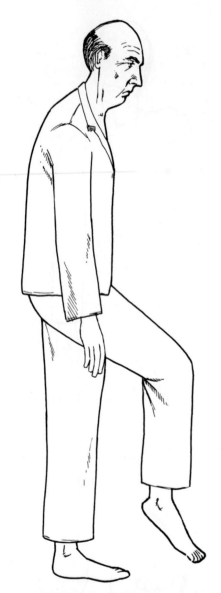

Fig. 9.4 The high-stepping gait in drop foot.

generalised polyneuropathy and can cause a high stepping gait in both legs.

Extrapyramidal lesions. A patient suffering from Parkinsonism will usually exhibit a slow, shuffling gait with each step being smaller than normal (Fig. 9.5). One of the early signs of the disease is an absence of arm swinging on walking. Some patients with Parkinsonism tend to take increasingly rapid steps forward in an attempt to maintain an upright posture. This is referred to as a festinant gait. Some patients with encephalitis lethargica or post-encephalitic Parkinsonism show odd interruptions of their forward progression. They may halt, spin around on their axis and then continue forward.

Cerebellar lesions. Patients with bilateral cerebellar disease walk on a wide base or in a drunken reeling manner.

Combinations of neurogenic gait disturbance may occur, one example being unsteadiness due to a cerebellar lesion combined with spastic stiffness of the legs in multiple sclerosis.

e. Psychogenic gait. Hysteria may be suspected if the gait is bizarre or if the patient appears to be strangely unmoved by the disability. The malingerer, on the other hand, is more likely to mimic a painful gait but usually fails to achieve the typical rhythm tending to linger on the painful limb creating an impression of great agony while doing so.

f. Prosthetic gait. When clothed, a patient with a below knee prosthesis is difficult to detect, but with an above knee prosthesis the patient hitches the whole leg forwards, snapping the knee into extension and bringing the foot heavily to the ground. This may be accompanied by the creaking of the prosthetic straps and hinges.

3. Initial examination of limbs and spine

Considered in conjunction with the history, this assessment will indicate that either all is well or that there is a local abnormality which will require more detailed review as described in Part 2 of this chapter. The methods used are inspection, measurement of joint movement, and palpation.

Inspection

Examination begins with the inspection of joints

(iii) Ankle and foot. Paralysis of the dorsiflexors of the foot results in the drop-foot gait. The abnormality will often be detected as readily by the ear as by the eye, for patients tend to lift the foot high to clear the toes from the ground and as it is returned there is a loud slapping noise (Fig. 9.4). Unilateral foot drop may be due to compression or division of the common peroneal nerve, or to a spinal lesion. Bilateral foot may be due to

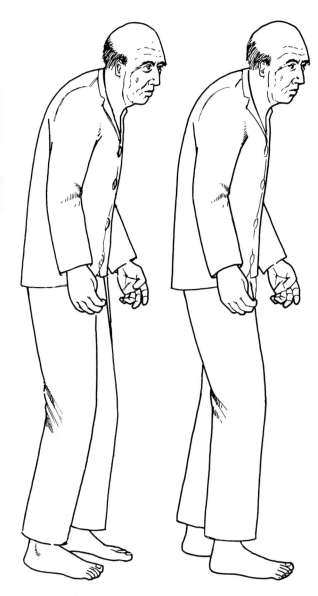

Fig. 9.5 The slow shuffling gait in Parkinsonism.

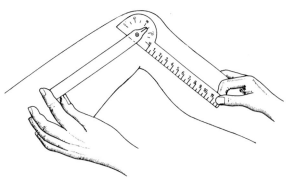

Fig. 9.6 Gonimeter.

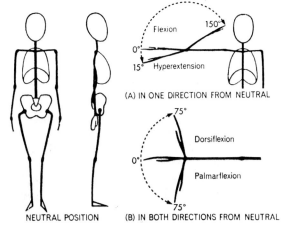

Fig. 9.7 Measuring movements of joints.

where note is taken of any deformity, swelling, discolouration or associated muscle wasting.

Measuring the movement of joints

Many students make the mistake of beginning by seizing the patient's limb and forcing it through a wide range of movements until halted by the patient's protest. Active movements are performed

and compared with those of the normal limb, or with the examiner's if both sides are affected. Movements of the limb joints can be measured directly and objectively by the use of a goniometer (Fig. 9.6). Such records are useful while description of movement such as good, fair or bad are useless for comparison. The neutral zero method is recommended as it is simple and generally accepted. In this method all the joints are considered to be in neutral position when the body is in the classical anatomical position with two exceptions. Firstly, the hands are flatly against the thighs in the saggital and not the coronal plane. Secondly, the feet are at right angles to the leg and are not plantar flexed (Fig. 9.7). In certain joints such as the elbow and knee, movement can normally occur only in one direction from neutral e.g. flexion 0°–

150°. Extension past 0° normally does not occur and when it does is therefore referred to as hyper-extension 0°–15°. In other joints such as the wrist and ankle movement normally occurs in both directions from 0° and in the wrist is defined as palmar flexion and dorsiflexion. Finally, certain joints such as the shoulders and hips allow movements in all directions from the neutral position. Such movements are defined as flexion, extension, abduction, adduction, internal and external rotation. Combined they result in circumduction.

Both the active and passive movements are measured and separately recorded if they differ. Where limitation of movement is present it is best described by the arc of movement present. For example, if a patient lacks 30° of extension of the elbow and can flex to 90° from that position, the range of movement is described as flexion 30°–90°.

Hands. These should be inspected as described on page 52 looking first at the dorsum of the hands. The patient is then asked to clench the fist, show the palms and spread the fingers (Fig. 9.8).

Wrists. After inspection the patient is asked to put the hands in the position of prayer and then lower the hands keeping the palms together. This demonstrates the extreme of dorsiflexion. The backs of the hands are then placed together and the arms raised to demonstrate the range of flexion, the two sides being compared. If these movements are normal, others need not be checked.

Elbows. The patient is instructed to bend and straighten both elbows simultaneously and limitation in this range is revealed by comparison of one side with the other. The patient is then asked to flex the elbow and pronate and supinate the forearm (see p. 269). Deformity or limitation of movement indicates the need for careful palpation of the joint.

Shoulders. The patient is asked to raise the arms forwards to their fullest extent and should be able to do so to the vertical. Abduction, external rotation and internal rotation of the shoulder are tested by the patient touching the back of the neck and then bringing the arms down to touch the small of the back keeping the arms in the coronal plane as they descend (Fig. 9.8). Any limitation of movement or painful arc of movement is noted.

Spine. Any deformity or abnormality of posture

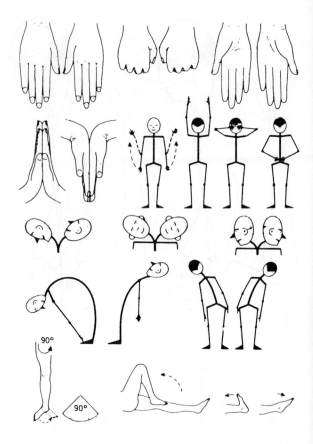

Fig. 9.8   Inspection of principal active movements.

will be noted on inspection. The patient is asked to touch each shoulder with the chin and then with each ear. The patient is then asked to touch the toes without bending the knees. The level which can be reached is noted and whether this movement is achieved by smooth general flexion of the spine. Protected spasm or structural change will be unmasked. If forward flexion is impaired, lateral flexion, rotation and extension should also be tested.

Hips. If rotation of the hip is unimpaired it is unlikely that other significant limitation is present. Rotation is measured by attempting to put the extended lower limb through the normal arc of 90° using the foot as an indicator. If rotation is restricted then the range of flexion, extension, abduction, adduction should be measured and recorded.

Knees, ankles and feet. Inspection of the knees is followed by requesting the patient to move the joints from full extension through a range of flexion. The ankle joints are similarly flexed and extended by the patient and the feet inverted and everted. Inspection of the feet will show any abnormalities such as flattening of the arches, callosities or deformities.

Palpation

This supplements the findings on inspection. Any points of tenderness should be localised by firm palpation and if possible the involved tissue identified by putting stress on the structure thought to be affected. The temperature of a swollen joint should be compared to that of the other limb. Active movements can be repeated while the joints are palpated to detect crepitus or clicks. Passive movements can then be assessed and compared with the active range. During these manoeuvres the patient should be asked to report any tenderness and the face should be watched for any indication of pain.

The interpretation of abnormal joint movement

The movements of a joint can be restricted or increased by changes in bone cartilage, synovial membrane, capsule, ligaments, muscles and related nerves. By the systematic examination of each structure in turn, the cause of the abnormal movement can be found.

Bone, articular cartilage and synovial membrane. Significant pathology, whether traumatic, rheumatological, degenerative or infective in nature, causes diminished movement in all

directions (Fig. 9.8). Tenderness, if present, is generally over the whole joint.

Complete lack of movement accompanied by pain is due to acute inflammation or recent trauma and these are differentiated by the history (Fig. 9.8). Complete lack of movement without pain indicates spontaneous fusion (ankylosis) or surgical fusion (arthrodesis) of the joint.

Capsule or ligament. A sprained or strained capsule or ligament is painful when stretched by active or passive movements towards the opposite side of the joint. Movement in this direction is restricted by protective spasm of muscles. Movements towards the side of the strained ligament relieves the painful tension and is not limited (Fig. 9.10). Tenderness is localised to the sprained area. An effusion may be present if the capsule is intact.

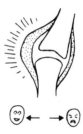

Fig. 9.10 Sprain of capsule or ligament.

A ruptured ligament is initially painful on movement towards the opposite side of the joint. This movement can be excessive in degree and any fluid in the joint escapes and causes a swelling over the ruptured ligament other than within the joint itself. Movement towards the same side 'closes' the joint and relieves pain (Fig. 9.11).

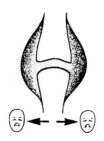

Fig. 9.9 Inflammation of a joint.

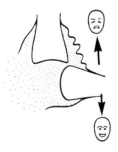

Fig. 9.11 Rupture of capsule or ligament.

Intra-articular structures. A structure such as a torn semilunar cartilage displaced in the joint is compressed by movement towards it. Pain is localised over the structure and that movement is restricted. Movement away from the pathology is not painful or reduced (Fig. 9.12). An effusion is usually present in the joint.

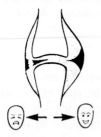

Fig. 9.12   Rupture of semilunar cartilage.

Muscle. With a painful lesion in muscle, active contraction, even with no movement, causes pain and is restricted. Passive movement in the same direction relaxes the muscles, relieves pain and is not restricted to the same extent. Both active and passive movements in the opposite direction are restricted by pain (Fig. 9.13).

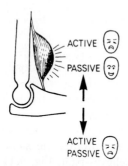

Fig. 9.13   Painful lesion in a muscle.

Pain arising in a muscle close to a joint can be distinguished from that due to a strained ligament. Contraction of the suspected muscle without movement of the joint (isometric contraction) will produce pain if the muscle and not the ligament is the cause. For example, in 'tennis elbow' passive extension of the elbow is painful, but this action stretches both the capsule of the elbow and the extensor muscle origin. The patient now clenches the fist without moving the elbow, thus contracting the synergistic extensor muscles and pain results localised to the extensor origin proving that this is the source of the pain.

When examining a muscle which acts over two joints, the same principles apply. Derangement of such a muscle is suspected when movement at one joint influences the range of movement at the neighbouring joint. For example, if there is a fixed equinus or flexion of the ankle joint when the knee is extended it could be due to changes in the ankle joint itself or to contracture of the gastrocnemius muscle or soleus muscle. Flexion of the knee relaxes the gastrocnemius muscle; if dorsiflexion is now possible the gastrocnemius muscle and not the ankle joint must have been the cause of the problem (Fig. 9.14).

Rupture or paralysis of a muscle. When a muscle is paralysed or its tendon divided, active movement towards the muscle is abolished but passive movement initially is unaffected (Fig. 9.15). Active and passive movement in the opposite direction is excessive and if no treatment is initiated the uncontrolled antagonist muscles will pull the related joint into an abnormal posture.

The nerves. The effect of paralysis on joint

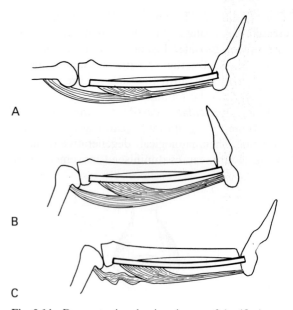

Fig. 9.14   Demonstrating that impairment of dorsiflexion at the ankle may be corrected by knee flexion if the cause is contraction of gastrocnemius muscle (B), but will not correct if the pathlogy is in the ankle (C).

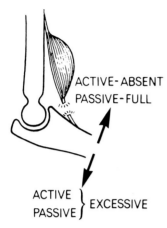

ACTIVE - ABSENT
PASSIVE - FULL

ACTIVE }
PASSIVE } EXCESSIVE

Fig. 9.15 Rupture of a muscle.

movement is discussed on page 259. Abnormal tension on a nerve will result in limitation of both active and passive movement which would increase that tension. The nerve stretching tests described on page 276 illustrate how such limitation of movement in the case of a prolapsed intervertebral disc can be differentiated from that caused by joint or muscle lesions.

PART 2
REGIONAL EXAMINATION

Another man, Adwyne by name, in the town of Dunwych, that dwelled on the sea shore, was so contracted that he could not use the free office of hand or foot. His legs were cleaving to the hinder part of his thighs so that he could not walk, and his hands were turned backward. Nothing could be done by them. The extremities of his fingers were so rigorously contracted in the sinews that he could not put meat to his mouth. In this grievous sickness he passed his young age.

Anon (quoted from Griffith E F 1951 Doctors by themselves. Cassell, London)

This twelfth century quotation is the earliest recorded account of the admission of a patient to St. Bartholomew's Hospital. It is a graphic but extreme example of the complexities which occur in the locomotor system in neglected patients. A very detailed and expert examination may be required

to elucidate the cause of each disability. However, the initial assessment may have to be carried out by any doctor. Undergraduates need not be overawed by what confronts them if their methods are based on an understanding of the anatomy and the pathology of the conditions commonly encountered in the various regions. A competent history will also do much to clarify the problem.

THE UPPER LIMB

THE HAND, WRIST AND FOREMAN

Some of the many abnormalities to be found in the hand have been outlined on pages 52–57, notably its involvement in arthritis and the changes of diagnostic value to be seen in the fingers (Fig. 4.1 p. 53) and in the nails (Fig. 4.2 p. 54). In this section the function of the hand is the primary consideration.

Hand function depends on mobility and sensitivity. The mobility depends upon the flexibility of the joints and the smooth gliding of tendons within sheaths. This makes it liable to a special group of friction syndromes involving tendons (tenosynovitis). The hands are extremely prone to injury for obvious reasons. Because of the intimate relationship of the skin, bones, joints and tendons, nerves and vessels, injury seldom involves a single structure. Open injuries often become infected and once established, infection may spread along the natural tissue spaces or the tendon sheaths.

Anatomical features

Skin and deep fascia. In the palm both structures are thickened and are bound together at the skin creases. On the dorsum the skin and deep fascia are thin and elastic. Because of these differences any generalised swelling of the hand will be more evident on the dorsum. The skin has a very abundant nerve and blood supply on both aspects of the hand.

Muscles. The muscles in the forearm are the power-house of the hand and wrist. Without the help of the intrinsic muscles of the hand however neither a proper grip nor fine movements are possible. If the intrinsic muscles are paralysed, the long muscles acting alone may cause curling of the fingers. Such a hand is useful only as a paper-weight or a hook.

Joints. The interphalangeal joints allow only flexion and extension. The metacarpal phalangeal joints allow flexion and extension and some abduction and adduction but only when extended. The wrist joint allows flexion and extension, radial and ulnar deviation and circumduction.

Rotation of the forearm. This movement depends upon the integrity of the superior and inferior radio-ulnar joints and on the concavity of the volar aspects of the shafts of the radius and ulna. In pronation these two concavities fit into one another and rotation will be limited if this curve is distorted as may occur after fracture.

Nerve supply. The radial, ulnar and median nerves are all involved in hand function. Variations in the distribution of nerve supply are very common particularly as a result of overlap between the median and ulnar nerves.

The *radial nerve* supplies the wrist and finger extensors and an area of skin sensation on the dorsum of the first interosseous space. Damage to the nerve is liable to occur in the spiral groove of the humerus resulting in 'drop wrist'. The grip is considerably weakened because the flexors now have no antagonist to steady the wrist.

The *ulnar nerve* supplies sensation to the ulnar border of the hand. Its motor contribution is most important in the hand where it supplies all the small muscles, except the short flexor, abductor and opponens of the thumb and the lumbricals to the index and sometimes the middle finger. The nerve may be damaged at the elbow or the wrist resulting in the claw-hand deformity (Fig. 4.3 p. 56). The ring and little fingers are clawed and the wasting of the muscles between the metacarpals is most evident in the cleft between the index and the thumb. The clawing-extension at the metacarpo-phalangeal joint and flexion at the interphalangeal joints is the result of the unopposed action of the long flexors and extensors.

The *median nerve* supplies the main bulk of the flexor muscles in the forearm and most of the small muscles of the thumb as well as the lumbricals to the index and middle fingers. The common site of damage is at the wrist where it lies superficially. Paralysis of the muscles supplied in the

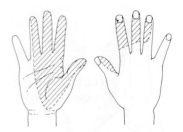

Fig. 9.16 The use of diagrams in case recording. Area of anaesthesia in a patient with a lesion of the right median nerve.

hand results and the muscles of the thenar eminence waste and the thumb falls into flat ape-like or simian deformity. Although this interferes significantly with hand function, the most disabling component of the injury is loss of sensation on the volar aspect of the index and middle fingers (Fig. 9.16). It is from this area that so much information is received about the environment during pinch grip. Activities such as dressing and sorting coins in the pocket can no longer be performed unless under direct vision.

Examination of the hand, wrist and forearm

This consists of inspection and palpation. Particular attention is paid to the assessment of the hand. The hand distal to any wound must be carefully examined. Any apparent trivial laceration may involve tendons, nerves or joints. Some authorities consider the thumb, others the index finger, as the first digit. In order to avoid confusion, therefore, the digits must never be numbered but must be specified by name — thumb, index, middle, ring and little finger. This may be tedious but it will reduce the risk of the wrong finger being treated or even amputated. Diagrams showing scars, amputated portions or other deformities make an accurate and easily understood record (Fig. 9.17).

Assessment of hand function

This involves examination of the active and passive movement of the wrist and digits. Any limitation of movement is assessed as described on p. 261 and the cause is identified. A long time may be

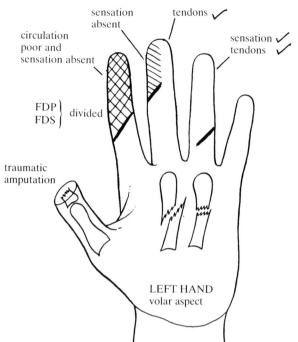

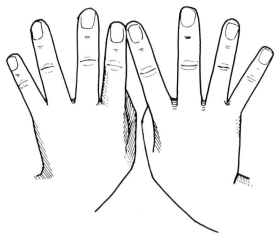

Fig. 9.18 Testing the dorsal interossei. Demonstrates weakness of the 1st dorsal interossei (abducter) on the left.

Fig. 9.17 The use of diagrams in case recording. This diagram summarises at a glance the following mass of information: (1) Traumatic amputation obliquely through the distal phalanx of the thumb. (2) Deep laceration of the index finger over the middle phalanx running obliquely from the radial side to the ulnar side of the finger. The digital nerves, arteries and both flexor tendons have been divided. (3) Deep laceration of the middle finger obliquely over the radial aspect of the middle phalanx. The digital nerve on the radial aspect has been divided. The tendons are intact. (4) Superficial laceration of ring finger over the ulnar aspect of the proximal phalanx without damage to tendons or nerves. (5) Closed fracture of the metacarpal of the middle finger obliquely through the mid-shaft with displacement. (6) Closed fracture of the metacarpal of the ring finger tranversely through the mid-shaft without displacement.

required to complete the examination of the whole hand and record the findings. The integrity of individual tendons is tested by observing if their normal reaction is present.

Flexor digitorum profundus is the only muscle which flexes the distal interphalangeal joint and its action is therefore tested by flexion of this joint while the finger is held in extension at the proximal joint.

Flexor digitorum sublimis flexes the proximal interphalangeal joints. When testing this tendon the action of profundus can be eliminated by holding

the remaining fingers in extension. The flexor profundus has a muscle belly action common to all fingers, and its action is therefore all or nothing. If three of the fingers are extended the muscle controlling the fourth finger will be unable to contract significantly. If the finger flexes at the proximal interphalangeal joint this is due to the action of flexor digitorum sublimis.

The lumbricals cause flexion at the metacarpophalangeal joint and extension at the interphalangeal joint. These are tested by asking the patient to actively extend the interphalangeal joints with the metacarpo-phalangeal joints held in flexion. The *interossei* assist the lumbricals with these movements and also abduct (dorsal interossei) and adduct (palmar interossei) the fingers from the midline of the middle finger. Abduction is tested by asking the patient to spread the extended fingers against resistance or pressing the side of the tip of the index fingers against one another. The finger with the weak interosseus muscle will be pushed towards the middle finger (Fig. 9.18). Adduction can also be tested by the ability to hold a card between the fingers held in extension.

The intrinsic muscles (interossei and lumbricals) frequently waste and become contracted in rheumatoid arthritis, producing an exaggerated version of their normal action. The metacarpophalangeal joints are flexed, the proximal interphalangeal joints extended and the distal joints

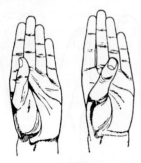

Fig. 9.19 Abduction and opposition of the thumb.

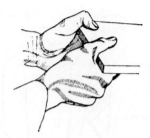

Fig. 9.20 Normal right and paralysed left adductor pollicis.

flexed — the 'swan neck' deformity. In the later stages of this disease, the metacarpo-phalangeal joints may become dislocated.

Thenar muscles supplied by the median nerve. The abductor brevis and opponens combine to produce opposition. This is tested by asking the patient to touch the terminal phalanx of the little finger with the thumb and maintain this position against resistance. Difficulty may be encountered at differentiating between opposition and adduction which is produced by the ulnar supplied adductor pollicis. Observe the nail of the thumb from the palmar aspect. On adduction (the ulnar nerve) it is seen in side view, in opposition it is rotated so that the plane of the nail lies in the plane of the palm (Fig. 9.19).

Thenar muscles supplied by the ulnar nerve. Paralysis of the adductor pollicis is accompanied by muscle wasting in the palm between the thumb and the index finger. The patient is asked to hold a thin book between the radial side of the clenched fingers and extended thumb. When the adductor is not functioning the thumb cannot be held extended and flexion occurs at the metacarpo-phalangeal and interphalangeal joints (Froment's sign). This is because the adductor is unable to hold the head of the metacarpal against the index finger (Fig. 9.20).

Extensor tendons. Assessment of paralysis is not difficult, but the tendons are liable to rupture at various sites. Separation may occur from the distal phalanx with or without fragment of bone. This results in mallet finger deformity. The central slip of the extensor which inserts to the bone of the middle phalanx may rupture producing a boutonniere deformity if the lateral bands slip

volarly along each side of the proximal interphalangeal joint. The proximal interphalangeal joint is then flexed and the distal joint is extended. The extensor pollices longus occasionally ruptures at the wrist after a Colles fracture or in rheumatoid arthritis with loss of extension of the thumb. The normal action of the extensor pollicis longus is to elevate the thumb when observed in side view. This is tested by asking the patient to place his palm on a flat surface and to lift the thumb off the flat surface like a hitch-hiker. Any apparent loss of the 'hitch-hiker's' thumb under these circumstances indicates loss of extensor pollicis longus function.

Trigger finger and thumb. Flexion is not limited but extension of the interphalangeal joint is until straightening of the finger suddenly occurs accompanied by a click, felt over the thickened portion of the mouth of the flexor tendon sheath. This lies at the level of the metacarpal head surface marked by the distal palmar skin crease. In babies the condition is often not noticed until extension at the interphalangeal joints is permanently limited. The thumb is most frequently involved at this age and the thickened flexor sheath is easily palpable over the metacarpal head. Triggering is produced by the thickened sheath causing a swelling on the flexor tendon. The finger locks in flexion as the tendon swelling jams in the narrow mouth of the fibrous sheath.

THE ELBOW

The humerus is not infrequently the site of acute osteomyelitis in the young. Fractures occur at all ages and the intimate relationship of the humerus with three nerves, the circumflex at its neck, the radial at the mid-shaft level and the ulnar nerve at the elbow, may result in injury to these nerves. Fracture at the supracondylar level may damage the brachial artery and cause ischaemic changes in the flexor muscles of the forearm (Volkmann's ischaemic contracture).

The elbow is not a common site of congenital deformity or degenerative change but next to the knee it is the most frequent site of osteochondritis dissecans. The reaction of the elbow to trauma is unpredictable. Minor trauma may be followed by complete stiffness, whereas gross disorganisation of the joint may be compatible with excellent function. One stiff elbow, provided it is not too extended is not a great handicap, but bilateral elbow stiffness can cause severe disability. Patients with sero-positive rheumatoid arthritis often develop nodules over the upper posterior aspect of the ulna.

Anatomical features

The joint is composed of two parts, that between the humerus, radius and ulna, and the superior radio-ulnar joint. The former allows flexion to a range of 150° and the latter allows rotation of the wrist through 180°. The forearm is abducted on the humerus to form a cubitus valgus. Where this angle is increased by fracture of the capitellum for example, the ulnar nerve can become stretched and its function impaired. The joint between the humerus, radius and ulna is stable and is not dislocated easily. The head of the radius, particularly in children, may dislocate.

Examination of the elbow

Inspection

With both arms exposed, deformities are detected by inspecting the elbow from behind with the arm flexed and extended. The relationship of the olecranon and the lateral and medial epicondyles in the abnormal joint is compared with that of the normal side. The hollow over the head of the radius is filled in when an effusion is present.

The patient should flex and extend both arms at the same time when the range of each can be compared. The patient is then asked to flex the elbow to a right angle and to tuck the elbow into the side while supinating and pronating both hands. Care must be taken to ensure that the elbow is kept to the sides when measuring pronation because the movement can be simulated by abduction at the shoulder.

Palpation

This is conducted for bony contour, local tenderness or signs of inflammation. In tennis elbow, tenderness is well localised in the region of the common extensor origin on the lateral epicondyle. Pain is reproduced by gripping, by resisted extension of the wrist and by passive extension of the elbow while the forearm is pronated and the wrist flexed. An effusion in the joint is most easily felt over the head of the radius and the postero-lateral aspect of the joint. Here the head of the radius lies almost subcutaneously and is easily palpated if the forearm is rotated at the same time. Loose bodies are seldom palpable as they tend to collect in the coronoid and olecranon fossae which are covered by muscle. The collateral ligaments can be tested only when the elbow is fully extended. The ulnar nerve is palpated in the post-condylar groove and compared with the normal side to determine any enlargement, tenderness or excessive mobility.

THE SHOULDER

The alignment of the upper limb has changed little from that of the reptile. Most of man's activities involve the use of the hands within an area limited above and below by the orifices of the alimentary tract, side-ways by little more than the breadth of the shoulder and forwards by the extent of the reach. The emphasis is on mobility rather than stability, despite which congenital dislocation of the shoulder is virtually unkown. In the young adult, dislocation readily occurs following injury and therafter the tendency to recurrent dislocation is very great. Osteoarthritis is relatively uncommon. However the joint has a marked tendency to become stiff because of little understood changes in the soft tissues. Whatever the cause, this condition conveniently and graphically described as 'frozen shoulder' is so common from early middle age onwards that it must be kept in mind when examining a patient suffering from any painful condition from the neck to the finger tips. The shoulder will stiffen if movement of the joint is not maintained for any reason, including pain in the neck or in the arm itself. It can occur after myocardial infarction or following hemiplegia. Subluxation is also very common following hemiplegia.

Anatomical features

Movements. Movement of the shoulder is a complicated synthesis of movement occurring at four joints. The glenohumeral and scapulo-thoracic joints each account for about half of the total range whereas movements at the acromio-clavicular and sterno-clavicular joints are relatively unimportant. Rather than define the range of movement and try to explain the complex relation-ship between rotation, flexion and abduction, the reader is invited to demonstrate these movements personally. The range of movement varies with the rotation of the arm. This can be shown with the elbow flexed to a right angle and the forearm act-ing as an indicator of rotation. Abduction can proceed only a little beyond 90° with the arm in neutral rotation. If the arm is then externally rotated full abduction is possible. When limitation of movement is present, the gleno-humeral and scapulo-thoracic contributions must be separated. This is achieved by holding the inferior angle of the scapula with one hand and abducting the arm with the other (Fig. 9.21). Rotation can be

demonstrated again by using the forearm as an in-dicator. With the arm by the side in neutral rotation and the elbow flexed to 90°, the forearm will be directed medially by some 20° and not lie in the sagittal plane. 90° of rotation should be possible from this position in both directions. The forearm cannot quite reach the coronal plane in external rotation but the patient should be able to touch the small of the back in internal rotation. With the arm in full external rotation and the elbow flexed at 90°, abduction of the shoulder will then bring the hand to the back of the neck.

Rotator cuff. This term is applied to the con-joint tendons of supraspinatus, infraspinatus and teres minor. These, with the tendon of sub-scapularis, form a hood-like structure covering the humeral head, holding it into the socket of the glenoid and initiating glenohumeral abduction. The rotator cuff, and especially the supraspinatus tendon, is the most common site of pathological change in the shoulder. When swollen and tender it affects the movement of the shoulder in a char-acteristic way. As abduction proceeds, the swollen portion becomes compressed under the acromion and causes pain. Once it has passed this point painless movement is continued. On clinical ex-amination the demonstration of this painful arc of movement is characteristic of an incomplete tear of the supraspinatus or of supraspinatus ten-donitis, perhaps associated with calcific deposition (Fig. 9.22).

When a rupture of the rotator cuff occurs at-tempts to abduct the shoulder produce only a shrugging of the shoulder as a whole, the arm barely leaving the side. The deltoid can only pull the humerus into its own axis up against the acromion. If, however, the humerus is passively abducted to 45°, the deltoid can now abduct the rest of the way. Patients learn trick movements to compensate for loss of the initial abduction often by leaning towards the affected side to initiate pas-sive abduction and then taking over with the deltoid to complete abduction. Soon after injury when the shoulder is painful, it is impossible to tell whether abduction is inhibited by pain or prevented by rupture of the rotator cuff. Abolition of the pain by injection of local anaesthetic may resolve the problem as the patient can then initiate abduction if the cuff is intact.

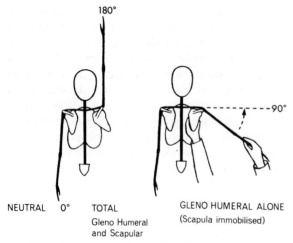

Fig. 9.21   Movements at the shoulder joint.

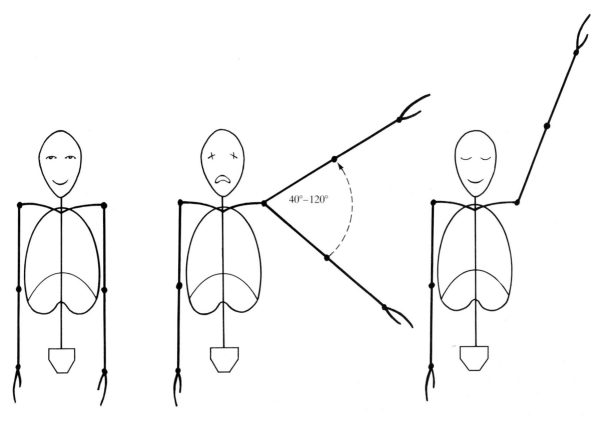

Fig. 9.22 Demonstrating painful 'arc' during abduction of the shoulder.

The long head of the biceps may be involved in lesions of the rotator cuff. This lesion is suspected when resisted flexion of the elbow causes pain in the shoulder.

Nerve supply. The spinal segments which supply the shoulder girdle also contribute to the phrenic nerve. In painful lesions affecting areas supplied by the phrenic nerve such as the central part of the diaphragm, pain may be referred to the tip of the shoulder in the area of C.4 due to the fact that the greater part of the phrenic nerve is derived from this root.

Special points in the history

Lesions in the neck, pericardium, pleura, the peritoneum and the central parts of the diaphragm may cause pain in the shoulder. Theoretically this should not present diagnostic problems because no limitation of movement or other abnormality should be found on examination of the shoulder. However, the picture may be confused by the tendency in the elderly to develop a frozen shoulder when mobility is reduced by pain from another site. Symptoms in the root of the neck, such as a cervical rib, tend to cause pain radiating down the inner side of the arm. The most sinister of these lesions is an apical bronchial carcinoma which can erode the neck of the first rib damaging the first thoracic nerve as it lies in close apposition to the bone at this point.

Occasionally ischaemic lesions of the heart cause shoulder pain, but clinical features of the pain, particularly the relationship with exertion. Should resolve any doubt about its true origin. Phrenic pain referred to the tip of the shoulder from the diaphragm may be aggravated by deep breathing. True shoulder pain tends to radiate to the insertion of the deltoid muscle and seldom below the elbow. Calcific deposits in the rotator cuff can produce pain which is so severe that an operation may be justified if injections of local anaesthetic and hydrocortisone fail to relieve the pain.

Examination of the shoulder

Inspection

When only one shoulder is affected much may be learned by simple inspection and comparison with the normal side. Anterior dislocation of the sterno-clavicular joint is not uncommon and except in the early stages after injury, does not interfere with the shoulder movements. Deformity caused by the prominent medial end of the clavicle is easily seen or palpated. Posterior dislocation is less common but is usually accompanied by severe pain and commanding symptoms including difficulty in swallowing and extreme pain on attempting to lift the head when supine. The deformity however, especially in the early stages, and especially when accompanied by swelling, may not be obvious even on radiological examination.

Fracture of the mid-shaft of the clavicle presents little difficulty in diagnosis. Dislocation of the acromio-clavicular joint may be confused with fracture at the lateral end of the clavicle as both cause a distinct step between the acromion and the upwardly displaced clavicle or medial fragment. Neither injury causes much disturbance to shoulder function, except in the early stages.

Anterior dislocation of the shoulder poses few diagnostic problems because the humerus displaces downwards as well as forwards. The normal smooth curved contour of the shoulder is replaced by an ugly angular projection of the acromion process. Posterior dislocation is frequently overlooked immediately after injury even with the help of radiological examination.

The contour of the shoulder is nearly preserved because the head of the humerus displaces directly backwards and not downwards. Inferior dislocation is rare, the patient being in a sorry plight of not being able to bring the arm to the side. This 'I am a tea-pot' posture may amuse the onlooker but not the patient.

Scapular movements. The ability to shrug the shoulders up, backwards and forwards is noted. Weakness of the serratus anterior will become ob-vious if the patient raises the arms forwards to press against the wall with both hands. The medial border of the scapula projects backwards producing 'winging' of the scapula.

Glenohumeral movements. The examiner stands behind the patient, immobilises the scapula by grasping the inferior angle and then puts the shoulder through both active and passive movements.

Total range of movements. The patient is asked to raise the arm forwards and upwards to the limit and then to the same end-point through abduction. Any limitation or painful arc of movement is noted.

Rotary movements. By flexing the elbow to a right angle, the forearm acts as an indicator. The shoulder is externally, then internally rotated with the arm at the side. The easiest way to demonstrate full range of rotation is to ask the patient to touch the back of the neck and the small of the back.

Palpation

Careful palpation may be required. Local tenderness must be accurately defined especially in lesions of the rotator cuff. The structure can be more fully explored if the patient clasps the hands behind the back during examination. Only occasionally in a lean subject a gap may be palpable where the rotator cuff is ruptured.

THE SPINE

Before considering the cervical, thoracic and lumbar segments separately, it is worth assessing the posture of the spine as a whole. At all times the normal spine should present as a straight line viewed from the front or rear. As seen from the side, the posture varies with the patient's age, depending mainly on the state of the intravertebral discs after maturity.

CERVICAL SPINE

The cervical spine is the most mobile section of the vertebral column. While the posture changes steadily throughout life, the neck is seldom in the same position for any length of time waking or sleeping. Degenerative changes are therefore common but are not necessarily accompanied by symptoms. This mobility is also a factor in the liability of this part of the spine to injury.

Anatomical features

In the cervical spine the transverse processes project laterally from the body of the vertebrae, protecting the more easily crushed cancellous bone of the body in the event of injury. The facet joints, however, lie more horizontally than at other levels of the spine thus forced flexion of the neck more often results in an anterior dislocation of the upper vertebrae than in a crush fracture. The neural canal is almost filled by the cervical enlargement of the spinal cord. The emerging cervical roots pass between the articular facets and the intervertebral discs. Prolapse laterally of a disc may produce compression. A central prolapse may produce pressure on the spinal cord itself. Osteoarthritic outgrowth is a common cause of root irritation in the lower cervical region, as in cervical spondylosis. Rotational neck movements take place mainly at the atlanto-axial joint, nodding of the head at the atlanto-occipital joint and flexion, extension and lateral flexion at mid cervical level.

Examination of the cervical spine

Because of the close relationship of the bones, joints, blood vessels, spinal cord and nerve roots, a lesion of the cervical region may produce both local and distant symptoms. Examination of the neck must therefore include a neurological examination of the upper limbs for lower motor neurone signs (see p. 248) and of the lower limbs for upper motor neurone signs (p. 248).

Inspection

Deformity is easily detected. Where a painful lesion is present the gait is characteristic. The patient walks with care to avoid jarring the neck, moving the whole body to look to the side. The chin may be supported by the hand. Torticollis (wry neck) is the most common deformity and is emphasised on movement. If this has been present

for several years asymmetry of the face will have developed.

The patient is asked to touch each shoulder in turn with the chin and then with the ear. Any limitation of active movement is noted and compared later with the passive range of movement. Forward flexion and extension are tested by putting the chin on the chest and by bending the neck backwards. Nodding tests movement at the atlanto-occipital joint.

Palpation

Bone contour is determined and tender spots are noted. These may be directly over the cervical spine or at some distance in the upper border of the trapezius. In the muscle the tenderest spots are often due to small areas of muscle spasm. Movements are repeated while palpation continues to detect crepitus. Passive movements are carried out if there is any impairment of active range. An accessory rib may obliterate the radial pulse when traction is applied to the arm, with it by the patient's side. Contraction of an abnormal scalenius anterior muscle may obliterate the radial pulse when the patient turns the head to the affected side and then takes a deep breath (Fig. 6.3 p. 134).

The foraminal compression test (Fig. 9.23) is performed if a cervical disc lesion is suspected. If pressure by the examiner's hand on the patient's head causes the characteristic pain, this confirms the presence of root compression.

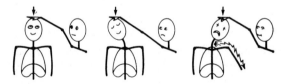

Fig. 9.23 Foraminal compression test.

THORACIC SPINE

This segment of the intervertebral column is least mobile and throughout life maintains a kyphosis. Congenital lesions are rare but developmental lesions, eg epiphysitis and infection, are common. Tuberculosis usually involves several vertebral bodies and before the introduction of specific chemotherapy, often resulted in gross destruction of the bodies producing an angular kyphosis. Idiopathic scoliosis or scoliosis secondary to paralytic conditions such as poliomyelitis may cause very severe deformity. The rotational element in scoliosis is best seen in the thoracic spine. At the apex of the lateral curve, the vertebral bodies no longer face ventrally but are directed towards the convex side of the curve. This vertebral rotation causes the ribs on the convex side of the curve to become directed dorsally producing a sharp angulation with a 'razor back' deformity. This results in narrowing and distortion of the chest cage and may interfere with the action of the heart and lungs. Although such patients experience little pain, they may have a limited expectation of life.

Young patients may suffer from ankylosing spondylitis which not only stiffens the thoracic spine but may also immobilise the ribs. In the older patient osteoporotic collapse of the thoracic spine can occur with the production of the characteristic 'Dowager hump' deformity.

Anatomical features

The movements of the thoracic spine consist of flexion and extension with a slight degree of lateral flexion and rotation. The range of movement is small and difficult to measure. Rib movement however is easily assessed by measuring chest expansion (p. 139).

Special points in the history

Pain in the thoracic spine is less common than in either cervical or lumbar spine. Disc lesions are infrequent but can occur and can be accompanied by girdle pain radiating into the chest mimicking the pain of cardiac disease. In the younger patient pain, infection of bone, pyogenic or tuberculous, has to be kept in mind, though it is much less frequently encountered in Britain than formerly. In middle and old age vertebral collapse associated with either osteoporosis or malignant disease, such as secondary carcinoma or myeloma, are common causes of pain.

Examination of the thoracic spine

Inspection

With the patient standing, the posture is inspected from the front, back and side and any deformity noted. Range of movement on forward, lateral flexion and extension are recorded. Particular note is taken of the effect movement has on any deformity present. If this is due to faulty posture it will correct on forward flexion. If due to structural changes it will be unaffected.

Palpation

The bony contour is first examined and areas of tenderness defined. Where local tenderness is not immediately obvious, gentle percussion with the fist or tendon hammer may elicit it.

LUMBAR SPINE

This segment of the spine falls heir to many infirmities. The lumbo-sacral region is a common site of congenital anomalies which seldom cause trouble. Trauma frequently results in damage at the upper end of the lumbar spine. The mobile lumbar segment joins with the less mobile dorsal spine. Ankylosing spondylitis, as its name implies, can cause marked limitation of movement (Fig. 4.12 p. 72). Osteoporosis may be marked in the lumbar spine and cause vertebral collapse, a condition that may be precipitated by steroids. Degenerative changes develop in the lower vertebral discs in the third decade, and osteoarthrosis in the facet joints by middle age. Although these changes and related ligamentous stresses provide the commonest explanation of low back ache this may also be due to gynaecological or psychological causes. Lesions in the lumbar spine may cause symptoms in the lower limbs without accompanying back pain.

Anatomical features

In the adult the spinal cord ends at the level of the second lumbar vertebra. Injury above this level may seriously damage the spinal cord which will not recover and the nerve roots which may recover. Below this level only nerve roots may be injured.

The transverse processes of the lumbar spine are analogous to the ribs and abnormalities are common at the upper end of the lumbar spine. Vestigial ribs may be mistaken for a fracture on X-ray examination. The sacrum is formed by the fusion of five segments of the spine. The last lumbar segment not uncommonly fuses partially or completely with the first sacral segment—sacralisation of the fifth lumbar vertebra. Conversely the first sacral segment may fail to fuse to the remainder of the sacrum—lumbarisation of the sacral segment.

The intervertebral disc contains a tough outer ring of fibrous tissue, the annulus, and a central nucleus with a surrounding jelly-like material with a high water content. The fit young adult may be 2 cm shorter by the end of the day due mainly to changes in the water content of the discs. By the third decade degenerative changes begin in the lower lumbar disc predisposing to disc lesions. These take the form of tears of the annulus with or without extrusion of the nucleus and are accompanied by pain and in permanent narrowing of the disc. The disc does not, however, slip in and out of place. The corresponding facet joints between the vertebrae develop osteoarthrosis. Such changes are 'normal' in most individuals by the fifth decade, but not always accompanied by symptoms. These individuals can achieve a 'do it yourself' spinal fusion of the vulnerable joints and this stiffness may result in the resolution of pain.

Pus from a chronic infection of the lumbar spine may collect in the sheath of the psoas muscle forming a palpable tumour in the iliac fossa before tracking further down the sheath of the muscle to present as a swelling or sinus in the groin. Deep infection causes spasm of the muscle and flexion of the hip. Active flexion of the hip aggravates the pain and passive flexion relieves it. This contrasts both with infection in the hip where all movements are painful, and with a lesion causing tension of the femoral roots (p. 278) where active and passive flexion of the hip relieves pain.

Pain not relieved by rest in younger patients suggests a lesion such as infection or spondylitis, and in the older groups primary or secondary malignant disease. However, if there is a long history of constant pain unrelieved by rest an organic cause is unlikely. Low lumbar or sacral pain may be due to pathological conditions in the pelvis, especially in the female.

Special points in the history

The mode of onset and pattern of lumbar pain are particularly significant. The pain of a disc protrusion usually comes suddenly when bending or on the day after such activity. This so overshadows the occasional backaches to which the patient has become accustomed during the preceding period of disc degeneration, that they are often not mentioned. A full enquiry will reveal the pattern of minor backache and acute episodes which settle with rest, followed by further aches, acute episodes or both. Disc lesions therefore cause episodic pain with periods of freedom from symptoms. Recurrences can often be related to stooping or lifting.

Osteoarthrosis in the lumbar region causes the usual pattern of pain and stiffness after rest, relieved by activity and recurring when the patient tires. Chronic ligamentous strain and spinal instability in contrast to osteoarthrosis, cause pain on standing and at the end the day, with freedom from pain at the beginning of the day. Ischaemia is a rare cause of gluteal pain and is usually accompanied by other features such as impotence. Spinal stenosis is discussed on page 256.

Examination of the lumbar spine

Inspection

With the patient standing the posture is observed from behind. The spine should be straight. The most common cause of deviation at this level is a lumbar disc lesion. The direction to which the patient deviates depends on the relationship of the disc prolapse to the adjacent root, not on which side of the midline the disc prolapse occurs. If the disc prolapse is lateral to the adjacent root, the patient leans toward the opposite side and the pain is aggravated by lateral flexion towards the same

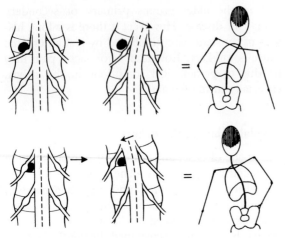

Fig. 9.24 Deviation of spine in prolapsed intervertebral disc.

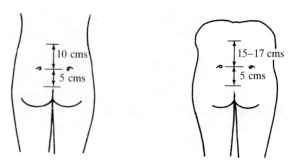

Fig. 9.25   Measuring forward flexion of spine.

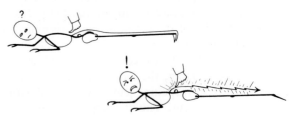

Fig. 9.26   Prolapsed intra-vertebral disc. Local and referred pain.

side as this pulls the root against the prolapse (Fig. 9.24). If the prolapse is medial to the root the patient lists to the same side as the lesion. The patient is then inspected from the side and the presence, accentuation, absence or reversal of the normal lordosis noted. If a painful lesion is present the lordosis is obliterated or even reversed. The patient is asked to bend forward and to each side. The level reached and the influence of movement on the lumbar spine are noted. Finally the patient is viewed in front.

Palpation

This is performed on the patient erect and prone and again the contour of the spine, the presence of tenderness and skin temperature assessed. If a measurement of spinal flexion alone is required, uninfluenced by the flexion of the hip joints, a mark is made on the skin at the lumbo-sacral joint level with the dimples of Venus. Other marks are made 10 cm above and 5 cm below this mark. On flexion, the distance in the normal spine to the upper mark, should increase by 5–7 cms and remain unaltered to the lower mark (Fig. 9.25). If firm pressure by the thumb is applied between the laminae over the prolapsed disc the pain will be aggravated and radiation of the pain produced (Fig. 9.26). This pressure may have to be maintained for some seconds. When positive this is known as the 'Doorbell' sign.

Nerve stretching tests

Sciatic roots. Usually the first sacral root is involved in a lumbo-sacral disc prolapse. Tension is put on these roots by flexing the hip with the knee straight, so-called *straight leg raising*. The test should be performed slowly and the patient told to report as soon as it becomes painful, and where the pain is felt. Normally 90° of flexion of the hip should be possible. Where the root is stretched round or over a prolapsed disc, straight leg raising will be restricted (Fig. 9.27A and B). When the limit of straight leg raising has been achieved further tension on the root is caused by dorsiflexing the ankle so pulling the posterior tibial component of the sciatic nerve round the ankle. If positive, the pain is aggravated and is felt in the back of the leg radiating into the lumbar region in some instances. (Fig. 9.27C). This test differentiates limitation of straight leg raising due to disc prolapse, from that due to short hamstring muscles or a lesion in the hip.

The Bowstring sign. This test is even more accurate and selective and may be useful in diagnosing malingering. Straight leg raising is performed as described above. At the limit the knee is flexed reducing the tension on the sciatic roots and the hamstrings. Unless the hip is stiff, further

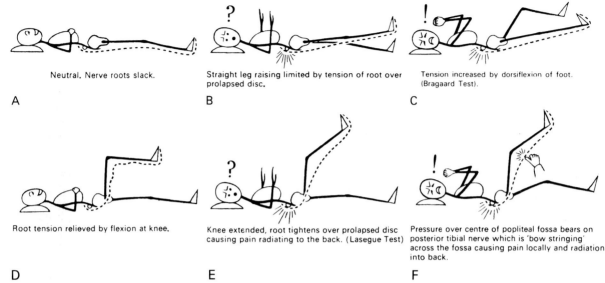

Fig. 9.27 Stretch tests — sciatic nerve roots.

flexion will now be possible. Having achieved more flexion at the hip the knee is again extended until pain is produced (Lasègue's sign). (Fig. 27D and E). At this stage the posterior tibial nerve is stretched like a bowstring across the popliteal fossa. Firm pressure is applied with the thumb, first over the hamstring tendon nearest the examiner and then in the middle of the popliteal fossa and finally on the other hamstring tendons. The patient is asked which caused pain, the first, second or third, and if the answer is the second, is then asked where the pain was felt. The test is positive only is the pain radiates from the knee to the back or down to the foot.

Flip test. This is a further test which can be carried out if it is suspected that the complaint may not be genuine. The patient sits with the hips and knees flexed to 90° and the knee jerks are tested. The knee then is extended ostensibly to examine the ankle jerk. Where there is genuine root tension the patient will flip backwards to relieve that tension. The bogus patient, distracted by attention to the ankle jerk test will permit full extension of the knee which is the equivalent of 90° of straight leg raising or forward flexion to the toes when standing (Fig. 9.28).

Femoral roots. Disc prolapse at high levels may involve the roots of the femoral nerve (L2/3). The femoral nerve passes into the thigh in front of the pubic ramus and straight leg raising will relieve any tension on these roots. They are stretched by extending the hip with the knee flexed. This is done with the patient lying prone. Where there is a large disc prolapse or a painful flexion deformity

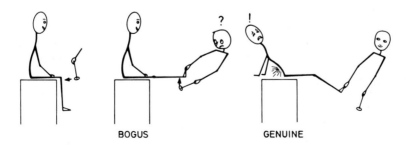

Fig. 9.28 Stretch test — sciatic nerve roots. In the 'flip test' when attention is diverted to the tendon reflexes the genuine patient will still not permit full extension of the leg.

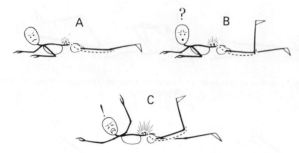

Fig. 9.29 Stretch test — femoral nerve. (A) Patient prone and free from pain because femoral roots are slack. (B) When femoral roots are tightened by flexion of knee pain may be felt in the back. (C) If still no pain, femoral roots are further stretched by extension of the hip.

in the hip, the patient may not be able to lie prone, but the test can then be performed with the patient lying on the unaffected side. In either case the knee is flexed. This may be enough to produce the pain and cause the patient to flex the hip to relieve the tension on the root. Where limitation of extension is due to the changes in the hip, knee flexion should have no afffect on the pain. If knee flexion alone causes no pain the hip is extended with the knee still flexed. If the test is positive it will cause pain radiating into the back (Fig. 9.29).

Neurological signs. Detailed examination of sensation, motor function and reflexes are a most important part of the examination when nerve root involvement is under consideration (Ch. 8).

SACRO-ILIAC JOINTS

Sacro-iliac joints are involved at an early stage in ankylosing spondylitis but other lesions are uncommon. Movement of the sacro-iliac joint cannot be measured on clinical examination, but the joints can easily be tested by firm compression and distraction of the iliac crests. Pain is produced in the region of the sacro-iliac joint if these are abnormal.

THE LOWER LIMB

Like the spine the posture of the legs varies throughout life. Congenital abnormalities are more frequently found in the lower than the upper limbs.

THE HIP JOINT

This large ball and socket joint is very vulnerable. The hip joint may dislocate at birth, be the site of epiphysitis (*Perthes disease*) or infection in childhood, may slip its femoral epiphysis at puberty, dislocate in the active young adult, develop spontaneous avascular necrosis with maturity, wear out in middle age, or fracture in the elderly as a result of osteoporosis or malignancy. Fracture can be complicated by the development of secondary avascular necrosis of the femoral head.

Anatomical features

Owing to the depth of the normal acetabulum the hip is a stable but remarkably mobile joint because the femur has developed a neck which is narrower than the maximum circumference of the head. In the adult the acetabulum faces outwards, downwards and slightly forwards. The neck of the femur is set on the shaft at an angle of 130° and is directed forwards or anteverted by some 30°. In the infant the acetabulum is directed forwards, the neck of the femur is set at a greater angle on the shaft, and is directed at least 70° anteriorly. The infant's hip is therefore most stable when flexed and abducted but is in danger if extended and abducted. In contrast the adult hip is most stable when the femur is extended and is more liable to dislocate when flexed and adducted, the posture adopted when sitting. This accounts for the high incidence of posterior dislocation of the hip in car accidents when the front of the knee impacts against the dashboard.

The femoral and obturator nerves supply sensory branches to the hip and the knee joint, explaining the frequent reference of pain to the knee from lesions of the hip joint.

Movements. As the hip is a ball and socket joint, flexion, extension, abduction, adduction, rotation and the combined movement of circumduction are all possible. The actual range changes throughout life as does the posture of the joint. As age increases the first movements to decrease are extension and internal rotation followed by abduction.

Special points in the history

Pain arising from the hip is most commonly situated in the groin, but may be felt over the greater trochanter or in the buttock. It may radiate down the thigh to the knee or be present in this joint alone. Any patient who cannot accurately localise pain in the knee should be suspected of having a disorder of the hip. Gluteal pain with a radiation of pain down the back of the thighs may suggest the spine as a source symptom.

Examination of the hip

Gait

This should be observed with the patient lightly clad, otherwise the disability from a stiff hip may pass unnoticed. When adequate inspection is possible it is obvious that the pelvis moves with the leg in this condition. The gait of gluteal dysfunction has been described (p. 259).

Posture

If the hip is mobile and one leg is short, the pelvis tilts down towards the shortened side and a scoliosis develops (Fig. 9.30). Alternatively the patient simply flexes the hip and the knee of the longer side to shorten this limb. A 'raise' under the short leg can correct the posture of the hips and the back (Fig. 9.30). A series of wooden blocks ranging form 2 cm to 6 cm in depth is used to determine the comfortable amount of elevation required by the standing patient to compensate for a shortened limb.

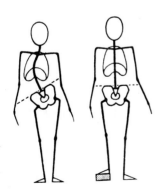

Fig. 9.30   Posture changes in short leg.

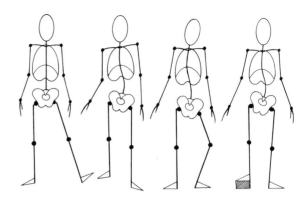

Fig. 9.31   Abduction deformity of the hip.

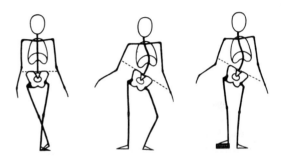

Fig. 9.32   Adduction deformity of the hip.

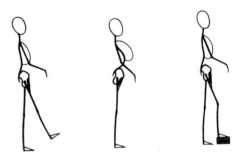

Fig. 9.33   Flexion deformity of the hip.

Fixed abduction deformity causes apparent lengthening of the leg because the pelvis tilts down on that side to bring the legs parallel. The patient can then adjust his posture by flexing the knee on the affected side in an attempt to shorten the limb or by wearing a raise under the normal but apparently short limb. Either way the scoliosis remains uncorrected (Fig. 9.31). Fixed adduction of the hip causes apparent shortening of the limb. The pelvis is elevated on that side to bring the legs parallel. Bending the other knee or using a raise on the affected side does not correct the scoliosis (Fig. 9.32).

A fixed flexion deformity will cause apparent shortening but the patient will be able to compensate by increasing the lumbar lordosis and no scoliosis will occur (Fig. 9.33). A single deformity seldom occurs. The most common combination is flexion and adduction of the hip.

Inspection of the supine patient

When the patient lies on the examination couch it is difficult to detect a deformity of the hip because the pelvis can tilt to compensate for a considerable malposition of the hip. The pelvis must first be positioned so that the iliac crest are on the same horizontal plane at right angles to the spine. Any fixed adduction or abduction will immediately be revealed. A flexion deformity will be masked partially or completely by the patient tilting the pelvis forwards and increasing the lumbar lordosis, (Fig. 9.34A and B). With a severe fixed flexion deformity the knee will be flexed but can be passively

extended, thus differentiating it from a fixed flexion deformity of the knee arising as a result of local knee pathology.

Inspection is completed by looking for swelling, signs of inflammation, muscle wasting or sinus formation. Although it is impossible to see distension of the hip joint when an effusion is present, the limb takes up the characteristic posture of slight flexion abduction and external rotation. If an infective process has caused destructive changes in the joint, flexion, adduction and internal rotation will develop.

Measurement of leg length

Accurate measurement can be achieved only by special radiological techniques but clinical examination gives a reasonable assessment of any discrepancy. Where a fixed deformity of the hip

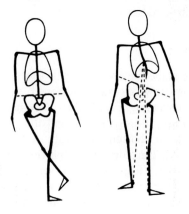

Fig. 9.35   Measurement of apparent shortening of the leg.

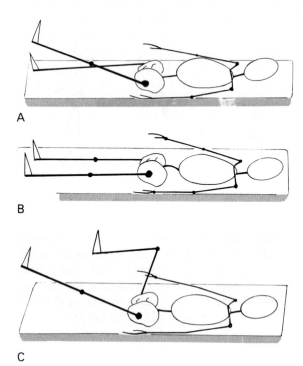

Fig. 9.34   Flexion contracture of the left hip (A), masked by lumbar lordosis (B). Unmasked by full flexion of right hip (C): Thomas hip flexion test.

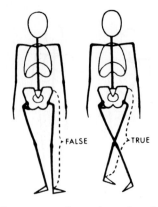

Fig. 9.36   Measurement of true shortening of the leg.

joint is present when the legs are brought parallel the limbs will apparently be unequal in length as shown in Figure 9.35. The amount of apparent shortening is measured between a fixed point such as the xiphi sternum or the umbilicus to the tip of the medial malleolus. True shortening is measured from the anterior superior spine to the medial malleolus (Fig. 9.36). The normal limb must be measured in a comparable position to the abnormal one in respect of adduction or abduction, if reasonable accuracy is to be achieved.

Palpation

In adults it is difficult to detect anything other than gross swelling around the hip joint. Palpation can localise tenderness and so give some indication of the source of the symptoms.

Measurement of movement

Flexion. The pelvis must be immobilised in order to be certain that the movement being measured is that of the hip alone and not also of the pelvis on the spine. The iliac crest is stabilised with one hand while the other grasps the leg (Fig. 9.37). The Thomas test is then carried out to determine if any fixed flexion is present. The examiner places one hand between the patient's lumbar spine and the examination couch. The lumbar lordosis is then obliterated by flexing the unaffected hip to its limit and continuing to push to straighten the lumbar spine (Fig. 9.34C). That this has been achieved is confirmed by the examiner's hand being squashed between the patient's spine and the examination couch. The af-

fected leg will then rise off the table revealing the amount of flexion deformity present. This test is performed first on the normal side and the range compared with the abnormal.

Abduction and adduction. Movements of the pelvis must again be eliminated. With the patient supine the examiner grasps the opposite iliac crest and lays that forearm across the pelvis over the anterior superior spine on the nearer side (Fig. 9.38). Abduction and adduction are then carried out. At each extreme the pelvis will be felt to tilt with the limb.

Rotation. This movement should be carried out with the hips first extended and then flexed. With the patient supine and using the feet as indicators, the legs are rolled on the couch and the range measured by excursion of the patellae. A more accurate method is performed with the patient prone. The knees are flexed to a right angle and the tibiae then act as indicators of the arc of rotation. The range of rotation of the flexed hips is measured by flexing both the hip and the knee to a right angle as the patient lies supine. Again the tibiae act as indicators of the degree of rotation.

The accurate measurement of rotation is particularly relevant if a slipped upper femoral epiphysis is suspected. An increase of external rotation at the expense of internal rotation is one of the earliest clinical findings. The teenager complaining of pain around the hip or knee should be asked to lie supine and flex the affected limb at the hip and the knee attempting to keep the knee in line with the ipsilateral shoulder while doing so. If the limb rotates externally as they are attempting to do this, then a slipped epiphysis must be excluded on X-ray examination. Conversely, con-

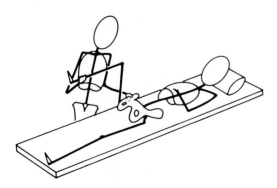

Fig. 9.37 Testing flexion of the hip.

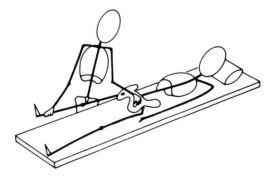

Fig. 9.38 Testing abduction and adduction of the hip.

genital dislocation of the hip is accompanied by more internal than external rotation.

Tests of the stability of the hip.

Instability is encountered in congenital dislocation in infants, slipped epiphysis in adolescence, traumatic dislocations in adults fractures of the neck of femur in the elderly, and in certain neurological and muscular disorders.

In infancy and childhood congenital dislocation of the hip must be diagnosed as soon as possible after birth, certainly many months before the child walks. The three most obvious features are:

1. Shortening and external rotation of the limb. The mother may remark that the child does not move the affected leg as much as the other.
2. Asymmetry of the fine buttock folds.
3. Limitation of abduction: 90° of abduction should be possible in both hips in an infant.

If any of these signs are present *Ortolani's test* should be performed. Indeed this test should be carried out on newborn infants as a routine. With the infant supine the hips are flexed to a right angle and the knees are brought together. Pressing gently backwards, the hips are then slowly abducted and extended. If the hips are unstable the first part of the manoeuvre will push the head of the femur out of the acetabulum. As abduction proceeds the head of the femur will be felt to click back into place (Fig. 9.39).

Testing for *telescoping of the limb* depends on an established dislocation, and is therefore a late sign. The term vividly describes the sensation of the limb apparently sinking into the trunk as it pushed in the axis of the limb towards the trunk.

Trendelenburg's sign demonstrates that hip abductor function is deficient or absent. It is useful in the later stages of congenital dislocation of the hip when the patient is walking. It is also used to assess the disability in paralytic disorders such as poliomyelitis affecting the lower limbs. In arthritic conditions there may be a painful limitation of abductor function. When the normal subject stands on one leg the glutei contract so that the opposite side of the pelvis is tilted up slightly to allow the opposite leg to clear the ground during gait. If the patient stands on the affected leg when the actions

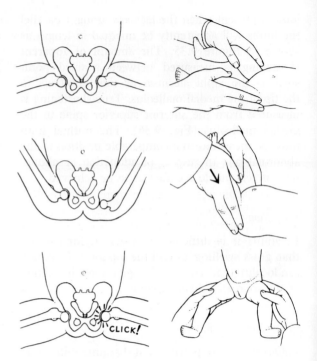

Fig. 9.39 Ortolani's test.

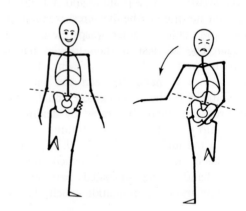

Fig. 9.40 Trendelenburg's sign.

of the glutei are deficient, the opposite side of the pelvis will tilt downwards and the balance can only be maintained by leaning over towards the side of the lesion (Fig. 9.40). This test is best performed with the patient's back towards the examiner. The patient stands on the normal leg and with the hip extended, flexes the knee of the other leg to a right angle. The pelvis usually tilts up slightly on the opposite side. The patient then stands on the abnormal leg and the pelvis tilts down on the opposite side. When walking the patient compensates for lack of abduction by leaning over to the opposite side so that the centre of gravity is moved over the affected hip. This causes the patient to dip or lurch towards the affected side; with bilateral abductor impairment the trunk leans from side to side producing a characteristic rolling gait.

In puberty and in adult life instability associated with slipped upper femoral epiphyses (adolescent coxa vara), traumatic dislocation of the hip and fracture in the region of the neck of the femur, is apt to occur within a particular age group and is associated with characteristic postures:

1. Slipped upper femoral epiphysis. This occurs at puberty. The limb is externally rotated, abducted and shortened.

2. Traumatic dislocation. This occurs only in mature patients. a. Posterior dislocation in which the limb is flexed, adducted and internally rotated, is the more common. b. In anterior dislocation the limb is flexed, abducted and externally rotated.

3. Fracture in the region of the neck of the femur. This is common in the elderly, especially women. The limb is extended, externally rotated, adducted and shortened. This is the same deformity as in slipped epiphysis because the same mechanism is involved.

THE KNEE

The knee is particularly prone to injury or twisting owing to the fact that stability through a range of movement of 150° is entirely dependent on the control of muscles and ligaments. In addition its exposed position renders it liable to direct injury. Repeated kneeling can produce a traumatic bursitis, with risk of direct infection of the joint by puncture wounds. Weightbearing often leads to degenerative changes, especially in the medial joint compartment, and inflammation such as rheumatoid arthritis commonly affects the knee.

Anatomical features

There is normally about 7° of valgus of the tibia on the femur when the knee is fully extended. Because of the shape of the condyles of the femur, the tibia externally rotates on the femur during extension. This in turn causes the collateral ligaments and the anterior cruciate ligament to become tight. In this situation the tibia is 'screwed home' on the femur and the joint 'locked' in full extension. In this position no abduction, adduction or rotation of the tibia on the femur is possible. This enables the individual to sustain the body weight using minimal muscle action. When the ligaments are tight in full extension they are particularly liable to injury. Within a few degrees of flexion external rotation is undone and the ligaments are relaxed and it is now possible to abduct, adduct and rotate the tibia on the femur or vice versa.

Semilunar cartilages, or menisci, are attached by their periphery to the capsule and are mobile structures. Although very resistant to compression forces they are very sensitive to loads applied in flexion and rotation. Under these circumstances the cartilages may be sucked between the bones to produce a variety of cartilage tears. The anterior, or more commonly the posterior horn, may be damaged to produce a 'parrot beak' tear. These are liable to be caught momentarily between the tibia and the femur and the patient is aware of a sensation of the knee being about to give way. Sometimes a longitudinal tear of a meniscus will occur resembling a 'bucket handle'. The 'bucket handle' fragment displaces medially and comes to lie between the condyles of the femur. The knee is then said to be locked because extension is obstructed to a varying degree. Cartilage tears are usually related to movements involving flexion and rotation whilst taking the body weight, e.g. while changing direction, running or twisting round when squatting.

The quadriceps is the most important group of muscles controlling the knee both in maintaining an upright posture and in the locking mechanism referred to above. When these muscles contract they tend to pull in a straight line from the trochanter to the tibial tubercle. Because of the normal valgus angle of the knee this tends to displace the patella laterally. The more valgus the knee the greater the tendency to lateral displacement. This tendency however is contracted by the important action of the obliquely disposed vastus medialis muscle.

Special points in the history

The anatomical features which have been discussed underline the importance of a detailed history of the mechanism of any injury of the knee. The menisci are liable to be torn by twisting injuries, especially when playing football. Possibly because of the greater valgus angle of the knee in the female, lateral dislocation of the patella, sometimes with spontaneous reduction, is not uncommon. The history may be identical with that of a medial cartilage injury and the differential diagnosis may depend on the clinical or radiological demonstration of patellar instability (see below). The knee itself responds differently according to the degree of injury. Severe violence results in bleeding within the joint which becomes distended due to the formation of a haemarthrosis. This develops immediately after the accident. 70% of these patients have ruptures of the anterior cruciate ligament. Some of the remainder may have fractures, and in these circumstances aspiration reveals fat globules within the aspirate. X-ray examination of the joint may be necessary to determine bony injury.

Very severe violence will also cause rupture of the collateral ligaments and although bleeding will occur, the blood will escape from the joint and present as swelling and bruising about the damaged side of the joint with no fluid being detected in the joint itself. Effusions tend to develop in relation to damage to avascular structures such as the menisci. The history will often differentiate between a large effusion and a haemarthrosis, as the effusion takes some hours or even a day to develop.

Arthritis is common in the knee joint and the pain and stiffness after sitting may be described as 'locking' by the patient. This underlines the importance of finding out exactly what the patient means by this description and not accepting such terms uncritically. Popliteal or Baker's cysts may form in association with arthritis. When these rupture the pain produced may be mistaken for deep vein thrombosis. (p. 98).

Pain may be referred to the knee, notably from the hip, as a result of almost any pathology affecting that joint. In these circumstances the patient is often unable to indicate its site accurately.

Examination of the knee

Inspection with the patient erect

The characteristic gait of a stiff knee is immediately evident (p. 258). Provided there is a reasonable control of the hip or foot, the patient can walk even when all the controlling muscles in the knee are paralysed, because of the locking mechanism.

Abnormalities of posture are most evident from the patient's stance. The most difficult problem is to determine when the degree of knock-knee (genu valgum) (p. 258) becomes abnormal in a 2–4-year-old child. The distance between the malleoli when the child stands with the feet parallel and the knees just touching is a useful measurement to record for comparison in the future. No absolute figure can be given for any particular age but in the majority the deformity corrects spontaneously by the age of 6–8 years. Thereafter separation of the malleoli by more than 5 cm is unlikely to correct itself. Before predicting that spontaneous correction will occur it is wise to inspect the parent's knees unobtrusively, because of the familial tendency to this condition. Asymmetrical genu valgum is abnormal at any age.

Inspection with the patient supine

Deformity can again be reviewed, and in particular the amount of genu valgum measured, as noted above. Wasting of the muscles and any swelling of the joint can now be more easily assessed.

Palpation

The bony contour is checked and signs of inflammation are sought. If wasting is present, muscle girth should be recorded in order to follow progress. The level above the patella at which this measurement is made should always be noted.

Tenderness must be accurately localised. With the knee flexed the medial and lateral joint lines must be found anteriorly and then palpated posteriorly throughout their length. Localised tenderness suggests intra-articular pathology. The whole extent of both collateral ligaments should also be palpated and the area of maximal tenderness defined.

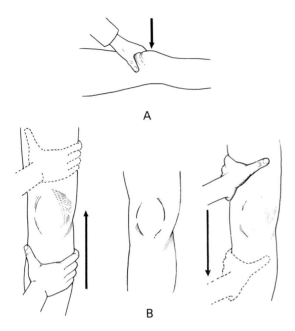

Fig. 9.41 Testing for an effusion (A) by the patella tap technique and (B) by the massage test.

Effusion. A *trace effusion* can be detected only by the massage test (Fig. 9.41). With the knee straight and the quadriceps relaxed, any fluid in the antero-medial compartment of the knee is massaged with the examiner's hand into the suprapatellar pouch. Then by applying pressure with the back of the hand on the lateral side of the joint and the suprapatellar pouch, the fluid is pushed back into the antero-medial compartment. A fluid impulse is observed on the medial side of the joint as the normal depression medial to the patellar tendon is seen to bulge as the fluid accumulates there.

A *moderate effusion* gives rise to a *patellar tap*. With the knee extended the suprapatellar pouch is emptied by pressure with the palm of the examiner's hand and with the fingers of the opposite hand the patella is then pressed sharply against the femur. If there is sufficient fluid to float the patella off the femur, it will be felt to tap against the femur.

A *large effusion* can be observed as a 'horseshoe' swelling immediately above the patella. This delineates the outline of the suprapatellar pouch as it extends a handsbreadth above the upper border

of the patella. Squeezing this swelling while palpating each side of the patella will demonstrate a fluid thrill, which differentiates the swelling from synovial thickening. Furthermore, synovitis usually produces a more boggy thickening associated with local increase in skin temperature.

Loose bodies. A careful examination of the knee is required when there is a history of locking. When its occurrence is unpredictable, locking is likely to be due to loose bodies. Under these circumstances the knee often unlocks very quickly as the loose body moves to the wider channels of the joint. Sometimes a loose body can be felt, especially in the suprapatellar region of the joint.

Movements of the knee

The normal range in the adult is 0–150° of flexion. In some subjects a few degrees of hyperextension is possible. This is found more frequently in females.

When only one knee appears to be affected, the active range is examined first in the normal and then the abnormal joint. The passive range is then performed in the same order and during this examination a hand is placed on the knee to detect the presence and character of crepitus. The site of any pain and its relation to a particular arc of movement are noted. Care is taken to detect even a few degrees of limitation in extension. When a 'bucket-handle' cartilage tear is displaced, passive extension of the knee is blocked. The sensation is of pushing against a firm rubber stop and the knee recoils as soon as the pressure is released. Sometimes difficulty can be encountered in distinguishing between true and apparent loss of extension due to spasm of the handstrings. True block to extension can be demonstrated by lying the patient prone with the legs projecting over the end of the examination couch, supported only by the thighs. The level of the heels provides an index of the degree of extension of the knees. With a

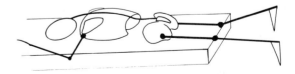

Fig. 9.42 Locked right knee.

true block, one heel remains higher than the other whereas with muscle spasm, both heels eventually come to adopt the same position (Fig. 9.42).

Tests of stability

To test the *collateral ligaments* the knee must be fully extended. The patient's ankle is held between the examiner's elbow and side, leaving both hands free to abduct and adduct the tibia on the femur while keeping the knee straight (Fig. 9.43). Normally no knee movement should be detected. Where a ligament is strained no movement occurs but pain is localised over the damaged ligament when it is stretched. When a ligament is lax the knee opens when pushed from the opposite side and is felt to close with a click when pressure is released.

The *cruciate ligaments* are tested with the knee flexed to a right angle. This position is maintained by the examiner sitting on the patient's foot (Fig. 9.44). The patient should be warned before doing

this because the polite patient withdraws the foot and the less polite complains. With both hands now free the examiner first checks by palpation that the hamstrings are relaxed otherwise the test is invalid. To test the anterior cruciate the tibia is grasped just below the knee and is drawn forwards. To test the posterior cruciate this movement is reversed. Starting with the normal knee the degree of antero-posterior glide of the tibia is noted as the normal for that patient. Movement in excess of this in the suspect knee is abnormal. Excessive anterior 'glide' or 'draw' is due to the laxity of the anterior cruciate, and posterior displacement is associated with laxity of the posterior cruciate ligament. Gross instability of a cruciate ligament is usually associated with laxity of one of the collateral ligaments and vice versa. When the collateral ligaments are intact with an isolated tear of the cruciate ligament, it is rarely possible to demonstrate an abnormal 'draw' sign.

The Lachman test. This is carried out with the knee in 20° flexion and is more likely to demonstrate rupture of the cruciate ligament when the collateral ligaments are intact. Here the examiner firmly grasps the lower end of the thigh and the upper end of the tibia. The lower thigh is pushed in one direction and the tibia pulled in the opposite direction and then the action reversed.

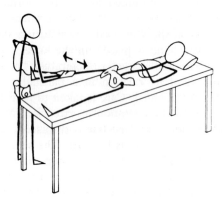

Fig. 9.43   Testing the collateral ligments of the knee.

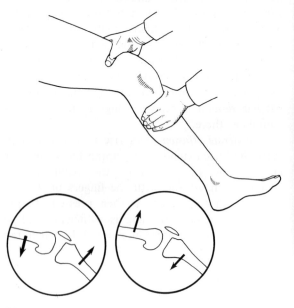

Fig. 9.45   Lachman's test.

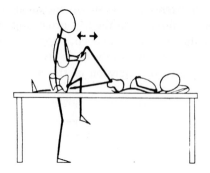

Fig. 9.44   Testing the cruciate ligments of the knee.

Difficulty can be encountered for those who have small hands, and it is not always possible to say precisely in which direction the laxity is occurring (Fig. 9.45).

Rotary instability. It is now recognised that there are various forms of complex rotary instability of the knee which can develop subsequent to injuries to the cruciate and collateral ligaments. Of these the most common follows rupture of the anterior cruciate ligament. In these circumstances the lateral tibial plateau is subluxed anteriorly beneath the lateral femoral condyle. At about 30° of knee flexion a sudden posterior shift of the tibia occurs with reduction of the anterior tibial subluxation. This can be demonstrated by a useful test known as the lateral pivot shift test, or the jerk test. The knee is examined with the patient supine and the knee extended. The examiner's hand holds the patient's hindfoot and applies an internal rotation force. The examiner's left hand applies pressure against the upper lateral aspect of the leg applying a valgus stress to the knee joint. As the knee is flexed from 0–30° a palpable and often visible reduction of the anteriorly subluxed lateral tibial condyle occurs (Fig. 9.46).

Stability of the patella. With the knee extended the patella is grasped and moved from side to side. An impression of excessive mobility may be gained and compared to the normal knee. If the patella has previously dislocated, the patella apprehension test is often positive. Here the knee is examined in 30° of flexion and pressure is applied by the examiner against the medial border of the patella. The attempted lateral displacement causes great patient apprehension when the patella is unstable (Fig. 9.47).

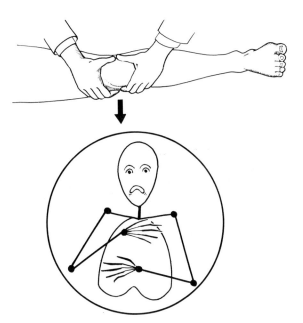

Fig. 9.47 Patellar apprehension test.

Stability of menisci. The most commonly performed and best known test of cartilage stability is the *McMurray test.* Although often applied generally to diagnose cartilage lesions, it was specifically intended to diagnose lesions of the posterior horn of the medial meniscus. The hip and knee are flexed to 90°, the examiner stands on the right side of the couch and grasps the patient's right heel with the right hand and steadies the knee with the left hand. The knee is flexed to the limit the patient will tolerate while pressing on the outer side of the knee with the left hand the knee is extended while the tibia is alternately internally and externally rotated by the right hand (Fig. 9.48). If positive, a 'clunk', accompanied by some discomfort to the patient, is felt over the displacing cartilage.

Tests for degenerative change in the knee

During active and passive movement of the knee the patient may detect crepitus or a grinding sensation if osteoarthrosis is present. The character of crepitus varies and fine crepitus can be due to soft tissue within the joint. Coarse crepitus suggests that there will be significant cartilage erosion.

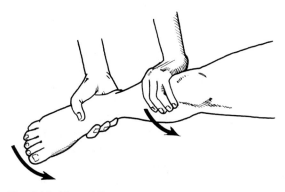

Fig. 9.46 Pivot shift test.

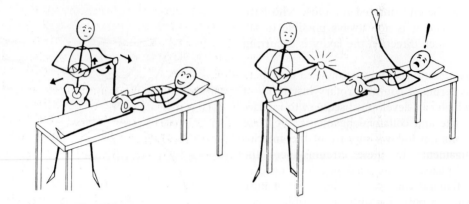

Fig. 9.48   The McMurray test of the semilunar cartilages.

With degeneration in the patello-femoral compartment coarse crepitus can be felt on palpating the patella during flexion and extension movements of the knee. Similarly if the patient contracts his quadriceps while the patella is restrained by pressure against its superior border characteristic patellar pain can be induced.

THE LEG, ANKLE AND FOOT

Many feet fail to achieve an ideal shape and the first metatarsal remains relatively short and deviated medially (varus). The phalanges then deviate in the opposite direction and hallux valgus results. This is only one example of many congenital defects found in the feet. In addition to this tendency to congenital abnormality, the feet have often to bear the stress of the bodyweight on hard unyielding surfaces, often cramped and confined by fashionable footwear. For these reasons many problems are encountered in the feet.

Anatomical features

The two feet placed side by side resemble an inverted soup-plate, each foot corresponds with half a plate. The inner border of the foot is raised to form the longitudinal arch. The outer border corresponding to the rim of the plate, lies on the ground. When the feet are placed together an arch lying across the midtarsal region is formed. When not weightbearing a further, but lesser, transverse arch lies under the metatarsal heads. The arches

of the feet and their associated ligaments and soft tissues act as shock absorbers when the feet take the bodyweight and give spring to the gait. The flattened outer border gives stability when standing.

When the patient is standing the long axis of the talus, navicular, medial cuneiform and first metatarsal normally lie in a straight line. This can only be seen accurately on radiological examination. Clinical examination will give some idea where this longitudinal axis is broken in foot deformity. As an aid to the understanding of various deformities the foot may be considered to have three main components: the talus, the calcaneus and the forefoot. The latter includes the navicular, cuboid, cuneiforms, metatarsals and phalanges.

Description of deformities. *Talipes* is derived form the words talus and pes, inferring that there is deformity involving the ankle and foot, and must be further qualified to have any meaning. *Talipes equinus* means the foot and ankle are plantar flexed, like the foot of a horse which walks on the tip of one 'finger'. *Talipes equino-varus* means that in addition the hindfoot is adducted and that the forefoot is also adducted or inverted at the midtarsal joint (Fig. 9.49). This is the typical clubfoot deformity. *Talipes calcaneus* indicates that the heel is dorsiflexed (Fig. 9.50). When combined with valgus of the other parts of the foot this becomes *Talipes calcaneo-valgus* and is the other common congenital foot deformity.

Any of these foot deformities may be associated with deformity of the longitudinal arch. A flat-

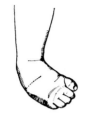

Fig. 9.49 Talipes equino varus.

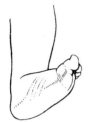

Fig. 9.50 Talipes calcaneus.

tened deformity is described as *planus*. A raised or increased deformity is described as *cavus*. It is possible therefore to have *talipes equinocavo varus* etc. *Pes* implies deformity involving the foot only and that the position of the ankle is normal. *Pes planus* means flat foot. The axis of the longitudinal arch may sag either at the talo-navicular, medial naviculo cuneiform joint or both. The most severe degrees of flatfoot are usually associated with the former. The normal heel is vertical when viewed from behind. In pes planus the heel is often valgus and the whole foot pronated.

In pes cavus the longitudinal arch is raised and the heel, as seen from behind, is often in varus. In this position the foot is supinated and the toes are usually clawed. This deformity may be associated with abnormalities of the central nervous system, such as spina bifida or Friedreich's Ataxia.

Claw toes may occur in isolation or more commonly in association with a pes cavus. The toes are extended at the metatarsophalangeal joints and flexed at the interphalangeal joints. All the toes are commonly affected and eventual dorsal dislocation occurs at the metatarsophalangeal joint.

Hammer toe often involves only the second toe and is not associated with other foor deformities. The metatarsophalangeal joint is extended, the proximal interphalangeal joint is flexed and the distal interphalangeal joint is extended. A painful corn often develops over the dorsum of the proximal interphalangeal joint.

Hallux valgus is probably the most common foot deformity. In addition to valgus deformity of the phalanges the metatarsal is often shorter than normal and deviated in the opposite direction, metatarsus primus varus et brevis. In *hallux rigidus* the big toe is often longer than the other toes and because of this develops degenerative change or osteoarthrosis in the metatarsophalangeal joint. Extension is diminished giving pain and difficulty with 'toe-off' while walking. In extreme instances the toe may become permanently flexed — *hallux flexus*.

Special features in the history

In children, pain in the feet directly related to the musculoskeletal structures is not common. When not associated with obvious deformity or inflammatory changes, the cause is usually epiphysitis involving the calcaneum, navicular or the metatarsal heads.

In the adult pain localised to the foot usually has its origin there, but pain arising in the foot may be referred up the leg. The character and pattern of the pain will give some indication of the cause. Osteoarthrosis has the familiar pattern of pain and stiffness after rest which is relieved temporarily by activity. Pain which gets gradually worse the longer the patient is standing suggests chronic ligamentous strain. Ischaemia of the feet can cause distressing pain at night (p. 86). Special enquiry should be directed at the condition of the feet in elderly patients as severe but remedial disability can be caused by minor abnormalities such as callosities or overgrowth of a nail (onychogryphosis).

Metatarsalgia (pain in the forefoot). This is commonly associated with claw toe deformity where the fibro-fatty pad normally present under the metatarsal head comes to lie under the toes leaving the metatarsal heads unprotected. The patient appropriately describes the pain as walking on pebbles or on glass. This situation also develops in rheumatoid arthritis. Other causes of metatarsalgia are stress fractures (march fractures of the metatarsal shafts) and epiphysitis of the second metatarsal head in adolescence (Frieberg's disease). A pain of a burning, tingling character radiating into the third and fourth toes of the foot suggest a digital neuroma in the cleft between these toes. The patient notices that removing the shoe relieves the pain and on examination there is tenderness between the third and fourth metatarsal heads and sensation is diminished in the same toe cleft.

Examination of the leg, ankle and foot

Gait

Stiffness without pain causes little alteration in the gait. Equinus deformity causes a high stepping gait in order to clear the ground. It can be distinguished from dropfoot (p. 260) in that it is fixed in the former, but loose and flapping in the latter. The gait of talipes calcaneus lacks spring — a peg leg gait.

Posture

Apart from the effects of congenital deformities already described, abnormal posture of the foot may result from poor general posture. Surprising correction of flat foot deformity can be achieved by correcting the typical slouching, knee flexed, pronated foot stance of the adolescent.

Inspection and palpation

This is best done with the patient sitting on the examination couch with the legs dangling over the edge. The calf is relaxed and the foot movement is freer when the knee is flexed. The examiner sits on a low stool in front of the patient. The colour, texture and temperature of the skin give useful information concerning the circulation and nutrition of the foot. The condition of the nails is noted. The toes are separated and the area between them is inspected for evidence of fungal infection in which condition the skin becomes thickened, whitish, sodden and fissured. Particular note is made of the site of any callosity as an indication of abnormal pressure. Tenderness or other signs of inflammation are accurately localised. Pulses of the dorsalis pedis and posterior tibial arteries are palpated.

Movement

While the patient is erect the ability to stand on the toes, on the heels and on the inner and outer borders of the feet is tested and active range of non-weight-bearing movement is then noted and finally the range of passive movement is reviewed.

Flexion and dorsiflexion of the ankle. The foot is in the neutral position when it is at right angles to the long axis of the tibia. In dorsiflexion the broader anterior surface of the talus is engaged in the ankle joint. In plantar flexion the narrow portion of the talus is engaged and some abduction and adduction can take place. In practice this cannot be differentiated from movement at the subtalar joint.

Inversion and eversion of the hindfoot. The examiner holds the heel of the foot at right angles to the leg (Fig. 9.51). The heel is then adducted and abducted. These movements take place mainly at the subtalar joint.

Inversion and eversion of the forefoot. The heel is held in one hand and the forefoot in the other and the forefoot is abducted and adducted in relation to the hindfoot (Fig. 9.52). These movements take place in the midtarsal joints between the talus and calcaneus posteriorly and the forefoot anteriorly.

Tarso-metatarsal movement. The range is so small that it cannot be accurately assessed by clinical examination.

Tests for stability

Tendo-Achilles. Diagnosis of a ruptured Achilles tendon may be missed, perhaps because it was not

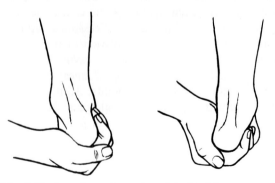

Fig. 9.51 Inversion and eversion of the hind foot.

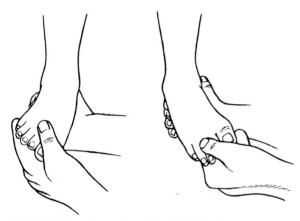

Fig. 9.52   Inversion and eversion of the forefoot.

realised that the foot can still be plantar flexed by the toe flexors. The classic signs are a palpable gap in the tendon about 5 cm above the heel. There is an inability to stand on tiptoe on the affected foot. However these signs may be difficult to assess because of pain and swelling at the time of injury but the squeeze test does not suffer from this handicap. With the patient prone or kneeling the calf is felt and gently squeezed just distal to its maximal circumference. Where the tendon is intact the foot plantar flexes. Where the tendon is ruptured no plantar flexion occurs. This test will also differentiate a ruptured tendo-Achilles from another common injury to the calf, avulsion of the medial head of the gastrocnemius muscle, as it causes pain at the site of the latter with retention of plantar flexion. There is no pain and no plantar flexion when the tendo-Achilles is ruptured.

Anterior ligament of the ankle. It is impossible on clinical examination to know if this ligament is ruptured because abnormal movement of the ankle joint cannot be differentiated from that occurring at the subtalar joint. Radiological assessment is required.

Footwear

An abnormality of gait may be suspected or confirmed by irregularities in the pattern of wear on the soles or heels of the shoes or boots. Unfortunately this information may not be available as patients often come to the doctor wearing their best and newest footwear.

FURTHER INVESTIGATION

Examination of the blood

Estimations of haemoglobin, leucocytes, ESR, plasma urate, and rheumatoid and antinuclear factors are used in the differential diagnosis of arthritis. Plasma calcium, phosphate and alkaline phosphatase provide information about the metabolism of bone, whilst estimation of vitamin D may assist in the diagnosis of clinical or subclinical osteomalacia. Acid phosphatase is elevated in carcinoma of the prostate with bone metastases.

Radiological examination and other imaging.

Radiological examination plays a very important part in the further investigation of abnormalities involving the locomotor system. It is essential for clinical and medico-legal reasons if a fracture is suspected. Two views must be taken in planes at right angles to each other to demonstrate the position of the bone fragments. If only one view is taken the fragments may appear to be in a good position when in fact they are overlapping and the bone ends are not in contact with each other. Two views may fail to show a crack fracture. When a fracture of the scaphoid is suspected at least four views are taken. If no fracture is visible but the clinical findings suggest that a fracture may be present, a plaster is applied and the radiological examination is repeated two weeks later. The alternative is to carry out a radionuclide bone scan before committing the patient to treatment.

In children the epiphyseal cartilage may be confused with a fracture especially in the elbow. Comparable views of the normal joint will clarify the situation.

When examining the X-rays of the skeleton the opportunity should be taken to look at the whole film for other abnormalities as, for example, at the apices of the lungs in antero-posterior views of the cervical spine. Similarly the examination of the lumbar spine should include a scrutiny of the soft tissue shadows of the psoas muscles, the abdominal viscera and the diaphram.

The extent of injury to the soft tissues can be demonstrated by special radiological techniques. Rupture of ligaments allows the related joint to sublux to a lesser or greater degree and this abnormal position may be demonstrated on a radiograph. For example, a sprained lateral ligament of the ankle cannot be clinically differentiated from a complete rupture of that ligament on clinical examination. An antero-posterior view of the ankle is required with the foot held in forced inversion. If the lateral ligament is ruptured the talus will be seen to be tilted within the ankle mortice as compared with the normal side. In recent injuries this may have to be performed under an anaesthetic.

If loose bodies are present in a joint more than routine antero-posterior and lateral views will often be required. For instance, in the knee additional intercondylar views are necessary. Special oblique views may be required for the adequate demonstration of certain joints, particularly in the spine, e.g. the sacro-iliac joints which are involved in the early stages of ankylosing spondylitis and the facet joints if spondylolisthesis is suspected.

Arthograms. These can demonstrate abnormalities in the intra-articular structures. Air, radio-opaque fluid or both are injected into the joint. This technique can be used in injuries to the semilunar cartilages in the knee, especially the posterior horn of the medial meniscus which is difficult to define on arthroscopy. It can also be used to define the position of the labrum of the acetabulum in congenital dislocation of the hip or the shape of the cartilaginous femoral head in Perthes disease.

Myelograms and *radiculograms* may be used to outline the spinal cord and nerve roots respectively (p. 246).

Discograms are occasionally helpful. A fine needle is inserted into the disc nucleus and a dye is injected. This outlines the disc and may also reproduce the patient's symptoms helping to confirm the diagnosis in some instances.

Radioisotope bone scanning (Fig. 9.53) can demonstrate fractures, avascularity, inflammatory and neoplastic lesions in bones and joints. This is approximately seven times more sensitive than plain X-rays and lesions can be demonstrated on bone scanning when they are not visible on X-ray examination.

Computed tomography can be used to define soft

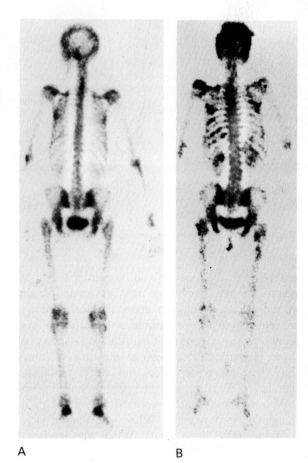

A   B

Fig. 9.53 Radioisotope scans (radionuclide imaging) as a diagnostic aid. Uptake of the radioactive tracer is a function of the rate of turnover of bone. In the normal (A) this is greatest in the weight-transmitting parts of the pelvis and spine and around joints (exaggerated in this patient's ankles by arthritis). The other patient (B) has multiple metastases in the ribs and elsewhere, Paget's disease of the skull and a calcific tendinitis of the left shoulder. A bone scan (scintograph) shows the presence of the abnormalities. Radiographs are necessary to make the differential diagnosis. (Courtesy of Dr M V Merrick.)

tissue abnormalities which are difficult to demonstrate by radiographs. It is also particularly useful to define lesions of the vertebrae and the extent and relationships of bone tumours prior to surgical excision.

Magnetic resonance imaging (nuclear magnetic resonance) promises to have particular application in the early detection of avascular necrosis in bone and in assessment of spinal pathology and bone tumours.

Other investigations

Synovial fluid. The properties of fluid aspirate from a joint are helpful in the diagnosis of traumatic, metabolic and inflammatory lesions. In the first, haemorrhage can be differentiated from an acute effusion and in the second, specific crystals can be seen in gout or pseudo-gout. In the third, leucocytes are found and the affecting organism and its sensitivity can be determined.

Arthroscopy. This is carried out under general anaesthesia and aseptic conditions and has greatly extended the accuracy of diagnosis in certain joints, especially the knee. Arthroscopy has largely superseded arthrography because, in addition to providing a more accurate inspection of the joint, it also allows biopsy and the removal of loose bodies and damaged menisci to be done at the same time.

Bone biopsy. In suspected metabolic bone disease the use of special needles allows specimens to be obtained, usually from the iliac crest. Using similar techniques many local lesions can be screened and biopsied, preferably under ultrasound imaging.

THE METHODS IN PRACTICE

BACKACHE

This example has been chosen mainly because it illustrates one way in which various tests may be integrated in order to cause the patient the minimum inconvenience and to economise on the clinician's time and motion. It also serves to exemplify some of the problems presented by malingering which is not uncommonly encountered with backache. In women, backache may be due to gynaecological difficulties which it would not be appropriate to discuss in this chapter.

History and examination

Some of the points of particular relevance have been discussed on page 255. After completing the taking of the history it is necessary to plan a comprehensive examination to include checking in particular posture, gait, spinal movements and neurological findings. Methods must be efficiently but rapidly executed as the majority of patients will have few or no signs. One effective sequence is shown in Figures 9.54–9.64. When positive findings are encountered the examination should be expanded as appropriate.

First the posture and spinal movements are inspected and next the gait when the patient proceeds to the examination couch (Fig. 9.54). Starting at the head and working downwards, the neck, breasts and abdomen are palpated to check the possibility of a malignant tumour causing metastases; then the sacroiliac joints are stressed and rotation of the hips tested (Fig. 9.55). Next sciatic and tibial nerve stretching, knee and plantar reflexes, sensation and peripheral pulses are examined (Figs. 9.56 and 9.57). The patient is then carefully observed on turning over on to the prone position (Fig. 9.58). The femoral nerve is stretched, the spine palpated for contour and local tenderness and active extension of the spine observed (Figs. 9.59 and 9.60). A rectal examination, if indicated, can conveniently be carried out at this stage (Fig. 9.61). If there is doubt about the patient's authenticity the 'flip test' (Fig. 9.28) is performed as the patient is about to descend from the couch (Fig. 9.62). Other tests in this category, for example the foraminal compression test (Fig. 9.23) can be carried out when the patient is again standing (Fig. 9.63). Finally when there are suspicions about ankle weakness, the patient is asked whether walking on the heels or on tiptoe makes the pain worse. The malingerer can do both but in apparent agony.

Interpretation of the findings

The history combined with the clinical signs will establish the diagnosis or indicate what further investigations are required. In the majority there will be few or no positive findings, for example in osteoarthrosis, spondylolisthesis, spinal stenosis and early malignancy, but the history will indicate the probable diagnosis.

In the minority there may be a plethora of clinical signs, for example in the presence of a prolapsed intervertebral disc, an abscess or an ad-

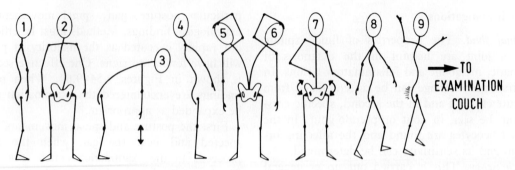

Fig. 9.54   Observe: posture — (1) lateral and (2) postero-anterior; (3) flexion; (4) extension; (5) and (6) lateral flexion; (7) rotation; (8) and (9) gait.

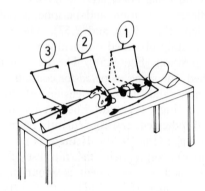

Fig. 9.55   (1) Palpate neck, breasts and abdomen. (2) Stress sacroiliac joints. (3) Rotate legs to check hip rotation.

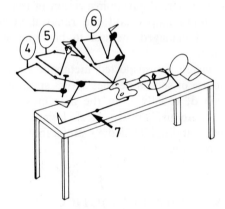

Fig. 9.56   (4) Knee jerks (5) Straight leg raising and ankle dorsiflexion test. (6) Posterior tibial nerve stretch test. (7) Check active straight leg raising.

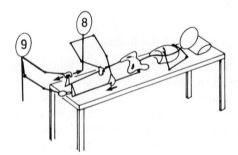

Fig. 9.57   (8) Test sensation from thigh to foot. (9) Plantar reflex; dorsi and plantar flexion of foot; peripheral pulses; girth of calf and thigh if wasting.

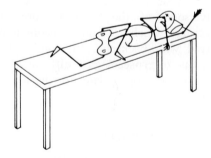

Fig. 9.58   Patient turns over; observe performance and posture — patient with femoral root tension cannot lie prone (first stage femoral stretch test).

Figs. 9.54 to 9.58   Backache: integration of examination. First stage.

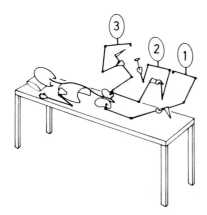

Fig. 9.59 (1) Flex knee (second stage of femoral stretch test). (2) Ankle jerks. (3) Extend hip with knee flexed (third stage of femoral stretch test).

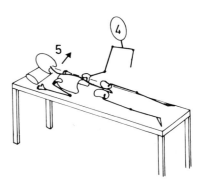

Fig. 9.60 4(a) Palpate spine in midline for contour and local tenderness. (b) Palpate asymptomatic then painful side for tenderness and 'door bell' sign. (5) Check active extension of spine.

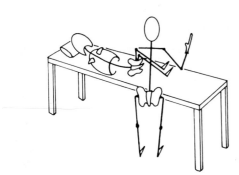

Fig. 9.61 Patient on left side for rectal examination if required.

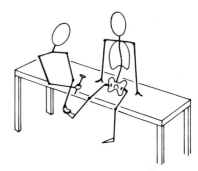

Fig. 9.62 Flip test to confirm authenticity of sciatic stretch tests.

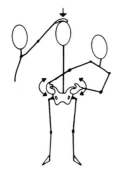

Fig. 9.63 Simulated rotation and axial compression in suspect patients.

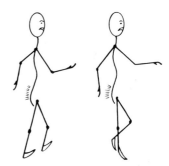

Fig. 9.64 Ask patient with suspect ankle weakness if walking on heels or tiptoe makes pain worse.

Figs. 9.59 to 9.64 Backache: integration of examination. Second stage.

vanced malignancy. They will present a consistent and anatomical pattern.

Hysteria and malingering may also produce a wealth of clinical signs, often easily recognised by their bizarre nature and inconstant and non-anatomical pattern. The affect of the hysteric is one of indifference while the malingerer is on the defensive and often aggressive. In the latter the typical history is one of prolonged continuous pain, even at rest, unaccompanied by any deterioration in general health (p. 256).

It is always important to maintain an impersonal and friendly manner throughout the examination especially when dealing with the last group of patients. Nothing is gained by attempting to brow-beat such individuals. Nevertheless all doctors must be aware of the existence of factitious illness. It is of course by no means confined to the locomotor system. Attention has been drawn to Munchausen's disease (p. 2), and to the sub-terfuges practised by drug addicts (p. 78). Other examples are puzzling fevers produced by thermometer manipulation and symptoms, such as persistent diarrhoea, due to drugs, self-administered with the intent of deceiving the doctor. The reason for such abnormal behaviour should be determined by an evaluation of the patient's personality as described on page 18.

ACKNOWLEDGEMENT

The technique of examination of backache described is that previously developed and demonstrated by Mr J.H.S. Scott, to whom my grateful thanks are due.

FURTHER READING

Apley A G 1982 System of orthopaedics and fractures 6th edn. Butterworths, London
Crawford Adams J 1985 Standard Orthopaedic Examinations 10th edn. Churchill Livingstone, Edinburgh
McRae R K 1983 Clinical Orthopaedic Examination 2nd edn. Churchill Livingstone, Edinburgh

10. The infant and child

H. Simpson

INTRODUCTION

General considerations

In previous chapters the emphasis has been on the acquisition of history-taking and examination skills in the adult. Though illogical chronologically, it is appropriate that students gain experience and confidence with adult patients before turning their attention to infants and children. An adult is, in the main, easier to deal with than a young child. The history can be obtained directly and cooperation during the clinical examination is usually assured. Physiological norms are also more constant than is the case during infancy and childhood. Obvious examples are respiration and heart-rates. More important, disease in adults occurs after the completion of growth and development whereas in children many acute and chronic diseases have a major impact on these processes. Meningitis in the first year of life may have a profound effect on both; nutritional deficiency and chronic infection, seen together in cystic fibrosis, have a predominant effect on growth. Similarly, the presentation of illness is influenced by the stage of development reaches — an apnoeic episode in a young child may indicate generalised seizure activity without the tonic/clonic features typical in older children and adults. The significance of clinical 'signs' also varies, for example, a liver palpable 1–2 cm below the costal margin in a 10-year-old will almost certainly be abnormal though normal in a toddler. For these reasons it is perhaps easier to learn first the standard methods of approach in adults and to adapt or modify them to take account not only of differences between adults and children but also of the wide variations that occur within infancy and

childhood. In this chapter it is assumed that the student will have gained preliminary experience with adults; the main emphasis will be placed on symptoms and signs peculiar to, or of special significance in, infancy and childhood.

1. the history is generally obtained from a second person;
2. the cooperation of the child cannot be taken for granted;
3. the predominant impact of disease may be on growth and development;
4. the expression of disease may be influenced by the child's growth and developmental status;
5. clinical norms may be different from those in adults;
6. clinical signs of disease may differ from those in adults with respect to occurrence, interpretation and significance.

Age periods

It is convenient to divide infancy and childhood into the following age periods.

Infancy	First year of life
Neonatal period	First month of life
Childhood	1–18 years
Pre-school child	1–4 years
School child	5–18 years

Interview setting

It is important to first introduce oneself to the parents and the child. A warm greeting and a friendly smile do more than anything else to allay anxiety and promote confidence. A complimentary remark about the child's clothing or possessions and a few words of conversation appropriate to the child's age, about school, sports, hobbies, etc, will help achieve the empathy essential for cooperation in the physical examination. At this stage, young children are usually eager to look at picture books or play with toys which should be in plentiful supply (Fig. 10.1). The history may then be obtained without too much interruption. Older children, on the other hand, may give the history unaided but more often prefer to let a parent (usually mother) provide the history and to contribute only when questioned directly or when they disagree with mother's account of events.

The limitations of obtaining a history through an intermediary must be appreciated. Parents may place their own interpretation on events rather than describe precisely what has occurred. They may also have failed to recognise misinterpretations which children put on words. For example, a young child may generalise from past experience and use a phrase such as 'sore tummy' to describe pain or discomfort in general, without this being appreciated by the parents. Similar problems may be created by previous medical advice. For example, unexplained fever — a common situation in childhood — may have been attributed in error to 'otitis' or 'tonsillitis'. It is easy to see how such misunderstanding can arise and although due

weight must be given to parental views, uncritical acceptance of interpretations offered for the child's symptoms is a common error in history-taking which must be avoided. Careful questioning and a shrewd appreciation of the degree of insight which parents have into the child's symptoms will enable the doctor to place such information in appropriate perspective.

THE HISTORY

The following approach is directed mainly towards infants and young children. It may be modified or adapted as appropriate for age and sex of the patient and for the reason for seeking medical advice.

Begin by noting the child's age, date of birth and sex and the source of referral. These details have usually been entered in the hospital records by the start of the interview.

Presenting complaint

The parent should then be encouraged to tell the story with a minimum of interruption while the clinician listens carefully. The history may be initiated by the question 'What seems to be the matter?' followed by 'When did the problem start?' when the first question has been answered. If difficulties arise in dating the onset of symptoms, it may be useful to ask 'When was . . . last totally well?' Obtaining a thorough chronological account of events without having to interrupt is ideal but seldom possible in practice. Intrusions may be necessary to avoid overemphasis on one aspect of the history or to clarify parental interpretation of events. Make a note of each complaint and its duration, of health immediately before the illness and of how the illness has progressed.

Present history

Once a brief account of the child's illness has been obtained, there are specific questions to ask designed to amplify and clarify the parents' description. These depend to some extent on the nature of the symptoms. For example, if vomiting has occurred, its amount and frequency should be

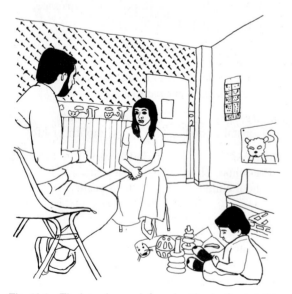

Fig. 10.1 The interview; an informal setting is often helpful.

ascertained. Is it effortless, forceful or projectile? Is it bile- or blood-stained? Similarly, when pain is the dominant symptom, enquiry must be made about its nature, severity and timing (p. 25). Does it interfere with normal activities? Is it constant or intermittent? Is it precisely located or is it of a general character? Does it radiate? Whatever the symptom, ask about aggravating and relieving factors? Has the child received medical attention and medicines before referral? In this way, information about each symptom volunteered is amplified. It is important also to enquire about associated symptoms and to record relevant negative data. For example the vomiting may have occurred in isolation or have been associated with abdominal pain, constipation, diarrhoea or abdominal distention. Pain, for example headache, may have been accompanied by vomiting, visual disturbance, motor dysfunction or incoordination. Such associations may be missed unless care is taken to extend the enquiry beyond the symptoms volunteered. Similar symptoms or illnesses currently affecting other family members or children in the same class at school are noted.

Systemic enquiry

To ensure that relevant information has not been forgotten a brief system review is also made. Its nature depends in part on the age of the child concerned. It is always useful to enquire about appetite, general activities, bowel habit, micturition and sleep routine. The child's behaviour and ability to relate to peers, siblings and other family members may be extremely relevant. When the main problems are behavioural or emotional, it may be best to postpone discussion on sensitive issues and to bring them up later in the absence of the child.

The nature and extent of systemic enquiry will depend on individual circumstances. It is helpful to consider symptoms in relation to the various body systems:

1. Alimentary Appetite, feeding, vomiting, diarrhoea, constipation, screaming attacks (or abdominal pain), jaundice, weight loss.
2. Respiratory Discharge from nose, eyes or ears, sore throat or earache, cough and its nature, respiratory noises — wheeze, stridor, grunting, snoring; apnoeic or cyanotic episodes.
3. Cardiovascular Breathlessness, tiredness and lethargy, slow feeding, poor weight gain, pallor or cyanosis.
4. Genitourinary Urinary incontinence (having previously been dry), increased urinary frequency, pain on micturition, abdominal pain, change in odour and appearance of urine, urine stream in boys, fever.
5. Central nervous Changes in activity, mood, behaviour, school performance, headaches or disturbances of vision, abnormalities of posture, gait or coordination, 'fits' — include detailed description.

While taking the history it is also important to form an opinion about the intelligence and reliability of the informant.

Previous history

The child's age and presenting symptoms will largely dictate the emphasis placed on the previous history. In general this will include:

Mother's health during pregnancy. Enquire about any illness or accident mother may have suffered during pregnancy, threatened miscarriage, contact with rubella or other infections, medication, drugs, smoking and alcohol consumption, nature of any employment, screening or diagnostic procedures undertaken (chorionic biopsy, amniocentesis, ultrasound examination), toxaemia and antepartum haemorrhage. This information may be supplemented from antenatal records.

The manner of birth may have a profound effect on subsequent health and development. The nature and duration of labour, mode of delivery, need for resuscitation at birth, gestation and birthweight are relevant, particularly in children who present subsequently with suspected developmental delay or with convulsions. Mothers may not remember the exact details and precise information may have to be obtained from the obstetric records.

Neonatal period. Information should be sought about the neonatal period. Were there convulsions, breathing difficulties, blueness, jaundice, vomiting, or any other abnormality? Was any special treatment required, for example antibiotics, oxygen therapy, phototherapy or mechanical ventilation? Were there feeding difficulties or poor weight-gain?

Post neonatal. Obtain details of feeding in the early months — breast, bottle or both, type, composition, volume, frequency of artificial feeds and the age at which solids were introduced. Note any problems relating to feeding, appetite and growth during infancy.

Previous illnesses. Record the nature, date, duration and severity of any previous illnesses or operations. Enquire specifically about previous measles, rubella, pertussis, mumps and chickenpox, and about recent contact with infectious illnesses. Obtain details also of immunisation procedures (primary and boosters) referring when necessary to pre-school health surveillance records. A knowledge of pets in the home and recent contact with animals may be relevant, for example in the presence of lymphadenopathy or unexplained fever due to toxoplasmosis.

Allergies. Note any history of allergic illness or allergic responses to drugs, for example penicillin.

Residence abroad. A history of periods of residence abroad or of recent travel indicates the possibility of imported diseases.

Developmental milestones. Knowledge of normal developmental milestones is important in diagnosis and evaluation of many childhood disorders (p. 351). Enquiry will depend on the child's age and individual circumstances. Ages of smiling, head control, fixing and following, sitting alone, crawling, standing, walking, talking (words and sentences) reading and hearing ability are noted. The result of the 8-month hearing test is recorded.

At what age was the child dry initially by day and during the night? Similarly, the age at which bowel control was achieved and any special difficulties in toilet training should be noted.

Progress at school, including the child's ability to mix with other children, academic ability and any special aptitudes are also recorded.

Family history

Ascertain the ages, present state of health, past health and possible consanguinity of the parents. The ages and sexes of other children in the family,

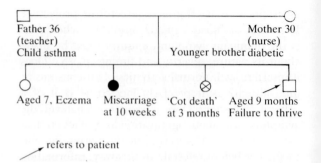

Fig. 10.2   A family tree.

the occurrence of any stillbirths or miscarriages should be noted. If any child in the family has died, record the age and cause of death. Note also past and present illnesses of siblings. It is helpful to construct a family tree that includes first-degree relatives (Fig. 10.2). Illnesses in other members of the family and close relatives should be recorded. Is there anything to suggest infection such as tuberculosis, emotional instability which may have led to child abuse, or an inherited illness? In genetically determined conditions, specific enquiries may be necessary about second and even third degree relatives. Any available medical history about the natural parents of an adopted child should be noted. Disorders within the family such as tuberculosis, allergies, diabetes, epilepsy, or a history of cardiovascular, neurological, renal or neoplastic disease may be relevant.

Social history

This embraces the home, the school and the provision for play and recreation. It is frequently the single most important part of the history, particularly in pre-school children. The parents' occupations, attitudes to each other and to their children, domicile, neighbourhood, financial means, whether together or apart and, if single, whether isolated or supported, may all be relevant. Who cares for the child if both parents work? Enquire about the size and conditions of the home, number of occupants and any special environmental circumstances of possible physical or psychological significance. Are there frequent changes of domicile?

Many disorders of the child have a psychological basis, commonly but not exclusively related to poverty or deprivation. An appreciation of the stresses of the environment which both home and school impose, the ability of the parents to cope, and the child's intelligence and capacity for survival are all relevant. Certain provoking situations occur, for example a new baby in the home, the death of an immediate relative, absence of one or other parent, first attendance at school, change of school class or new teacher, change of residence to another district with loss of playmates, bullying at school, scholastic difficulties and too rigid enforcement of a desired pattern of behaviour.

Summary

It is helpful to precis the main points in the history at this stage and to consider a provisional or differential diagnosis. These impressions guide the approach to the clinical examination. For example:

Helen is a three-year-old girl who presented with a history of recurrent cough and wheeze from the age of six months when she was admitted to hospital with a severe chest 'infection'. Her symptoms are usually precipitated by upper respiratory infections and tend to be worse at night-time and in the winter months. She has been admitted to hospital twice in the past three months with severe wheeze and breathlessness. These symptoms have usually responded to treatment with beta 2 agonists. Her father has asthma, an older sibling hay-fever, and a six-month-old brother infantile eczema. In other respects she has been healthy. Birth, history, growth and developmental progress have been normal and she has been fully immunised. There are no adverse social factors.

Impression: Bronchial asthma. The original illness may have been acute bronchiolitis.

PHYSICAL EXAMINATION

General approach

The scheme of examination of children is broadly similar to that adopted in adults apart from the difficulties and differences peculiar to infants and young children. It is not possible to describe an all-embracing technique appropriate to every situation that may arise. The patient may be an inconsolable infant, a toddler clinging to his mother and burying a tearful face in her lap at the slightest approach of the examiner, a defiant 5-year-old boy who will resist all attempts to remove his clothing — particularly his trousers, a retarded hyperactive child intent on destroying toys and furniture or an apprehensive schoolgirl who just retains her self-control during questioning but recoils in terror when a sphygmomanometer or ophthalmoscope is produced. In contrast, many children cooperate fully without being alarmed in any way. Understanding, sympathy, patience, and at times finesse and subtlety enable most problems to be overcome.

Growth measurements

The height and weight of children attending paediatric outpatient departments will have been measured before the interview. These measurements are recorded on centile charts (p. 353) and provide 'advance' information on whether height/weight are within the normal range for age and sex. Accurate measurement and precise recording are essential — do not rely solely on clinical impressions.

Weight

The most useful single measurements of physical development in infancy and childhood are weight and height. A comparison between actual and expected weight should be routine in any examination. Expected weight according to age can be calculated in a number of rough and ready ways or may be determined more accurately from tables. In the early weeks of life the average infant should gain approximately 30 g per day after the tenth day, at which time the birthweight should have been regained. Thus at six weeks the expected gain in weight should be almost 1 kg. By five months of age the birthweight should have doubled and by a year should have trebled. For the next few years the expected weight in kilogrammes can be calculated approximately from the formula — age in years plus four, multiplied by two. It should be remembered that the average is not necessarily the normal for any individual. The normal weight for a child of small parents may be well below the average. Thus weight in the individual child must be interpreted against a number of background factors. Changes in weight of the individual child have a more specific significance.

Length

Length is the other valuable parameter of growth. It can be measured as standing height in toddlers and older children and as crown-heel length in infants. The same considerations concerning 'normal' and 'average' apply as with weight.

A correlation normally exists between height and weight. A knowledge of the expected weight for any particular height and an appreciation of any dissociation between these measurements may be of value. In hypothyroidism, for instance, height may be reduced and weight normal. In a wasting disorder height may be normal and weight reduced, in obesity height normal and weight increased.

Head size

The occipito-frontal circumference is recorded routinely in infants and young children. It is measured by a non-stretch tape from the frontal bones (just above the eyes) in a horizontal plane. Variations in this, both above and below normal, may have considerable significance in respect of childhood disease. Values for different ages are given in Table 13.1 p. 352.

Pubertal development grading

This is not assessed routinely but may be of crucial importance when problems of growth and maturation are suspected in later childhood. The stages of physical sexual development — related to age and sex, are given in Table 13.3 p. 355. For each of the indices considered, stage 1 is fully infantile and stage 5 fully adult. Only stages 2, 3 and 4 need be remembered.

Preliminary observations

The examination really starts on first meeting the child and parent(s). These impressions are reinforced during history-taking by observation of the child's appearance, general demeanour, state of alertness, play activities, speech, posture and perhaps gait. The interaction between child and parent should be observed. Some parents dominate the situation and will not allow the child to answer a question independently, others constantly correct the child or demand inappropriately high standards of conduct and behaviour. Hopefully, by the time the history has been completed, the child will have accepted the examiner's presence and may be showing signs of trust and friendship.

Guidelines

1. Young children, particularly toddlers, must be allowed to take stock of their surroundings. If kept occupied and interested while the history is being taken, they are usually ready for attention when it has been completed.
2. Rapport should have been established with the parent before starting the examination. Children are quick to sense any lack of empathy between parent and doctor.
3. Infants under six months may be examined lying on a couch. Those over six months and very young children are best examined on their mothers' laps.
4. Preschool children may be examined on a couch. Ask parent to sit the child on the couch and to remain in close attention at the head end.
5. Undressing may be gradual and staged. It is not necessary to undress children completely as a preliminary step.
6. A relaxed unhurried approach is essential. Let the child handle instruments, such as the stethoscope, or 'blow out' the auriscope light, to distract attention from the examination.
7. Warm the hands and, if necessary, the head of the stethoscope before touching the child.

General examination

Certain observations are made without disturbing the child. The facies and expression may reveal whether the child is well or ill, relaxed or apprehensive, at ease or in pain. An impression is gained about the child's growth, development, nutritional status and hydration. The breathing rate is best counted by observing movements of the abdomen and the pulse rate counted at the wrist while the child holds the parent's hand. Table 10.1 lists some additional information that may be gained by careful observation of the head and face. The presence of bruising, skin rashes or blemishes, e.g. cafe au lait spots, will also be apparent (Figs 10.3 and 10.4).

A purely systematic approach to examination is seldom possible in young children. Information is gleaned as the opportunity presents and examination proceeds from one area to another without rigorous adherence to 'system'. During examination the following guidelines are helpful.

1. Observation always precedes palpation, percussion and the use of the stethoscope.
2. Speak quietly to the child before touching and explain what you are doing.
3. Examine by region and not strictly by system.
4. Talk to the parent and indicate how s/he may help.
5. Be gentle at all times.
6. Be continually aware of the child's response.
7. Pause immediately if the child becomes upset or cries.
8. Improvise when necessary to ensure cooperation.
9. Leave until the end any uncomfortable procedures, such as examination of the ears, mouth, throat and hips.
10. Do not lose the opportunity to examine the infant or young child if he/she goes to sleep.
11. Sometimes, in fractious children, examination may have to be postponed.

EXAMINATION OF SYSTEMS

For ease of presentation, the examination of the various systems is described briefly. This sequence is followed more closely in the examination of schoolchildren; at a younger age examination by region is more appropriate.

Respiratory system

In infants the cross-section of the chest is roughly circular. The ratio of the antero-posterior to the transverse diameter of the chest falls from unity at birth to the adult value of 0.75 by the age of 3. Most of the young child's respiratory movement is diaphragmatic and produces quite marked abdominal movements and little apparent chest movement.

It is important to remember that in infants and young children, extensive lung disease may be present when the physical signs obtained by auscultation or percussion, may be absent or minimal.

Inspection

Before examining the chest note the child's colour (whether pink or blue), count the breathing rate, and observe the pattern of breathing. Look for any flaring of the alae nasi or discharge from the eyes, nose or ears, and listen for cough and 'noises' (wheeze, stridor, grunting) associated with breathing. Look next at the chest for evidence of deformity (pectus carinatum, funnel chest, Harrison's sulci or scoliosis). Observe anterior neck muscle activity, the presence of hyperinflation or asymmetry of chest movements and of indrawing (suprasternal, supraclavicular, intercostal and subcostal).

Palpation

Check the degree of symmetry of chest movements, and note whether wheeze is palpable. Identify the apex beat and the position of the trachea. Tracheal deviation is unreliable as a clinical sign in young children.

Auscultation

Normal breath sounds in infants and children are often more intense and expiration more prolonged than in adults, giving the mistaken impression of bronchial breathing. They are often described as bronchovesicular. In young children with lower respiratory tract infection, for example pneumonia, the sequence is also different. Instead of the normal adult respiratory cycle — inspiration, expiration, pause — expiration is first, followed immediately by inspiration and then a pause. Confusion may arise unless the abdominal

Table 10.1   Head and neck

Area	Observation	Abnormality	Associations
Cranium	Size and shape	Plagiocephaly	Prematurity
		Microcephaly	Mental retardation
		Brachycephaly	Down's syndrome
		Scaphocephaly	Sagittal suture stenosis
		Oxycephaly	Coronal suture stenosis
		Hydrocephalus	Neural tube defect
	Hair	Loss	Acrodermatitis entero-pathica
		Coarse, plentiful	Mucopolysaccharidosis
		Dry, brittle	Hypothyroidism
		Low line posteriorly	Turner's syndrome
		White forelock	Waardenberg's syndrome
	Fontanelles	Delay in closure	Raised intracranial pressure
			Rickets
		Premature fusion	Impaired brain growth
		Depression	Dehydration
		Tense, bulging	Meningitis
	Sutures	Premature fusion	Craniostenosis
		Separation	Raised intracranial pressure
	Bones	Bossing	Rickets
		Craniotabes	Prematurity
		Maxillary prominence	Thalassaemia major
		Bruit	A–V malformations
Ears	Setting	Low set	Pierre Robin syndrome
	Development	Dysplastic	Potter's syndrome
	Configuration	Malformations	Renal abnormalities, hearing defects
		Tags	Treacher Collin's syndrome
Face	Expression	Anxiety, fear	Emotional status
		'Dead pan'	Neuro-muscular abnor-mality
	Movements	Asymmetrical	Facial nerve palsy
		Involuntary	Tics
	Appearance	Characteristic grouping of abnormalities	Down's syndrome
	Forehead	Prominent, narrow re-ceding, bossed	Varied
Eyes	Setting	Mongoloid slant	Down's syndrome
		Ante-mongoloid slant	Treacher Collin's syndrome
	Interpupillary Distance	Hypertelerism	Oesophageal abnormality
	Lids	Epicanthic folds	Down's syndrome
		Periorbital oedema	Nephritis, nephrosis
	Conjunctiva	Colour	Jaundice, blue sclerae
	Iris	Heterochromia	Wilm's tumour
	Lens	Opalification	Galactosaemia
	Cornea	Cloudiness	Mucopolysaccharridoses
	Movements	Squint	Raised intracranial pressure
			Intraocular diseases

Table 10.1 (cont'd)

Area	Observation	Abnormality	Associations
Nose	Shape	Depressed ridge	Hypothyroidism
	Alae nasi	Movements	Lower respiratory infection
	Nostrils	Discharge	Infection
	Mucosa	Pallor	Allergy
Lips	Appearance	Swelling	Allergy
		Fissuring, ulceration	Infection, e.g. candida
	Colour	Blue	Cyanotic congenital heart disease
		Pallid	Anaemia
Jaw	Size	Small	Cleft palate
Mouth	Size and shape	Small oral cavity	Down's syndrome
	Mucosa	Dryness	Dehydration
		Ulceration	Herpes simplex infection
		Adherent 'curd'	Candidiases
		Koplik's spots	Measles
	Tongue	Macroglossia	Glycogen storage disease
	Gums	Bleeding	Gingivitis
	Teeth	Number, shape, size colour, caries	Varied
	Tonsils	Redness	Tonsillitis
	Oropharynx	Swelling and redness	Pharyngitis

inspiratory movements are observed during auscultation. If breath sounds are more harsh on one side of the chest than the other, the harsher side is probably normal. Listen carefully for crepitations (crackles), rhonchi (wheeze) and for a pleural rub. Accompaniments related to localised pathology may be heard on both sides as sound is readily transmitted through the chest wall of the young child.

Percussion

In young children percussion follows auscultation. Percuss lightly to compare corresponding areas on the front, sides and back of the chest. Percussion may be helpful in detecting diminution of cardiac dullness when the chest is over-inflated, or dullness due to collapse, consolidation or a pleural effusion.

Cardiovascular system

Inspection

First observe the child from a distance. Is the child ill or undersized? Is the breathing rate increased? Is there grunting or wheezing? Is the child blue around the lips or the extremities? Is there puffiness of the face, sweating, or clubbing of the fingers and toes? Distinguish between central and peripheral cyanosis.

Thereafter the sequence will vary according to the age of the child. In infants and young children it may be best to start by examining the precordium. Asymmetric prominence of the left anterior chest wall usually indicates cardiac enlargement. A thrusting impulse at the apex is characteristic of left ventricular hypertrophy and pulsation at the lower left sternal border or xyphi-sternum indicative of right ventricular hypertrophy.

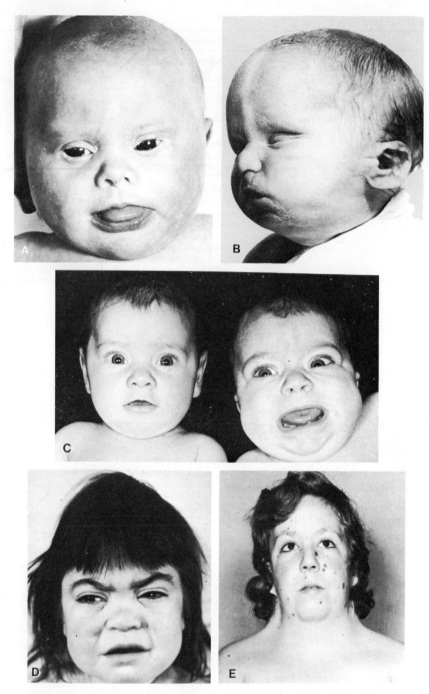

Fig. 10.3   The face as a diagnostic aid. (A) Down's syndrome — palpebral fissures sloping laterally upwards and elongated prominent protruding tongue associated with small mouth. (B) renal agenesis — small jaw, flattened nose, low set ears. (C) Cretin with normal twin — large tongue, coarse features, bloated cheeks and double chin due to myxoedematous change. (D) Mucopolysaccharidosis — wide nose with depressed bridge, prominent supraorbital ridges and eyebrows. (E) Webbing of neck in Turner's syndrome. Pigmented naevi also present.

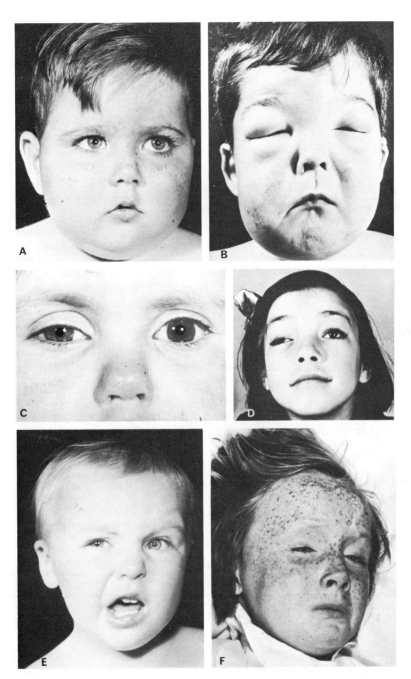

Fig. 10.4 The face as a diagnostic aid. (A) Mooning of the face induced by corticosteroid therapy. (B) Facial oedema in the nephrotic syndrome with peri-orbital involvement almost preventing opening of the eyes. (C) Right-sided Horner's syndrome — smallness of pupil (miosis) enophthalmos and a narrow palpebral fissure. (D) Ptosis (more marked on right side) in myasthenia gravis. (E) Left-sided facial palsy. (F) Risus sardonicus in tetanus; marked freckling of skin.

Palpation

Locate the apex beat. Sometimes one or both heart sounds are palpable. A palpable second heart sound in the pulmonary area suggests increased pulmonary arterial pressure. If a thrill is palpable, its site of maximum intensity should be localised either by the palm of the hand or by the finger tips.

Auscultation

Auscultate early in the examination while the child is cooperative. Provided the room is quiet and the child lies reasonably still, the heart sounds are easily heard. The first heart sound is single and the second is generally split with widening of the two components during inspiration and narrowing during expiration. The two components are usually of equal intensity. Splitting is usually best heard at the second left intercostal space. The third heart sound, best heard at the apex, is common in healthy infants and young children. The presence of murmurs — site(s), timing and quality, intensity, propagation and variations with positional change, are noted. Most murmurs in children are innocent. In distinguishing between innocent and organic murmurs, account must be taken of the child's overall state of health and other physical findings. Innocent murmurs are not accompanied by thrills and tend to disappear more readily with changes of position than organic murmurs. There are several varieties:

1. A musical vibratory systolic murmur, best heard at the left third interspace. It disappears with the valsalva manoeuvre.
2. A soft pulmonary ejection murmur, best heard when the patient is supine. It usually disappears when the patient is upright.
3. Venous hum. In the sitting or erect position it is a medium-pitched humming systolic/diastolic murmur audible over the base of the heart. It can usually be obliterated by pressure over the jugular veins or by lying the child flat.
4. A pleuro-pericardial systolic murmur may be heard at the apex or lower left sternal border. It varies with respiration and is usually secondary to a pleuro-pericardial adhesion.

The murmurs associated with a number of congenital heart lesions are summarised in Table 10.2.

Percussion

Percussion of cardiac borders is sometimes useful in children in determining heart size but does not distinguish between left and right ventricular hypertrophy. An increased area of cardiac dullness indicates cardiac enlargement or a pericardial effusion.

Pulses

Many children have sinus arrhythmia and extrasystoles are not uncommon. In suspected congeni-

Table 10.2 Murmurs associated with congenital heart disease

Lesion	Nature of murmur	Maximum site	Other features
Ventricular septal defect	Pansystolic	L. lower sternal border	Mid-diastolic mitral valve flow murmur may be heard
Pulmonary stenosis	Ejection systolic	2nd L. intercostal space	Split 2nd heart sound
Atrial septal defect	Ejection systolic	2nd L. intercostal space	Fixed splitting 2nd heart sound, mid-diastolic tricuspid valve flow murmur may be heard at apex
Patient ductus cutenosus	Continuous	2nd L. intercostal space and under L. clavicle	Collapsing peripheral pulses.

tal heart disease, both radial and brachial pulses should be palpated for rate, rhythm, quality and amplitude. The average resting pulse-rate ranges from about 120/min in infants to 80/min in older children. There is a wide variation in normal values at all ages. Be sure to compare upper and lower limb pulses. When the femoral pulse is absent, weak or delayed in comparison with the brachial pulse, coarctation of the aorta must be suspected.

Arterial blood pressure

Blood pressures should be measured at the arms and legs. The auscultatory method is usually easy in children over the age of 3. Cuff dimensions are important — a ratio of 2:3 (cuff width upper arm length) is necessary. A cuff that is too narrow will produce spuriously high blood pressure and vice versa (see p. 91).

In infants palpation of the pulse distal to the occluding cuff provides an approximation of the systolic blood pressure. The flush method is useful in small infants. A cuff of appropriate size is applied round the upper arm or thigh. The area distal to the cuff is blanched by squeezing or by wrapping an elastic bandage around it. The cuff is then inflated, following which the compression of the limb is released. Flushing corresponds to a value approximately that of the mean systolic pressure.

Recently the Doppler ultrasonic method has been employed. This combines a small ultrasound transducer with earphones and a sphygmomanometer. Cuff dimensions remain critical.

Average blood pressure readings mmHg $\pm$ 20% in infancy or children are as follows:

Newborn 60 (flush method)
Infancy 80/55 (auscultation)
Pre-school child 90/60 (auscultation)
Schoolchild 100/65 (auscultation)

Venous pressure

The level of the distended jugular vein above the suprasternal notch when the child is at 45° angle is a measure of venous pressure in older children. In infants and young children the neck tends to be short and fat and the method unhelpful.

Extremities

Central cyanosis with bluish discolouration of the lips and tongue is usually indicative of cyanotic congenital heart disease. Clubbing of fingers or toes is present in cyanotic congenital heart disease but seldom appears before the age of 1 (see p. 133).

Oedema of the legs is characteristic of right ventricular heart failure in older children and adults. In infants and young children, however, peripheral oedema is more likely to affect first the face and then the presacral area and eventually the legs. Enlargement of the liver is an important sign of right heart failure in infants and children. The spleen may also be enlarged in long standing congestive cardiac failure. However, limb oedema, liver and splenic enlargement are all late signs of the cardiac failure in congenital heart disease. They are usually preceded by wheezing, grunting, tachypnoea or tachycardia.

Alimentary system

In young children it is best to leave the examination of the mouth, tongue, teeth and gums to the end. Abdominal examination is usually carried out when the patient is supine and relaxed. This may not always be possible. The young infant may be examined on mother's lap, while feeding or sucking the teat. In the toddler age-group the abdomen may be examined for tenderness and masses while the child sits facing mother with the legs straddling her lap. Similarly, in fractious infants, do not lose the opportunity to examine the abdomen if the child is lying temporarily quiet in the prone position. This may provide the only opportunity to confirm the diagnosis of intussusception. The abdomen cannot be examined adequately while a child is crying.

Inspection

Observe the size and contour of the abdomen. It may be distended or scaphoid. Movements with respiration, the state of the skin, the presence of visible peristalsis, umbilical hernia (common in the first two years of life), sepsis, distended veins and any groin swelling are noted. The rounded contour of a full bladder may be obvious.

Palpation

Remember:

1. If abdominal pain has been present the child should be asked to point to the area most affected and to indicate whether the pain has moved.
2. Position yourself at the appropriate level, either by kneeling or sitting, at the cot-side. A hand (previously warmed) should be placed flat on the abdomen.
3. Light palpation, especially for the spleen, is more informative than deep palpation.
4. Start remote from the site of any pain.
5. Look at the child's face during palpation.

The technique of palpation does not differ from that in the adult (p. 169). The liver is normally palpable 1–2 cm below the right costal margin in the first two years of life. In older children the spleen becomes palpable in the left hypochondrium and enlarges towards the right iliac fossa, while in infancy it is more laterally placed and enlarges towards the left iliac fossa. The kidneys can often be felt by bi-manual palpation in normal children and especially in the newborn. The bladder, when distended, is felt as a rounded pyriform swelling in the suprapubic region. A full bladder can interfere with palpation (Fig. 10.5). Other masses of varying size, site and consistency may also be felt. Faeces may be palpable along the descending colon. Mesenteric nodes may be felt. Tumours, such as neuroblastomas or Wilm's tumour are likely to be easily felt.

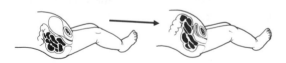

Fig. 10.5 Palpation of abdomen. An example of a remediable problem. Children with full bladders resist palpation; rectal 'rocks' become easily palpable once the bladder is empty.

The soft sausage-shaped tumour of an intussusception in the right upper quadrant may be much more difficult to feel. It may be associated with a detectable emptiness in the right iliac fossa. For swellings in the groin, distinguish between herniae, lymph glands, cryptorchidism and hydrocoele in boys.

When congenital hypertrophic pyloric stenosis is suspected a pyloric tumour must be sought. The examiner sits on the infant's left and places the left hand flat on the abdomen, the fingers directed towards the right hypochondrium with the tips below the liver-edge and lateral to the rectus muscle. The tumour tends to harden intermittently and can be felt by gentle depression of the tips of the fingers. The infant is best examined when feeding though the tumour may be most easily felt when the stomach is empty immediately after vomiting.

In examining males for suspected maldescent of the testes, start in the inguinal area and work downwards towards the scrotum. This avoids the testes being pushed upwards during examination or being retracted due to a brisk cremasteric reflex. Note any abnormalities of the penis remembering that the foreskin is not normally retractile before the age of 2–3 years. In females vaginal discharge, labial adhesions or hypertrophy of the clitoris may be noted. The need for more detailed examination will depend on clinical circumstances. In both sexes pubertal changes may be apparent.

Percussion

Light percussion from resonant to dull areas may help to confirm enlargement of liver and spleen and define the nature of any abdominal mass present. It is essential in detecting shifting dullness.

Auscultation

Tinkling or crackling bowel sounds are normal. As in adults they will be accentuated when there is increased peristalsis and diminished or inaudible in the absence of peristalsis.

It is unnecessary to perform rectal examination routinely. It is however essential in children with acute abdominal pain and in any cases of suspected sexual abuse. Observation may reveal irritation, fissuring or prolapse of the anus. When indicated, rectal examination should be performed by slowly inserting the little finger. Muscle tone, character of stools, tenderness or the presence of masses are noted.

Nervous system

Examination of the nervous system in the older child can be conducted with the same precision as in the adult. Chapter 8 covers the neurological examination as applied to such children. With the younger child or infant neurological examination requires a somewhat modified and more flexible approach. The central nervous system is not fully developed and full cooperation is not possible at this stage of maturity. Age and cooperation are the variables which make most demands on the patience, sensitivity and skills of the examiner.

Inspection

Observation is of key importance. During history taking the child's activities, alertness, attention span, creativity and demeanour whilst at play provide clues about intelligence, developmental status and emotional stability.

Record any disorder of posture or movements. What position does the child adopt voluntarily? Is posture appropriate for age? Is there local or generalised limitation or asymmetry of movements? Clear hand or foot preference before the age of 3 may indicate a defect on the contralateral side. Is there obvious peripheral nerve damage — facial palsy, wrist drop or Erb's palsy? Are there involuntary movements of the trunk (salaam attacks), limbs (tremor, choreoid, athetoid, myoclonic, twitching), face (tics) or eyes (rolling, nystagmus).

Note any unsteadiness while sitting or walking and any incoordination in reaching for toys. Is the gait abnormal — broad-based and unsteady (ataxia), stiff-legged (spasticity), scissoring (diplegic), or accompanied by an outward fling of the leg with paucity of ipsilateral arm movements (hemiparesis)?

Cry and speech may be abnormal. The cry may be high-pitched, as in cerebral birth injury or meningitis. The speech may lack intelligibility to a varying degree (cerebral palsy), disappear (aphonic chorea), be monotonous and lacking in expression (certain post-traumatic states) or accompanied by stammer (psychological disturbance). Delay in onset of speech may indicate deafness, mental retardation or infantile autism. The range of vocabulary, language and reading and writing ability give further indication of mental and cerebral functional status.

Level of consciousness may be closely related to neurological disease. Hyper-excitability, drowsiness, unresponsiveness, or loss of consciousness may accompany such disorders as meningitis, encephalitis, post-epileptic state, and cerebral palsy. Assessment of the unconscious child is similar to that in adults (p. 251).

An impression will now have been gained of the child's mental and developmental status. General inspection may also be helpful. Abnormalities of growth, head size or shape may provide important clues of neurological abnormality. Observation of the hair, nails and skin can sometimes give diagnostic information, for example depigmented areas of skin in tuberous sclerosis. Similarly, disturbance of breathing rate or pattern may indicate brain stem abnormalities or neuromuscular weakness. Asymmetry of growth or hemihypertrophy suggest the presence of neurological disorder, e.g. neurofibromatosis.

It is conventional to document the findings starting with the cranium and spine and then in turn with the cranial nerves, motor and sensory function and tendon and superficial reflexes. In practice, proceed as circumstances permit.

Cranium and spine

Evaluation involves inspection, palpation, percussion and auscultation. Note any abnormality of shape or size of the head and measure its occipital frontal circumference (Fig. 10.6). Midline defects over the cranium, spine and lumbo-sacral area include encephalocoele, meningocoele, dermoid cysts, and dermal sinuses. The fontanelles may be open or closed. The anterior fontanelle usually closes between 15 and 18 months. It may be large, small, bulging in raised intracranial pressure or

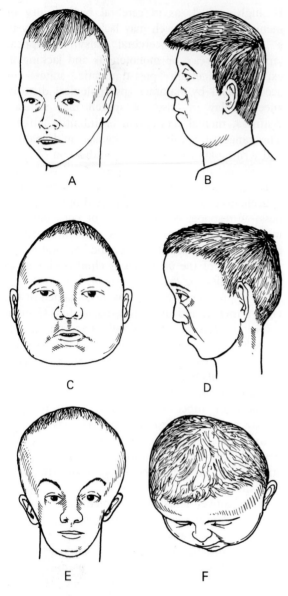

Fig. 10.6 The cranium as a diagnostic aid. (A) Okycephaly or turricephaly — elongated skull with prominent vortex. (B) Brachycephaly — short cranial vault. (C) Microcephaly — small cranial vault. (D) Scephocephaly — long narrow skull. (E) Hydrocephalus — large cranial vault due to enlarged ventricles. (F) Plagiocephaly — asymmetrical skull.

depressed with dehydration. Venous distention over the scalp or a crack pot sound on percussion may indicate raised intercranial pressure. Transillumination of the infant's skull may help in indicating focal or diffuse abnormalities of the brain. Cranial bruits are not uncommon in healthy infants and children, and sometimes indicate an underlying vascular malformation. Note the spinal contour, particularly any exaggeration of the lumbar lordosis or thoracic scoliosis. Localised tenderness over the spine may indicate infection of the epidural or intervertebral disc spaces.

Cranial nerves

During routine examination the cranial nerves are seldom examined in full detail. The younger the child the greater will be the limitation imposed by age.

Cranial nerve: 1. Specific appreciation of smell does not develop until later childhood.

2. Vision is probably present at birth. At about 4 weeks infants will watch the mother. By 6 weeks they will follow moving objects but the arc of visual movement will not be more than 90°; by 8 weeks they will fix, converge and focus and by 12 weeks the arc of movement will be approximately 180°. Thus, by 6–8 weeks defects in visual perception and from 12 weeks disordered eye movements begin to be evident. The ability of the young child to follow or pick up very small objects is a rough indication of visual acuity. Visual fields are more difficult to test — a rapidly approaching object (the examiner's hand) from either side at eye-level will elicit a blink if temporal fields of vision are normal. Examination of the fundus may reveal a wide range of disc and retinal abnormalities (See Ch. 8).

3, 4 and 6. A full range of eye movements depends on the integrity of these nerves. In infancy, horizontal and vertical movements can be assessed by spinning the infant through 360° of arc and by tilting the vertically-held infant in a semiprone position. In late infancy the infant's ability to follow attractive objects in vertical, horizontal and diagonal directions can be tested, and the presence of nystagmus noted.

Squint is a common problem. A certain amount of transitory squinting occurs in the early weeks of life. Squinting after that age is always significant and may be paralytic (non-concomitant) or nonparalytic (concomitant). In the former, the paralysed eye will constantly fail to move in one or more directions when a slowly moving light is being followed. Thus, the angle between the axes of the eyeballs will vary according to the direction in which the child is looking. For example, in paralysis of the right sixth nerve, the squint will be evident on looking to the right and will disappear when looking straight ahead or to the left. In a non-paralytic squint the two eyes maintain the same relative position in whatever direction the child looks. It is not necessarily persistent and is often more obvious at the end of the day when the child is tired. The squinting eye can be determined by asking the child to look at a distant object and covering alternately one and then the other eye. When the dominant eye is covered, the squinting eye will deviate to look at the object but its gaze will move away from the object when the dominant eye is uncovered. The dominant eye will remain fixed on the object when the squinting eye is covered and uncovered. Check the pupillary responses to direct and consensual light.

5. Corneal reflex and facial sensation can be tested in infants and children. Absence of the corneal reflex may result from a sensory deficit (cranial nerve 5) or a motor defect (cranial nerve 7). Testing in the latter situation results in lacrimation. Muscle power (temporalis, masseter, pterygoids) and jaw jerk are easily tested in older children.

7. Facial asymmetries are common in young children and do not necessarily imply weakness of the seventh cranial nerve. Lower motor neurone lesions cause weakness of the upper and lower face whereas upper motor neurone lesions involve only the lower face. In cooperative children, wrinkling the forehead, frowning, raising the eyebrows, maintaining the eyes closed against resistance, and smiling, indicate an intact facial nerve. Taste on the anterior portion of the tongue can also be tested in cooperative children.

8. Testing of hearing is vital in early infancy as corrective measures at that stage may result in normal speech development.

Hearing can be assessed crudely in early infancy by observing the response to a loud auditory stimulus presented to one or other ear. In the newborn hearing loss may be detected using an acoustic cradle that measures the motor responses of the baby to auditory stimuli. It is not yet a routine screening method but can be applied to babies at high risk of deafness — positive family history, low birthweight, birth asphyxia or severe neonatal jaundice, intrauterine infection or malformation of ears or face.

The distraction test is a screening procedure carried out in 7–8-month-old infants by Health Visitors (Fig. 10.7). The child sits on mother's knee, the distractor in front of the child, and a third person who introduces the test sounds behind the child. The child's attention is aroused by holding up an attractive object which is then removed. A test sound is then made about three feet from the baby at the same level as the ear and the child's reaction noted by the distractor. The test is repeated on each side using high- and low-frequency sounds.

The variety of performance tests can be used subsequently in children who either fail the distraction test or are judged to be at increased risk of deafness, for example, post-meningitis or head injury; at school entry, the 'sweep' test is widely used for auditory screening. Parents' views on children's hearing ability must always be considered carefully.

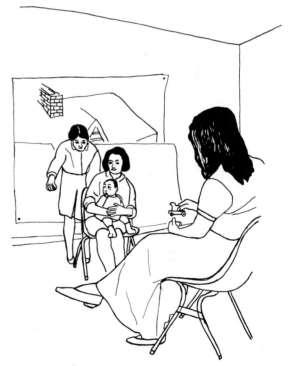

Fig. 10.7 The distraction test to assess hearing.

9 and 10. Involvement of the lower cranial nerves indicates disorders of the lower brain stem. When intact there will be normal palatal and pharyngeal gag reflexes. Inspiratory stridor may be a sign of abnormality of the 10th cranial nerve causing weakness of vocal cord abduction.

11. The strength of the trapezius and sternomastoid muscles can be assessed in young children.

12. The movement of the tongue and any associated tremor or wasting can be observed directly.

Motor system

Observe muscle size, contours and outlines. Handling the child will give a general idea of muscle tone. Hypotonia will be indicated by softness of the muscles, floppiness on handling or excessive laxity of the joints, and hypertonia by excessive firmness of the muscles and stiffness in movements of the limbs, for example, thigh adductor spasm in spastic diplegia.

Muscle power may be inferred by observing children at play. Loss of power is deduced from lack of activity or limitation of movement without obvious cause. In cooperative children, power can be systematically assessed in the limbs, neck and trunk, including flexion, extension, abduction, adduction and rotational movements.

Fine movements can be tested by asking the child to carry out specific movements, for example picking up small objects, by finger-to-nose testing, rapidly alternating pronation and supination of the hands, assessing the child's ability to stand with the eyes closed, or to walk in a straight line. Intention tremor, nystagmus and ataxia, sometimes accompanied by muscular hypotonia, indicate disturbance of cerebellar function.

Careful examination of infants and children while they are relaxed and quiet and again when they are moving will help to differentiate various forms of movement disorders. In general, spasticity becomes more marked when a child runs whereas extrapyramidal signs lessen. Reference has already been made to gait. A decreased swing of the arms may reflect a mild hemiparesis. A waddling gait may be due to weakness of the pelvic girdle musculature, and disinclination to walk a sign of pain.

Sensation

Sensation is difficult to test reliably and consistently in infants and young children. Most children over 3 years will cooperate for testing of peripheral modalities including light touch, pinprick, vibration and movement of the joints. Testing of cortical sensory function becomes possible in children over 5. Proprioception can be assessed by asking the child to close the eyes and to touch the nose with a finger and to stand erect with feet together.

Reflexes

Tendon reflexes may be elicited at all ages. Any increase or decrease in resting muscle tone will influence tendon reflex responses. In infants, evaluation of the symmetry of reflex activity must take into account resting muscle tone and the positioning of the head.

Superficial reflexes are present from birth. The abdominal reflexes show the adult pattern of response throughout childhood. A plantar flexor response is seen in children over 1 year of age. Under 1, an equivocal response with fanning of the toes is normally obtained. The anal reflex consists of constriction on stroking the perianal skin. In certain disorders, for example meningomyelocoele, it may be lost. The cremasteric reflex is active in boys from the age of 6 months.

So-called 'infantile' reflexes are normally present in young infants during the early months of life. With cortical development they are progressively inhibited; persistence beyond the normal time of disappearance suggests diffuse cerebral dysfunction. They include sucking and swallowing, rooting, Moro, grasping and tonic neck reflexes.

Sucking and swallowing reflexes. These are present in all normal full-term infants and persist until voluntary control of these activities is achieved.

Rooting reflex. When light contact is made with the infant's cheek, the infant turns towards the point of contact. This reflex is present in normal infants and helps them to find the mother's nipple.

Moro reflex. The infant is held in the supine position with the shoulders, back and buttocks supported in one hand and arm of the examiner and the head (occiput) in the other. If the head is allowed to fall back about an inch while the body remains supported, the arms rapidly abduct and then come together with an embracing movement.

Grasp reflex. This is elicited by placing the examiner's forefingers in the palm of the infant's hand. The baby's hand closes around the examiner's finger.

Tonic neck reflex. This is elicited with the baby in the supine position. Rotation of the head to one side produces increased tone and partial extension of the arm of the same side accompanied by flexion of the knee on the contralateral side.

Tests of meningeal irritation

Neck stiffness and a positive Kernig's sign (see p. 238) may be present in meningitis. Their absence in young infants does not exclude meningitis.

Locomotor system

The principles underlying examination of the locomotor system and the techniques involved have been described in Chapter 9. The examination of the nervous system will inevitably have involved some examination of the locomotor system. More specific examination may reveal other defects. Congenital and inherited defects and growth disturbances of the musculo-skeletal system figure more prominently in children than in adults. The possibility that bony injuries are non-accidental must be considered (see Fig. 10.8).

Generalised skeletal disorders

Each of these conditions is rare and is usually recognised soon after birth. Infants with the severe type of osteogenesis imperfecta present with recurrent fractures and develop bony deformities and growth retardation. In Klippel-Feil syndrome, the neck is short and stiff, the hairline low and the ears often low-set. Multiple spinal abnormalities may be present with hemivertebrae and scoliosis. A high scapula (Sprengel's deformity), renal anomalies and deafness are common associated defects. Conditions such as achondroplasia and osteochondro-dystrophy are readily recognised by their characteristic skeletal effects.

Deformities of trunk and neck

These should be sought with the child standing erect. They may take the form of scoliosis, kyphosis or lordosis. Torticollis, suspected by the characteristic tilting of the neck to one side and slight turning of the head to the other, is excluded by checking the range of head movement. In the lumbo-sacral area, a tuft of hair may be visible overlying a palpable spina bifida occulta.

Deformities of the limbs

In the upper limbs a number of deformities may be evident. There may be an increased carrying angle at the elbow as seen in Turner's syndrome. In the absence of the radius, severe flexion and lateral twisting of a hand occur at the wrist. There may be absence of part of the arms or fingers,

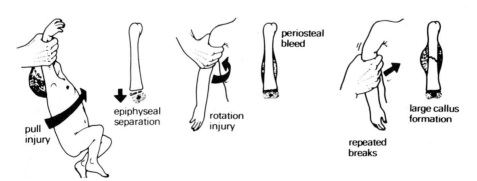

Fig. 10.8 Examples of non-accidental bone injuries. (Courtesy of Professors A D Milner and D Hull.)

extra digits (polydactyly), fusion of digits (syn-dactyly) or a variety of other abnormalities. Functional deformities, such as the dinner-fork deformity at the wrist with the hands outstretched (as in chorea) may be elicitable.

In the lower limbs examples of deformity include absence of part of the limbs, talipes equino varus (club foot), metatarsus varus, shortening or unequal development, for example hemiatrophy or hemihypertrophy. Pes planus is best observed with the child standing. Eversion of the foot and flattening of the normal plantar arch will then be evident.

Muscles

The muscles should be examined for evidence of general or local wasting and for absence of individual muscles. Enlargement of the calves may be noted in the Duchenne type of muscular dystrophy. Assessment of muscle power and tone has been described on page 218.

Joints

Examination of a joint will assess its range of movement, the presence or absence of deformity, swelling, tenderness, pain on active and passive movement and any local rise of temperature. Enquire about the presence of pain before touching or moving the joint. Swelling may be seen in a variety of conditions, e.g. the large joints in haemophilia and the small joints in juvenile rheumatoid arthritis. The diagnosis of congenital dislocation of the hip in the newborn is described on page 282.

Growth disturbances

Idiopathic scoliosis is about five times more common in girls than in boys. Its presentation and assessment has already been described (p. 274). Remember to examine the back in adolescents presenting for routine physical examination at school.

Slipped femoral epiphysis must be considered in otherwise healthy children who present with a painful limp. Pain is often referred to the side of the knee. Be sure to examine the hip-joint in any

child complaining of knee-pain, particularly in adolescence. Physical examination reveals limitation of internal rotation. This condition must be distinguished from transient synovitis of the hip by appropriate radiological investigation.

Other conditions — genu varum (bow legs), genu valgum (knock-knees), tibial torsion, femoral anteversion and a range of foot problems (flat foot, claw toes, etc) — are not uncommon in young children. Diagnosis and treatment demands a knowledge of the normal changes that occur during growth.

Fractures

These may be suspected because of bony deformity, local pain and tenderness on attempted movement. Crepitus may be present but should never be actively elicited. Bony tenderness and swelling may also be present in other conditions, for example osteomyelitis. In non-accidental injury a range of bony injuries may occur (Fig. 10.8).

Potentially uncomfortable examinations

Throughout this section it has been emphasised that procedures that are likely to be disturbing or uncomfortable should be left until the end. These include examination of the ears, mouth, neck and hips.

Ears

Infection in the ears is common in childhood, and auriscopic examination is an important procedure (Fig. 4.7). The child may be held as shown in Figure 10.9. The speculum used should be appropriate to the size of the auditory canal. Wax or purulent discharge should be noted and also any other obstruction such as a boil. Further inspection may not be possible until wax has been removed by a loop, or discharge by dry mopping with cotton-wool on an orange stick. The drum should be examined for colour, bulging, retraction and perforation. It will appear dusky and injected in the presence of acute infection and there may be distortion of the cone of light normally extending forward from the tip of the handle of the malleus. A bulging drum appears to be displaced towards the examiner and the light reflex is usually lost. With retraction, the malleus is unduly prominent. Perforation may occur in any part of the drum but is more likely to be present in the upper part.

Mouth

A child may open the mouth voluntarily. Refusal is likely to be encouraged where there is too much display of shiny instruments and too obvious an indication of intent to use them. Most children will react more willingly to the request to, 'Let me see your teeth', than to, 'Open your mouth', or, 'Show me your throat'. The demonstration of the teeth is more likely to be a matter of some childhood pride. Physical force should be avoided as it breaks the confidence built up between patient and clinician and will make subsequent examinations very difficult.

With a willing child, inspection of the mouth may reveal possible abnormalities in the *state of the mucosa* — dryness, abnormal colour, ulceration, purpura; the white adherent curd-like lesions of thrush which leave bleeding points when scraped off; Koplik's spots in measles, and disorders of the gums.

The *teeth* should be observed for number, whether of the primary or secondary dentition,

size and shape, caries, enamel defects and discolouration. For example, a yellow colour occurs in the primary dentition of prematurely born children who have suffered from severe neonatal jaundice, or in children whose mothers have been given tetracycline during pregnancy. The time of eruption of the teeth may be an index of normal development (p. 352).

Defects in the *palate* will also be evident. *Tongue* size (large in cretins), shape (elongated and thin in mongols) and surface will be noted. The ease with which the tongue can be examined does not justify the over-importance which in the past was attached to its appearance.

The *tonsils* should be observed for size (varying with age and maximal at the age of 7–8 years), colour, exudate or pitting, and the peritonsillar region for swelling and inflammation. The posterior pharyngeal wall should be observed for inflammation, swelling, postnasal discharge and the presence of lymphoid tissue.

Oropharynx. At this point, if not earlier, the examiner will probably require to introduce a spatula into the child's mouth in order to see the throat clearly. Some children in saying 'Aah', will depress the tongue sufficiently to avoid the need for assisted depression. In others a spatula will have to be used. As the child says, 'Aah' the spatula should be placed on the back of the tongue. If the child continues to co-operate, depression of the tongue will reveal the oropharynx. If tense or actively resistant the child will arch the tongue and defy depression of it. It is at this point that the examiner elicits the gag reflex. By advancing the spatula to touch the posterior wall of the pharynx gagging will be induced, the posterior part of the tongue will be actively depressed and the throat exposed. The exposure is short-lived and the examiner must take every advantage of it. One gag should usually be enough, as repetition will upset the child.

Sometimes examination of the mouth will have to be performed in a child who remains uncooperative in spite of coaxing. The infant or toddler should either be seated on the knee of the assistant or laid on a couch. Movement of the arms should be prevented by wrapping the child in a blanket. If the child is held on the knee, the assistant should place one arm round the child's body to prevent movement of the arms and trunk

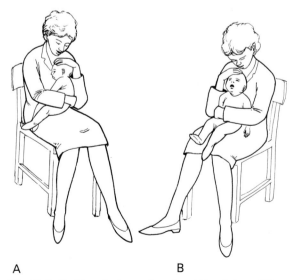

A   B

Fig. 10.9 Positions for inspection of ear (A) and throat (B).

and the other round the head, holding the forehead (Fig. 10.9). If the child is lying on a couch, the assistant should hold the child's head between two hands and the examiner should restrain movement of the child's arms. The examiner should introduce a wooden spatula between the teeth at the side of the mouth and advance it slowly by gentle levering towards the posterior pharynx. It is possible to do this even although the child is clenching the teeth. When the tip of the spatula reaches the posterior pharyngeal wall the child will open the mouth and gag. In this brief moment, the examiner will have to observe all the features of the mouth which have been mentioned above.

Neck

Limitation of flexion (neck stiffness or rigidity) may be an important sign of meningeal irritation due to infection or haemorrhage. It can be tested passively with the patient lying supine on a couch, the examiner placing a hand behind the occiput and gently raising the head. The infant or child may then resist flexion and cry, or the whole trunk may be raised. An older child may be asked to bend forward with the knees drawn up and to put the nose on the knee.

Abnormal swellings such as enlarged lymph nodes should be sought in the anterior and posterior cervical triangles and over the occipital region. Cystic hygromata are soft and trans-illuminable, while abnormal thyroid swellings are confirmed by palpation and by observing movement on swallowing. A sternomastoid tumour is a firm nodule or swelling in the sternomastoid muscle seen in infancy. Branchial cleft remnants may also be found.

When cervical lymph glands are enlarged, other groups should be palpated. In palpating the axillary lymph nodes the child's arm should first be held at right-angles to the trunk to allow adequate access of the fingers to the axilla, and with the fingers in position the arm returned to a position beside the trunk. In generalised lymphadenopathy, the epitrochlear, inguinal and femoral lymph glands may be enlarged. The significance of enlarged lymph nodes is influenced by the findings on examination of the liver and spleen.

Hips

In the newborn, the diagnosis of congenital hip dislocation depends upon demonstrating instability of the joint. The infant is placed supine on a hard surface. The examiner's forefinger is placed over the greater trochanter and the thumb over the inner aspect of the thigh. Both hips are flexed 90° and then slowly abducted from the midline. With gentle but firm pressure an attempt is made to lift the greater trochanter forward. A feeling of slipping as the head goes into the acetabulum is a sign of instability (Ortolani's sign) (p. 282). If the hip is more stable, pressure is applied with thumb on the medial side of the thigh as it is again abducted. It may cause the hip to slip posteriorly accompanied by a 'clunk' as the hip dislocates (Barlow's sign). These signs of instability are the most reliable criteria for diagnosing congenital dislocation of the hip in the newborn period. They become less obvious in the early weeks of life. Limitation of abduction of the hip then becomes the main sign of abnormality. Normally the hip should abduct fully to 90° on either side during the early months of life. When testing for symmetry of abduction the pelvis should be held level. If dislocation remains undetected until the child walks a painless limp may be present with a lurch to the affected side. In bilateral dislocation the gait is waddling. Treatment is most effective when the diagnosis is made in the newborn.

Temperature

In the presence of any constitutional upset one of the most common observations made either in the home or in the hospital is that of temperature. For most purposes skin temperature is adequate, but the site selected should not have been unnaturally cooled by exposure or heated by any artificial means. In infants the groin is probably the best site with the thigh held flexed on to the abdomen; in older children the axilla is more suitable. Some prefer the rectal temperature in infants. Where the temperature does not record on a standard clinical thermometer, as for instance in so-called neonatal cold injury, special low-reading thermometers covering the range from 30° to 40°C should be used. The accepted dividing line between normal and abnormal temperatures, namely 37°C, is appropriate for infants and children; where a skin temperature is taken the normal rectal temperature would be higher by about 0.25°C. Somewhat lower temperatures are normal in premature infants.

Developmental diagnosis

The progressive acquisition of the various body movements and motor skills which characterise normal development is closely related to the maturation of all systems and especially to that of the nervous system. A knowledge of how children develop and of the normal variations that occur is necessary for the identification of those in whom development is delayed or deviant. The identification of such children is an important activity of Community Child Health services.

In assessing whether development is 'normal', motor, linguistic, social and adaptive achievements are considered. Clinically, a convenient sequence is to observe in turn posture and gross body movements, visual perception and fine motor movements, speech and hearing, and social adaptation and play. A summary of age-related developmental attainments is given in Appendix 1 (p. 351). It is no more than a general guide as the age at which normal infants acquire individual skills varies widely. Sequential observations over a period of months are often more informative than a single evaluation. It is important to remember that developmental screening is largely a community activity carried out in apparently well children — it has no place during acute illnesses. Table 10.3 is a summary of the screening programme recommended in the Court Report.

FURTHER INVESTIGATION

Collection of biological samples

Time must be spent explaining any diagnostic or therapeutic procedure to the parents and the child. Encouragement and reassurance at this stage help allay anxiety and fear and greatly increase the likelihood of success. The need for patience, adequate preparation and, during the procedure,

Table 10.3 Programme of development screening (Court Report)

Age	Main objectives and assessment
6–8 weeks	Discuss feeding problems and immunisation Exclude congenital abnormalities, e.g. dislocation of hip(s), cataracts Carry out simple neurodevelopmental check
8–9 months	Carry out distraction hearing tests Ensure sitting unsupported Assess manipulation Assess vision and test for squint
18 months	Ensure walking well Assess language and hearing Assess fine motor skills
3 years	Assess letter matching Carry out vision testing using Snellen charts Carry out word discrimination hearing test Assess speech and language Assess fine motor and performance skills

Plot indices of growth regularly on a centile chart.

proper positioning and restraint cannot be over-emphasised.

Collection of urine

A plastic bag with a round opening surrounded by an adhesive surface that adheres to the skin may be used. In boys the penis is placed in the plastic bag and the adhesive surface is applied to the surrounding skin; in girls the opening of the bag is placed around the external genitalia. After voiding the bag is removed and emptied of urine. Even with careful cleansing before application, culture is frequently positive due to contamination. Bags with a catheter outlet from which urine may be periodically removed are useful for collection of 24 h urine specimens. The average daily output of urine at different ages is as follows:

Days	Volume
1st and 2nd days	30–60 ml
3rd to 10th day	100–300 ml
10th day to 2 months	250–450 ml
2 months to 1 year	400–500 ml
1 to 5 years	500–700 ml

A mid-stream urine sample may be needed for

bacteriological purposes. The external genitalia are carefully cleansed and during voiding an uninterrupted mid-stream specimen can be obtained and sent to the laboratory. This method is most useful in toilet-trained children but is also of value in infancy provided the attendant has the time and patience to wait.

Suprapubic percutaneous bladder aspiration is indicated in selected cases when it is essential to obtain an uncontamined urine sample. It is particularly valuable in the newborn infant in whom the bladder is high and easily accessible. A full bladder must be confirmed by palpation or percussion above the pubic bone before any attempt is made to aspirate urine. The skin is carefully prepared with an antiseptic solution whilst the child is held by an assistant in the frog-leg position (Fig. 10.1). A sterile needle (22 or 25 gauge) is inserted through the skin and abdominal wall at the midline 1–2 cm above the pubic symphysis with the needle at right-angles to the skin. The plunger is gently withdrawn whilst advancing the needle. The appearance of urine in the syringe indicates a succesful tap. Finally, the needle is withdrawn swiftly and the area covered with a dressing. Potential dangers include the introduction of infection, transient haematuria and puncture of the bowel.

Collection of blood samples

Venepuncture is more difficult in infants than in older children due to plumpness of the limbs and the smaller size and greater mobility of the veins. If available, an antecubital vein or the superficial dorsal veins of the hand and wrist should be used; alternatively puncture of the external jugular vein is a safe procedure in infancy. The infant should be wrapped in a sheet securing the arms, and held lying on one side. The neck is flexed laterally and the child held by the nurse. The external jugular vein is brought into prominence as it crosses the sternomastoid and its distension will be increased by crying. The needle is most readily inserted from below upwards (see Fig. 10.11).

Whatever the method, the overlying skin should be cleansed adequately. A number 20 or 22 gauge needle or number 21 scalp-vein needle with attached tubing may be used. Exert gentle suction throughout. When blood has been obtained, remove the needle and exert firm pressure over the vein.

Femoral vein puncture and internal jugular vein puncture are not recommended as routine procedures. Capillary blood may however be obtained from fingertip or heel (small infants). The earlobe is a less satisfactory site as excessive bleeding is more likely to occur. After warming the skin and cleansing with alcohol, a stab is made with a lancet. Free-flowing blood is collected into capillary tubes or an appropriate container. Applying pressure with sterile cotton-wool usually ensures haemostasis. The site should be checked periodically for persistent oozing of blood.

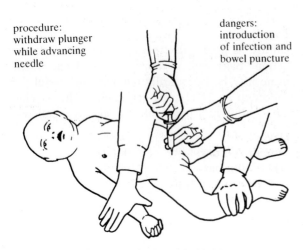

procedure:
withdraw plunger
while advancing
needle

dangers:
introduction
of infection and
bowel puncture

Fig. 10.10   Suprapubic aspiration of the bladder.

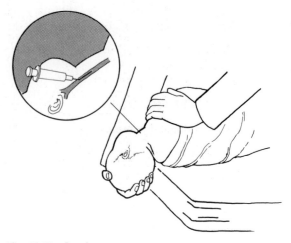

Fig. 10.11   Jugular venepuncture.

Collection of nose, throat and lower respiratory tract secretions

Nasopharyngeal secretions are frequently collected for virological studies in respiratory tract infections. An ordinary polyvinyl feeding tube attached via a sterile container to a syringe is introduced into the nostril and nasopharynx and gentle suction applied with the syringe.

A throat swab may be obtained by visualising the oropharynx (p. 317) and swabbing the tonsils and pharynx. A cough or per nasal swab may be taken to obtain a sample for bacteriological examination, for example when whooping cough is suspected.

Sputum is more difficult to obtain as it is generally swallowed and not expectorated. Early morning gastric washings may be of value when tuberculosis is suspected.

Collection of gastrointestinal secretions

In babies the passage of a fine polythene tube into the stomach through the nose or mouth is easy as active swallowing is not necessary. Infants and older children who are unable to cooperate may require to be restrained in the supine position before passing a nasogastric tube. Following its insertion the child is placed on the left side allowing the stomach to assume a dependent position. The posture selected for gastric aspiration depends on the circumstances. When the danger of pulmonary aspiration is great, the patient should be placed with the head dependent. When consciousness is impaired, tracheal intubation with a cuffed tube should precede gastric aspiration. When indicated for the treatment of ingestions, a large-bore orogastric tube is essential. The appropriate tube length is determined by measuring the distance from the bridge of the patient's nose to the xyphisternum and adding 7–10 cm.

Methods are available for the collection of bile, duodenal and pancreatic secretions. A standard feeding tube used to aspirate the stomach can be passed through the pylorus into the duodenum. The child is placed on the right side and the tube advanced 1–2 cm per hour. The appearance of bile, change in pH of the aspirated material or X-ray visualisation confirms the proper positioning of the tube.

Faeces

Specimens of faeces should be collected in sterile containers using a spoon or spatula to transfer the specimen from the pot or the napkin. Where a specimen is not obtainable a rectal swab may be taken for bacteriological examination. An ordinary throat swab is introduced gently into the anus for about an inch for this purpose.

Cerebrospinal fluid

Lumbar puncture is the procedure most frequently used for obtaining cerebrospinal fluid for diagnostic purposes. The infant or child is restrained in the lateral recumbent position. The skin around the lumbar area is carefully cleansed and sterilised. The needle is inserted into the subarachnoid space through the L3–4 interspace identified by the point where an imaginary line between the iliac crests crosses the lumbar spine. Local anaesthesia is used.

With the child restrained and the operator comfortably positioned, a 22 gauge lumbar puncture needle with stilette in place is inserted in the midline at right-angles to the body (see Fig. 10.12). The needle is gently inserted and in older children a distinct give is felt when the dura is pierced. This may not be appreciated in newborns or young infants. To check, remove the stilette and look for the appearance of fluid. Once adequate fluid has been obtained the needle is removed with a single movement and pressure applied to the puncture site for several minutes with a sterile swab. Before attempting lumbar puncture it is essential to exclude raised intercranial pressure.

Bone marrow aspiration

This procedure is indicated in the diagnosis of blood dyscrasias, neoplastic disease, and certain storage disorders. The anterior and posterior iliac crests may be used at any age, the tibia or femur up to 2 years and the sternum from 6 years onwards.

In performing anterior iliac crest aspiration the child is placed supine. Sedation is usually necessary and in children who have repeated bone marrow aspirations general anaesthesia is preferable. The skin is throughly prepared and the

procedure:
check fundi
position back
glove and clean skin
identify L3, 4
local anaesthetic
advance needle
no 22 gauge at right-angle
to spine

dangers:
introduction of infection
coning

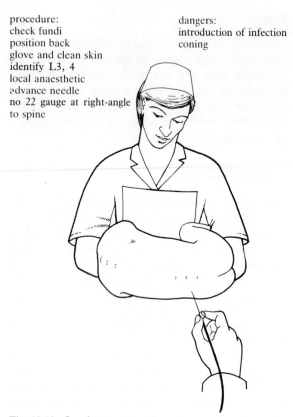

Fig. 10.12   Lumbar puncture.

procedure conducted under conditons of surgical sterility. In non-anaesthetised children the skin is infiltrated with local anaesthetic in an area approximately 2 cm below and behind the anterior superior iliac spine. A bone marrow needle with obturator is inserted perpendicular to the skin and to the periostium. The needle is pushed through the cortex using a firm steady screwing motion. It can usually be felt to enter the marrow and to be firmly in place. The marrow is obtained by moving the obturator and fitting a 20 ml syringe onto the needle and applying strong suction for a few seconds. After aspirating 0.5–1 ml of marrow, smears are prepared for subsequent staining and counting (see p. 348). After replacing the obturator the needle is removed and local pressure exerted for several minutes until bleeding has stopped. A dry sterile dressing is then applied.

Collection of sweat

The diagnosis of cystic fibrosis depends almost en-

tirely on the accuracy with which sweat tests are carried out. The collection and analysis of sweat is now a specialised laboratory procedure requiring a high degree of technical proficiency. It comprises three stages — stimulation of the sweat glands, collection of the sweat sample, and analysis of the sweat. The pilocarpine iontophoresis method is the most widely used and is reliable in all age-groups except the newborn. Stimulation of sweat production is maintained over a 5–6 minute period, the arm then rinsed with electrolyte-free water and pre-weighed filter-paper applied. It is covered with plastic and sealed with plastic tape to avoid evaporation. The filter-paper is removed after 30 minutes and the amount of sweat collected determined by re-weighing the filter-paper. The sample is then analysed for sodium and chloride. The minimum weight of sweat needed for accurate testing is 100 mg. Normal children under 14 usually have sweat chloride concentrations below 40 mEq/l. A level over 60 mEq/l strongly supports the diagnosis of cystic fibrosis but should be confirmed by repeat testing.

THE METHODS IN PRACTICE

The example chosen supplements as well as exemplifies what has been discussed in this chapter.

EXAMINATION OF THE NEWBORN INFANT

All newly born infants should be medically examined. An abnormality may be obvious on casual inspection, or encountered only after a thorough examination. The principles and practices described throughout this chapter apply in the main to the newborn infant but clinical examination at this age has its limitations. Underlying disease may be present but the signs by which it can be recognised may not yet have developed. For example a gross congenital cardiac defect may be present without murmurs, cardiac enlargement, cardiac failure or cyanosis (which may occur later). Vision has not developed; gross mental defect may be impossible to recognise; hypothyroidism may be present without any of the signs of cretinism. These limitations are offset to some extent by the important positive information that can be gleaned, for example the diagnosis of instability of the hip(s) which allows effective preventive measures to be introduced as early in life as possible. As the methods have been largely described already, this section will indicate mainly the breadth and scope of the neonatal examination rather than the technique. Information from parents and/or nurse, and additional details from mother's obstetric records, may be of crucial importance to the diagnosis and management of any abnormality.

History

Routine examination of the apparently normal term newborn infant is usually carried out without the benefit of a detailed history, though this information becomes essential if any abnormality is detected. A thorough history is always required in those infants with obvious major abnormalities such as cleft lip and palate, or who may develop symptoms, e.g. cyanotic episodes, or are about to be admitted to a Special Care unit.

The history of previous illness consists largely of the birth history (p. 300). This should include information on fetal distress, for example slowing of the fetal heart-rate, or meconium staining of the liquor; early rupture of the membranes; induction of labour; prolonged or rapid labour; difficulties of delivery-forceps at delivery or caesarian section; maturity; birth rank; birthweight; asphyxia such as that associated with delayed onset of respiration; grunting or irregular respirations; respiratory distress with increased respiratory effort and costal margin recession; twitchings and convulsions or disturbances of consciousness; jaundice, pallor or cyanosis.

The medical history of parents and other relatives is relevant in disorders that have a strong hereditary tendency such as haemophilia, cystic fibrosis or Duchenne muscular dystrophy, and those with a weaker but definite hereditary tendency such as cleft lip and spina bifida. The history of mother's pregnancies may indicate recurring factors such as prematurity or post-maturity. Her age may be important, for example Down's syndrome is more common in the elderly mother. Diseases such as rubella, cytomegalovirus infection, toxoplasmosis or HIV may have affected the mother during pregnancy with potentially profound effects on the fetus.

Drugs administered early in pregnancy, for example phenytoin, may be related to the occurrence of congenital abnormalities. Maternal smoking and alcohol consumption may also be important. Enquiry about siblings may reveal familial disease such as mental retardation, thalassaemia or adrenogenital syndrome. Mother's age, parity, previous pregnancy history and health during the present pregnancy should be considered. Maternal diabetes, recurrent urinary tract infection, hypertension, vaginal bleeding, hydramnios or prolonged leaking of liquor may be relevant. Similarly, any previous genetic counselling or diagnostic tests carried out during pregnancy (chorionic biopsy, amniocentesis, ultrasound) should also be known.

Examination

The minimum information the examiner will possess will be the infant's birthweight, length (crown–heel) and head circumference. If available, the weight charted from the time of birth is also valuable. The examination should be carried out in a warm room, free from draughts, with the infant fully undressed and lying on a nappy.

Inspection

The following are a few examples of abnormalities which when present will be obvious in most cases:

1. Defects of body covering, for example meningomyelocoele or gastroschisis.
2. Abnormalities in cranial shape and size such as hydrocephalus, caput succudaneum, excessive moulding, or cephalohaematoma.
3. Abnormal facies, such as that of Down's syndrome, or the flattened nose and low set ears of renal agenesis.
4. Deformities of the limbs such as talipes equino varus or hemimelia (arm ends abruptly above or below elbow).
5. Abnormalities of extremities, for example absent or supernumerary digits.
6. Tumour masses such as sacrococcygeal teratoma.
7. Areas of local swelling such as umbilical hernia or a cystic hygroma should also be obvious.

Skin. The skin is elastic and pink in the healthy infant but may be cracked and parchment-like in placental insufficiency, abnormally pallid as a result of foetal exsanguination, cyanosed with asphyxia or severe congenital heart disease, jaundiced in hepatobiliary and haemolytic disorders, loose and inelastic in prematurity, dry and inelastic in dehydration, blemished with superficial angiomata or milia (pinpoint white spots due to retention of sebacious material) or infected with pustule formation. Oedema may be present especially in premature infants. The character of the umbilical cord and the presence of umbilical bleeding or infection should be noted. There may be skin rashes such as erythema toxicum, haemangiomas or Mongolian blue spots usually over the buttocks or lumbar sacral area, skin defects, or areas of fat necrosis (hard subcutaneous plaques) where there has been previous trauma, e.g. forceps blades. If the skin feels cool temperature is checked with a low reading rectal thermometer.

Cranium. Obvious abnormalities will have been apparent. The size and tension of fontanelles, (Fig. 10.13) the degree of separation or overriding of sutures, and the presence of defects or areas of thinning and softening of the skull (craniotabes) are recorded. The eyes are examined for abnormalities of size or shape, discharge and cataracts. An increase in size and haziness of the iris may be due to congenital glaucoma, and absence of the red reflex to retinoblastoma.

Misting of the shiny end of the stethoscope held under the nostrils suggests that the nares are patent. The mouth is examined to exclude an isolated cleft palate, drying of the mucous membrane, ulceration and infection. A small mandible provides a clue to the Pierre-Robin syndrome.

Spine. The entire midline including the cranium and the back is examined for the presence of a cyst, naevus, dimple or hairy patch. Aplasia of the lumbo-sacral area may occur in infants of diabetic mothers. At this stage it is helpful to look also at the limbs — to count fingers and toes and to detect any positional deformities (varus and valgus positions of the ankles). Examination of the hips is left to the end (p. 318).

Central nervous system. The infant's posture and the state of consciousness will have been observed. The unresponsiveness of severe apnoea or the open eyes and hyperactivity of cerebral irritation may be evident together with the response to stimuli such as pinching of the skin. The amount of spontaneous movement may be significant. Convulsive movements where present may be localised or generalised. Look for paresis, for instance, on one side of the face in facial palsy or of legs in the presence of spina bifida. The Hemi syndrome is characterised by diminished movement on one side of the body. The Moro and grasp reflexes may be absent in the presence of acute cerebral injury. The character of the cry may be helpful — the high-pitched cry of cerebral irritation or the 'cri du chat' syndrome. Muscle hypotonia or hypertonia frequently indicate cerebral disturbance.

Abdomen. The newborn abdomen often seems protruberent but is not taut or over-distended. A scaphoid appearance suggests herniation of the abdominal contents into the chest or high bowel atresia. Peristaltic waves may be obvious in intestinal obstruction. The abdomen should be palpated for enlargement of the liver, spleen, kidneys, bladder, and for abnormal masses. Feel for inguinal herniae and examine the anus for position and patency. Enquire about the passage of meconium. It may be advantageous to watch the infant while feeding for vigour and coordination of sucking and character of swallowing. The genitalia are examined for conditions such as hydrocoele, undescended testes and hypospadias in the male, or for labial fusion and clitoral enlar-

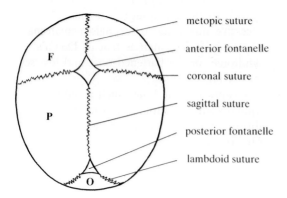

metopic suture

anterior fontanelle

coronal suture

sagittal suture

posterior fontanelle

lambdoid suture

Fig. 10.13 Cranial bones, sutures and fontanelles. (F) Frontal; (P) Parietal; (O) Occipital.

gement (as in adrenogenital syndrome) in the female.

Respiration. The shape of the chest, the respiration rate, the pattern of respiration, the presence of grunting or indrawing, mucus at the mouth, and abnormalities in auscultation may be important. Tachypnoea in the neonate may have a wide range of causes including respiratory distress syndrome, meconium aspiration, cardiac failure, hypovolaemia, anaemia, neurological dysfunction, and metabolic acidosis.

Heart. The heart will be examined for position, for the presence of any abnormal precordial pulsation and for murmurs. The radial and femoral pulses should be palpated and, if indicated, the blood pressure measured in the arms and legs (Doppler method).

The performance of certain basic activities in the newborn, such as sucking, swallowing and crying, and a normal sleep pattern (about 20 hours of sleep and 4 hours awake) are dependent on the integrity of the nervous system. Any deficiency in these activities or disturbances of pattern raise the question of brain damage. Examination should include observation of the infant's ability to suck and swallow and an appreciation of the pattern of sleep and wakefulness.

Meconium and urine. Inquire about the passage of meconium and whether urine has been passed. The character of stools passed subsequently should be noted. Where indicated, urine is examined chemically and bacteriologically.

Futher investigations

Screening tests for phenylketonuria and hypothyroidism (TSH/T_4) are carried out in all infants after feeding has been established. Additional investigation — haematological, biochemical, bacteriological and radiological, are seldom indicated in the absence of symptoms. These investigations are frequently performed in Intensive Care Neonatal units together with repeated estimations of blood gas tensions and pH, and ultrasound examination of the head to detect intracranial bleeding.

Conclusion

The examination of the newborn infant exemplifies fundamental clinical principles even although they are being applied at a time of life when many manifestations of disease are different from those found later. The fact that presenting symptoms in eary life are less specific than in adulthood underlines the need for a full clinical examination in all infants who appear unwell. Diagnosis is based on minimal and not gross signs. Thus, in the newborn period, a potentially devastating condition such as meningitis must be considered and excluded in any infant with fever, poor feeding, irritability or unexplained vomiting. To delay investigation, in this instance lumbar puncture, until more definite conventional signs appear, could be a grave error.

REFERENCES

Forfar J O, Arneill G C 1984 Textbook of paediatrics, 3rd edn. Churchill Livingstone, Edinburgh
Gill D, O'Brien N 1988 Paediatric Clinical Examination. Churchill Livingstone, Edinburgh

11. The use of the ophthalmoscope

R. E. Cull

Modern ophthalmoscopes are so constructed that attention to a few simple details of technique will suffice to enable the student to see the fundus without difficulty. In different subjects, the colour and form of the visible structures vary like complexions and faces; familiarity with the range of normal appearances is therefore essential. Inspection of the fundus should be included as part of the routine clinical examination.

Serious or life-threatening conditions, such as diabetes mellitus, accelerated hypertension, raised intracranial pressure, miliary tuberculosis, or melanoma may be revealed by ophthalmoscopy. Fundal examination may lead to the diagnosis of such problems as glaucoma and retinal detachment which can cause loss of vision.

The ophthalmoscope

The principles of operation of the ophthalmoscope are simple. A beam of light is defleted through a right angle by an angled mirror at the top of the instrument. The observer looks through a small hole in the mirror along the pathway of the light, through the pupil, so that the structures of the eye, including the fundus, are illuminated, and can be inspected (Fig. 11.1). Lenses of graded focal length may be placed behind the hole in the mirror and are moved by a milled wheel, conveniently placed so that it can be controlled by the index finger of the hand holding the ophthalmoscope. There is a series of lenses marked with a '+' which are convex or with a '−' which are concave. Each lens also bears a number which corresponds to its focal length expressed in dioptres. One dioptre is the refractive power of a lens whose focal length is one metre, while two

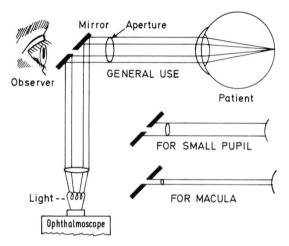

Fig. 11.1 Ophthalmoscopy: basic principles. Some models have a changeable aperture to narrow the beam of light, e.g. for inspection of the macula. Others also have an auriscopic attachment (p. 62).

dioptres corresponds to a focal length of half a metre and twenty dioptres to one twentieth of a metre. These lenses are used to compensate for hypermetropia or myopia (p. 329) in the examiner's or patient's eyes and for the inspection of opacities lying in front of the retina.

Technique in the use of the ophthalmoscope

During a routine examination, the fundus may be inspected through the untreated pupil. However, for a thorough examination of the fundus, the pupil should be dilated with a short acting mydriatic. Tropicamide (0.5% drops from a single dose capsule) is best; it is effective in about 20 minutes, maximum within an hour and lasts less than 8 hours. Alternatively 1% cyclopentalate may be used but its effect persists for about 24 hours.

Mydriatics should not be used if consciousness is impaired or when there is a suspicion of developing intracranial disease, since pupil reflexes will be lost or rendered unreliable as physical signs. Mydriatics should also not be used if the patient is known to suffer from glaucoma. Rarely, dilatation of the pupil by mydriatics may precipitate an attack of acute (closed angle) glaucoma in those patients who have a shallow anterior chamber. An effective estimate of the depth of the anterior chamber may be made fairly simply by shining a light from the margin of the cornea across the iris; if the anterior chamber is of normal dept, the iris will glow around its whole circumference. If the patient has a shallow anterior chamber, only that half of the iris near to the light will be illuminated. If there is any doubt about the depth of the anterior chamber, expert ophthalmological assessment should be made before mydriatics are employed. If this precaution is observed, it is not essential to constrict the pupil after the examination; a drop of 1% pilocarpine will do so if this is thought desirable..

The procedure for the use of the ophthalmoscope itself is as follows:

1. The patient should be examined in a darkened environment.

2. If the examiner has a refractive error, the ophthalmoscope may be used wearing spectacles. Preferably they should be removed and an appropriate correcting lens selected.

3. The ophthalmoscope should be held in the right hand and the right eye should be used to examine the patient's right eye. The examiner's left hand and left eye are used to examine the patient's left eye. If however the clinician experiences difficulty in using the non-dominant eye, an alternative is to examine the patient from above (Fig. 11.2).

4. The patient should be asked to look straight ahead, to keep an eye fixed on a selected, distant object and to keep both eyes open. Blinking does not interfere with the view. Considerate beginners and patients tend to hold their breath. This is unnecessary when the recommended position is adopted.

5. Vision in the eye not being examined should not be obstructed by the examiner's head; otherwise the patient's gaze tends to wander (Fig. 11.3).

6. The ophthalmoscope should be held steady by pressing it against the side of the examiner's nose and superior orbital margin. The examiner's eye should be placed as close as possible to the ophthalmoscope; this enables a greater area to be visualised through the sight hole — as when one looks through a keyhole.

7. The examination should begin with the ophthalmoscope held 20–30 cm away from the patient's eye with the light directed into the pupil. The pupil will then appear to glow uniformly red in normal circumstances. This is the red reflex.

8. The ophthalmoscope and the examiner's head are moved closer to the patient's eye and during this procedure opacities, appearing as black or glistening silhouetted gaps in the red reflex, may be seen. The ophthalmoscope should come as

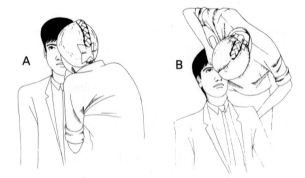

Fig. 11.2 Ophthalmoscopy: correct methods. (A) The patient's gaze can be fixed on a distant point. (B) Using the right (dominant) eye to inspect the patient's left eye from above by an examiner who has difficulty in using the left eye. The patient's gaze is not obstructed.

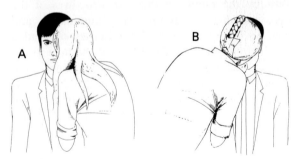

Fig. 11.3 Ophthalmoscopy: wrong methods. (A) The examiner's hair obtrudes. (B) The patient's view is obstructed and the gaze cannot be fixed on a distant point.

close as possible to the patient's eye, without touching the eye lashes or cornea.

9. The examination of detail is possible only if the instrument is steady. This is best achieved by resting the middle and ring fingers of the holding hand against the cheek of the patient. If in addition the ulnar border of the other hand rests on the patient's forehead, its thumb can be used to steady the upper end of the ophthalmoscope, while the fingers form a useful shield to shade the eye. If the eyes are closed voluntarily or involuntarily, the thumb can be used to raise the patient's upper lid gently clear of the pupil.

10. The fundus should be brought into clear focus, using correcting lenses if necessary. Inexperienced observers often accommodate for near vision because of the closeness of the examiner's eye to the patient. Practice at 'looking into the distance' will enable the observer consciously to prevent this accommodation.

11. The light should always be directed at the patient's pupils even when it is necessary to make lateral movements of the ophthalmoscope. A clear view of the fundus may be hampered by light reflected back from the patient's cornea. This can be obviated by a slight tilting of the ophthalmoscope.

Opacities and errors of refraction

Opacities causing interruptions of the red reflex may lie in the cornea, the lens or the vitreous . The site of any opacity should be determined. Corneal opacities due to scarring are revealed if a light is shone obliquely on the cornea. Opacities behind the cornea are better defined by use of convex (+) lenses behind the sight hole of the ophthalmoscope. There may be opacities in the lens due to cataracts which are prone to develop in diabetes and in patients receiving corticosteroids but are extremely common in the elderly.

Opacities in the vitreous are commonly due to irregular, spider-like, drifting black masses. These are known as vitreous 'floaters'. These are extremely common, particularly in myopic patients and the elderly; they are due to precipitation of the vitreous proteins and do not indicate any serious lesion. Vitreous opacities may also be due to haemorrhages and occasionally to persistent

fetal hyaloid vessels or their vestiges which lie between the optic disc and the posterior pole of the lens.

Opacities of the refractive media may be localised by slight lateral movements of the ophthalmoscope. Opacities in the cornea will then appear to move in the direction opposite to that of the light of the ophthalmoscope. Opacities of the lens will not move at all. Opacities in the vitreous seem to move in the same direction as the light.

Errors of refraction. If there are no opacities, close in to the normal position and adjust the lenses if necessary until the retinal vessels are in sharp focus. If the observer's and the patient's eyes are both normal, emmetropic, then no lens ('0') is required; the fundus, although only about 3 cm from the examiner's eye, is in perfect focus owing to refraction by the cornea, lens and vitreous body amounting in all to about 60 dioptres (Fig. 11.4.). The need to employ a plus lens to focus on the fundus indicates hypermetropia, while a minus lens is required for a myopic eye (Figs. 11.5, 11.6.). Myopia is common, and in very short-sighted persons it may be necessary to use a −20 lens or more before a clear view is obtained. Many ophthalmoscopes have no

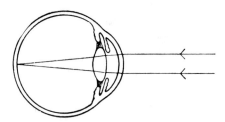

Fig. 11.4 The emmetropic (normal) eye. The retina is in focus without a lens in the ophthalmoscope.

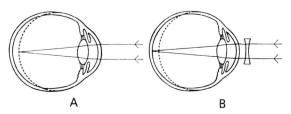

A   B

Fig. 11.5 The myopic (short-sighted) eye. (A) The eye is too long and the retina is not in focus when no lens is used. (B) The use of a concave (minus) lens brings the retina into focus.

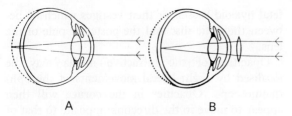

Fig. 11.6 The hypermetropic (long-sighted) eye. (A) The eye is too short and the retina is not in focus when no lens is used. (B) The use of a convex (plus) lens brings the retina into focus.

more than a −20 lens so that exact focus may not be possible unless the patient wears suitable spectacles or contact lenses.

The cornea, vitreous and the lens combine to magnify the features of the fundus. In an emmetropic eye the optic disc appears about four times its true diameter. If the lens of the eye has been removed for cataract it will be noted that the retina of a previously emmetropic eye is now in focus with a +10 lens, a large area of the fundus is in view, the disc and vessels look very small and the inevitable little movements of the patient's eye do not have the usual adverse effect on one's ability to see the fundus. On the other hand, in a myopic eye, a strong minus lens is required, only a small area of the fundus may be in view, the disc and the vessels appear very large, and any little movement is magnified. A very myopic patient can be asked to wear spectacles while the optic disc and the central parts of the retina are examined; the features are more readily seen. Unfortunately, the reflection off the glass makes it impossible to examine the peripheral parts of the retina in the usual way . A good area may, however, be examined by asking the patient to look up, down, to the right and to the left, though patches are liable to be missed.

Gross astigmatism may also cause some difficulty. If the curvatures of the cornea and the anterior and posterior surfaces of the lens of the eye are segments of perfect spheres, the fundus is magnified without distortion. However, there is commonly some degree of astigmatism, a term applied when the curvature of any of these surfaces varies in different planes. The effect of severe astigmatism is to distort the image just as one sees distortion on looking through a window pane that

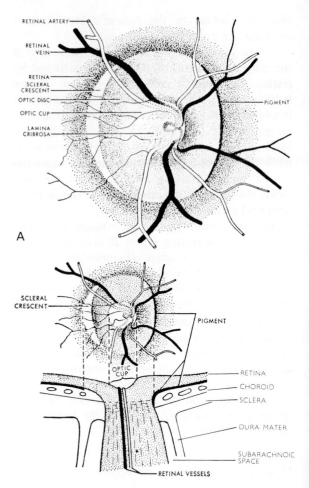

Fig. 11.7 The normal right optic disc. (A) Details. (B) Underlying structures.

is slightly defective. Particular difficulty then arises in trying to recognise segmental narrowings of the retinal arterial blood columns.

Inspection of the optic fundus

It is important to adhere to a fixed routine when examining the fundus of the eye.

1. The optic disc should first be inspected (Fig. 11.7). It lies slightly to the nasal side of the optical axis of the eye and looks paler than surrounding retina. It can be located by following the course of an artery or vein. The acute angle between a main vessel and its branches or tributaries points towards the disc.

2. The arteries and veins should be inspected next. Note whether they are straight or tortuous and examine their width and colour, the light reflex along the centre of the arterioles and the appearance at arteriovenous crossings. The artery usually lies on the vein and blood columns should not be distorted by the crossing. The light reflex is normally the only evidence of the vessel wall. If the ophthalmoscope is quite steady, it is possible in most subjects to see pulsation of the retinal veins as they lie on the optic disc. Absence of this venous pulsation is not necessarily abnormal but is sometimes an early feature of raised intracranial pressure.

3. The appearance of the fundus background should be studied systematically by radiating from the disc to the periphery right round the fundus in a clockwise or anticlockwise manner. The position of any abormality such as alteration of pigment, or haemorrhages, exudates, tubercles or underlying choroidal changes should be noted as if the fundus was a clock with the optic disc as its centre.

4. Finally the macula and its surroundings should be examined. Unless the pupil is dilated, it is probable that a narrow beam will be required for inspection of the macular area (Fig. 11.1). It can be seen at once if the patient looks directly into the light. The macula is situated about two discs' width to the temporal side of the lower pole of the optic disc. It appears as a dull red patch, darker than the remainder of the fundus. In the centre there is often a little glistening white dot which is due to reflection of light from the fovea. Lesions in this area tend to cause serious loss of vision.

Interpretation of ophthalmoscopic appearances

The optic disc and its immediate surroundings

Attention should be paid particularly to the colour of the optic disc, the physiological cup and the disc margin.

A normal optic disc (Fig. 11.7) is a variable shade of pink because of the interlacing capillaries which lie among the translucent nerve fibres. There are fewer capillaries over the temporal half of the disc which in consequence tends to look paler than the nasal half. Capillaries covering the

base of the optic cup are sparse and the cup, therefore, appears whiter than the rest of the optic disc. The surrounding retina is a duskier shade of red than the disc owing to the mass of interlacing choroidal blood vessels underlying the pigment layer.

The physiological cup, recognised by its pallor, varies in depth and diameter in different individuals. It usually occupies about a quarter of the area of the optic disc. Although in some normal people it may extend almost to three quarters of the disc's area, enlargement and deepening of the physiological cup are characteristic of chronic glaucoma (Plate III). In the depths of the cup lies the lamina cribrosa which often can be seen as a very faintly chequered appearance (Fig. 11.7). In about 15% of normal people, especially in hypermetropes, the physiological cup cannot be seen.

The margin of the optic disc is usually well demarcated from the rest of the retina. Sometimes, in normal people, the periphery of the nasal side of the disc lies slightly above the level of the surrounding retina and this leads to obscuring of the disc margin in this area. There is commonly a line of pigment around part of the disc's edge which is of no pathological significance (Fig. 11.7).

In myopia the optic disc appears large and the stretching of the inner coats of the eye frequently cause degenerative changes in the choroid which expose white sclera around part or the whole of the disc (myopic crescent); pigment may be seen in or at the edges of these white areas.

In hypermetropia the disc appears small and may also look a deeper shade of pink than is normal. This makes the disc less easily distinguished from the surrounding retina sometimes leading to a mistaken diagnosis of papilloedema.

In papilloedema (Plate III) the swelling of the optic nerve head is not only associated with hyperaemia of the disc but also with obliteration of the optic cup, congestion of the veins and, if the changes are of recent, acute occurrence there may be haemorrhages radiating out from the disc. Swelling of the optic nerve head may be a manifestation of raised intracranial pressure when it is called papilloedema; it may arise from an intrinsic lesion of the optic nerve when it is known as papillitis. The ophthalmoscopic appearances of these two conditions are indistinguishable. They are differentiated by associated changes in visual acuity and in the visual fields. Papilloedema of recent onset usually produces little or no change in visual acuity, but the visual field of the affected eye may reveal enlargement of the blind spot. With more profound and prolonged papilloedema there is often concentric constriction of the whole visual field. On the other hand papillitis due to intrinsic lesions of the optic nerve, such as a retrobulbar neuritis, is attended by severe diminution in visual acuity; if the visual fields can be delineated, a central gap (scotoma) will be demonstrated.

In optic atrophy the disc is abnormally pale. The pallor is due to gliosis in the optic nerve head together with an associated loss of some small blood vessels. There is confusion in the terminology which is applied to optic atrophy. Primary optic atrophy is generally used to describe a pathologically pale disc with well defined margins. Secondary optic atrophy usually refers to a pathologically pale disc with irregular or blurred margins. Some people, however, subdivide this latter group into 'secondary' and 'consecutive' categories. Consecutive optic atrophy is then the label given to a pale disc of irregular outline associated with disease of the retina or choroid; secondary optic atrophy is applied when these changes are the sequel to a period of raised intracranial pressure. Unfortunately these two terms are used in directly contrary ways by other authorities, one person's 'secondary' is another's 'consecutive ' and vice versa. It is best to describe the disc's appearance and then deduce from the history or other features the likely nature of any antecedent condition. There is usually some loss of visual acuity associated with optic atrophy. This is not necessarily of severe degree. When there is marked loss in visual acuity due to optic atrophy, this is reflected in an impaired direct pupillary response to light on the affected side.

The normal pallor of the temporal half of the disc is sometimes mistaken for partial optic atrophy as are myopic crescents, large optic cups, and myelinated nerve fibres abutting on to the disc. The last is a congenital abnormality of no pathological significance. The fibres are opaque and white, display irregular edges and usually lie contiguous to the disc margin. Rarely, they may be seen in more peripheral parts of the retina.

Blood vessels

In the retinal arteries and veins only the blood is visible. Light is reflected as a thin bright white line down the centre of the blood column, its width being proportional to the thickness of the vessel wall.

Thickening of vessel walls is mainly recognised by narrowing of the blood column. The arterioles may show pallor and diffuse or segmental narrowing, widening of the light reflex and sometimes sheathing due to hypertensive sclerosis (Table 11.1). Sometimes a vessel may be white. This is due to extreme thickening so that the blood column can no longer be seen, or to total occlusion. Atheroma is rare; it shows as a dense yellowish-white opacity obscuring part or the whole of the blood column and sometimes projecting beyond it.

Emboli are sometimes seen in retinal arteries. Glistening spots which seem to lie on the arterial wall are due to cholesterol emboli. A platelet embolus appears as a white spot in an artery, obstructing blood flow; it often breaks up and disappears within a few hours.

Dilatation of the veins appears especially in chronic respiratory failure, papilloedema and diabetes. A ratio of 2:3 between the normal artery and vein is approximately valid but only when branching of the vessels is comparable as in the superior temporal quadrant of Figure 11.7. Changes in the ratio may be due to narrowing of the arteries or dilatation of the veins.

Table 11.1 Retinal changes in hypertension

Grade	Change	Comments
I	Arterial tortuousity and change in calibre; inc. light reflex	Features of arteriosclerosis rather than hypertension; not of prognostic importance
II	Arteriovenous nipping; right angle A.V. crossing	Apparent nipping produced by arterial wall thickening; only observed when artery crosses anterior to vein
III	Haemorrhages, flame shaped. Exudates, hard and soft	A feature of accelerated hypertension
IV	Papilloedema	Associated with cerebral oedema

Arteriovenous crossings. The artery and vein share their media and adventitia at these crossings. Hypertensive sclerosis tends to cause the artery to cross the vein more closely to a right angle than is usual and therefore commonly distorts or obscures the venous blood column which appears to be 'nipped'. Senile arteriosclerosis with thickening of the adventitia may cause similar appearances so that the arteriolar changes already described provide the more direct evidence of hypertension. However, distension of the vein distal to the crossing usually indicates arteriosclerosis; it is apt to be complicated by venous thrombosis.

The background

The red background of the fundus is due largely to blood in the massive meshwork of choroidal vessels whose detail is fogged by the pigment layer on which the rods and cones lie. If the pigment layer is missing, as in the albino, or is thin, as in some fair haired people, then the choroidal vessels will be clearly seen lying on a white background of sclera. In contrast, dense pigment, commonly present in dark skinned or black haired people, is often arranged in streaks between the main choroidal vessels and gives a tigroid appearance to the fundus. The pigment also tends to become finely granular with advancing years, and the retina loses the shiny appearance seen in the child and young adult.

Nerve fibres, interspersed by their cell nuclei, run vertically from the light receptors in the deepest layers of the retina until they reach the internal limiting membrane where they turn horizontally and converge upon the optic disc. The retinal vessels lie in the anterior horizontal layer of nerve fibres and nourish the inner third of the retina while the choroidal vessels supply the outer-two-thirds. Consideration of these facts explains the shapes of haemorrhages according to their depth.

Background abnormalities may be red, white or black.

Red lesions. These are due to haemorrhages, microaneurysms or new vessel formation.

Haemorrhages. Superficial haemorrhages are linear, or fan- or flame-shaped because they track along the horizontally arranged nerve fibre layer.

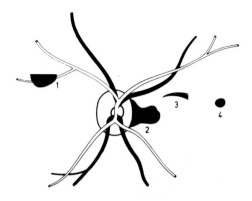

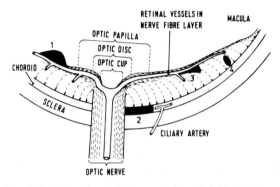

Fig. 11.8 Sites of retinal haemorrhages. (1) Subhyaloid haemorrhage. (2) Choroidal haemorrhage. (3) Haemorrhage in nerve fibre layer.(4) Deep haemorrhage in diabetes mellitus.

This type of haemorrhage predominates in arterial hypertension (Fig. 11.8 and Plate IV). Haemorrhages which lie in the deeper layers of the retina, where the tissues are arranged vertically, do not spread laterally and so appear as small dots or blobs, a particularly common feature of diabetic retinopathy (Fig.11.8 and Plate IV).

A choroidal haemorrhage is less common; it is often large with a wavy, map-like margin, and dark owing to the fact that it lies beneath pigment of variable density (Fig. 11.8). It may be mistaken for a melanotic tumour but, like all other haemorrhages in the fundus, it tends to disappear without trace in a few weeks.

A subhyaloid (preretinal) haemorrhage bulges forward and lies between the retina and the vitreous. A light reflex may be seen somewhere near its centre. Roundish at first, it usually sediments to give a flat topped lesion (Fig. 11.8). The blood may burst into and mix with the vitreous, and obscure the fundus by total darkness. Alternatively it may cause streaky pools in the vitreous which are seen to lie in front of the retinal vessels. Vitreous haemorrhages may become organised by fibrous tissue. A subhyaloid haemorrhage is most often seen in company with subarachnoid haemorrhage, especially one arising from the anterior communicating artery, but may also be observed in almost any other condition in which retinal haemorrhages occur.

Occlusion of a retinal vein is accompanied by masses of linear haemorrhages and sometimes also by patches of oedema in the affected segment (Plate III).

Microaneurysms. These are dark red, small, dense, well circumscribed 'dots' which may rupture to form 'blot' haemorrhages (Plate IV). They are persistent in contrast to haemorrhages of comparable size which disappear within two weeks. Microaneurysms have been shown to arise on the venous side of the retinal capilliary network. They occur characteristically as an early feature of diabetic retinopathy but they may also be found with arterial hypertension and macroglobulinaemia or following occlusion of a retinal vein.

Neovascularisation. New vessel formation may be seen in diabetes mellitus, first as fine tufts of delicate vessels forming arcades on the surface of the retina expecially on or around the disc. These vessels are fragile and readily leak, causing retinal, preretinal or vitreous haemorrhages. Later a connective tissue reaction (retinitis proliferans) is seen first as a white cloudy haze among the network of new vessels. This extends to obliterate the vessels and cover the surrounding retina in a dense white sheet. At this stage bleeding is less common but retinal detachment occurs. In Britain diabetic retinopathy is the single most common cause of blindness in the middle aged.

RETINAL CHANGES IN DIABETES

Background
Micro-aneurysms
Blot and dot haemorrhages
Venous dilatation & variability in calibre
Hard exudates [especially perimacular]
Soft exudates

Proliferative
New vessel formation
Glial proliferation — may lead to retinal detachment

White or whitish lesions. These are due to exposed sclera, exudates, colloid bodies, miliary tuberculosis, fibrous tissue and other causes.

Sclera is exposed in albinos, in congenital and myopic crescents around the disc, and in choroidal lesions such as congenital gaps (colobomata) or post-inflammatory or degenerative changes (Plate III)

Exudates are white lesions. They are usually described as hard or soft. The terms refer to visual appearances which suggest degrees of hardness.

Soft exudates (Plate IV) are fluffy and ill-defined and look rather like small pieces of cotton wool. Although usually associated with areas of retinal ischaemia and infarction, the soft exudates themselves are due to hold-up of axonal transport in retinal nerve fibres, with accumulation of subcellular organelles which reflect light. They often displace or obscure retinal vessels indicating that they lie superficially. Soft exudates occur in arterial hypertension, diabetes mellitus and other microvascular diseases such as systemic lupus erythematosus; they are also seen in severe anaemia. Soft exudates often disappear within a few weeks.

Hard exudates which are small, intensely white, spots lie deeply and consist of lipid deposits. They are a common feature of diabetic retinopathy.

The arrangement of nerve fibres has a bearing on the distribution of exudative lesions. In the peripheral retina a single nerve fibre is distributed to about 80 light receptors. In the macular region each cone has its own nerve fibre; the number is so great that the fibres have to radiate outwards from the macula before turning towards the optic disc. The deeper inter-connecting fibres which run perpendicularly elsewhere, here lie nearly horizontally. This accounts for the star-like pattern of exudative lessions in this area (Plate IV and Fig. 11.8).

Colloid bodies are hyaline deposits in the deepest layer of the retina; they appear with advancing years and are common in elderly subjects.

Miliary tubercles, which usually lie in the

choroid, are rare in Britain but are important because of their diagnostic significance in cryptic miliary tuberculosis.

Fibrous (glial) tissue occurs, especially in diabetic retinopathy in association with neovascularisation, and the prognosis for vision is poor. In contrast a patch of myelinated nerve fibres is a harmless congenital anomaly (p. 332). Thick or occluded blood vessels show as white streaks (p. 332).

Black lesions. The tigroid fundus and the deposits of pigment at the disc edge have been described (p. 333). Occasional black spots of congenital origin occur which are comparable with benign melanomas of the skin. Other pigment disturbances indicate choroidal or deep retinal lesions. Choroidal degeneration in myopia or in healed choroiditis causes irregular clumps of pigment patches on or around a white background of sclera (Plate III). In the hereditary disorder, retinitis pigmentosa, characteristic pigment patches giving the appearance of bird's footmarks occur in the midzone, while visual acuity relentlessly deteriorates. Lastly, the rare but very malignant melanoma is also sometimes determined by a dominant inheritance.

Fluorescein angiography

Some abnormalities may not be clearly diagnosable by unaided ophthalmoscopy; this may be then augmented by angiography. Fluorescein is injected intravenously and the fundus is photographed at frequent intervals while the dye passes through the vessels. Abnormal permeability of vessels is demonstrated by leakage into the tissues, leaving persistent fluorescein. This technique provides a precise way of confirming the presence of papilloedema when the ophthalmoscopic appearance of the optic disc is equivocal, and can be used to identify areas of retinal vascular disease more precisely.

Conclusion

Although there is no real substitute for direct experience, modern colour photography has much to offer and the student is advised to study an atlas of ophthalmoscopy as an introduction to the clinical appreciation of this field. A few examples have been reproduced in Plates III and IV.

FURTHER READING

Kritzinger E E, Beaumont H M 1987 A colour atlas of optic disc abnormalities. Wolfe Medical
Lim A S M, Constable I J 1987 Colour atlas of ophthalmology. Wright, Bristol

Pitts Crick R, Trimble R B 1986 A textbook of clinical ophthalmology. Hodder & Stoughton

12. The examination of urine and blood

N. C. Allan   J. F. Munro

A clinical examination is not complete until observations have been made on the patient's sputum (p. 127), urine and, in appropriate circumstances, on the blood, vomit (p. 156) and faeces (p. 161).

EXAMINATION OF THE URINE

A fresh sample of urine should be tested from every patient and this is conveniently performed immediately before or after the physical examination. Significant renal disease may develop without specific symptoms or physical signs but is almost invariably accompanied by urinary abnormalities. Other conditions, which do not primarily affect the kidney, may be diagnosed by the presence of abnormal constituents in the urine; for example, glycosuria in diabetes mellitus. Simple and convenient tests using commercially prepared strips containing the necessary reagents have become established as reliable methods for examining urine. This development has resulted in urine testing becoming an important way in which early diagnosis of some diseases may be achieved by screening at risk groups.

When tablets or reagent strips are being used, the manufacturer's instructions should be followed exactly. Strips are available for testing for specific gravity, pH, protein, glucose, ketones, bilirubin, urobilinogen, nitrate (bacteriuria) and blood, either separately or in various combinations in a single strip. Combined reagent strips should not be held upright when reading them because urine may run from one square to the next mixing the reagents and producing errors.

In special circumstances, urine can be submitted to a large number of additional biochemical or biological investigations.

Volume of urine

Measuring the volume of urine is important in many clinical circumstances both as a guide to the state of hydration and as a means by which oliguria or polyuria may be recognised. In some circumstances, as for example after severe injury or prostatic operations or during cardiogenic shock, it is necessary to monitor the urinary flow hourly. This is conveniently done by using a calibrated urimeter attached to a bladder catheter.

When the urine is being collected over 24 hours, the patient should empty the bladder at a convenient time immediately before the start of the period, e.g. 8 a.m. All the urine passed in the next 24 hours up to and including the same hour next day is collected in a clean polythene or glass bottle. For some collections a reagent may be required in the container, e.g. HCl for the estimation of catecholamines and their metabolites in the diagnosis of phaeochromocytoma. For others, such as screening for porphyrins, it is necessary to use a dark bottle. It is often more difficult in hospital than in the home to collect the total output of urine over a period of 24 hours; nurses may empty the bedpan, domestics may remove the urinal, and through failure of communication or memory, specimens are lost. Whenever possible the close cooperation of the patient should be enlisted.

Appearance of urine

Normal fresh urine is clear, but its colour varies greatly and dyes in some sweets may make the urine green and it may become pink after eating beetroot. Certain colour changes should be confirmed by appropriate qualitative tests.

These changes include:

Bile	Brownish 'like beer' with yellow froth.
Blood, haemoglobin or methaemoglobin	Red, brown or 'smoky'.
Porphobilinogen	Red on standing if the urine is acid.
Melanogen	Urine darkens on standing.
Homogentisic acid (Alcaptonuria)	Urine darkens on standing.

The colour of urine may also be altered by the presence of certain drugs or their derivatives as follows:

Tetracyclines and riboflavin	Yellow.
Phenindione	Orange.
Phenolpthalein purgatives	Reddish orange, colour disappears on acidification.
Methyldopa	Dark grey.
Iron (intramuscular)	Grey or black.
Rifampicin	Pink.

The urine may be cloudy and a sediment may be present because of the presence of mucus, pus or blood, or because of precipitation of some of its constituents on standing, e.g. phosphates or urates. The nature of such deposits can best be determined by microscopic examination (p. 342). A milky urine may indicate the presence of fat globules as in chyluria.

Smell of urine

Most people are aware of the peculiar odour of concentrated urine. An ammoniacal smell is the result of bacterial decomposition and is commonly present on babies' napkins or in urine which has been standing for many hours. Food and drugs may cause distinctive smells. For instance, asparagus causes a characteristic odour, while turpentine was consumed by Cleopatra to give her urine the scent of violets. A fishy smell is caused by infection with *Esch. coli*.

Specific gravity of the urine

The specific gravity of the urine is usually measured by a clinical hydrometer which is a relatively inaccurate instrument. Errors are less if the urine is allowed to cool to room temperature as hydrometers are calibrated to read at 15°C. The hydrometer should be pushed deeply into the urine and gently rotated, care being taken to see that it floats freely without contact with the wall of the container.

A guide to the specific gravity and osmolality of the urine can also be included in multiple test strips.

For most clinical purposes and in the absence of glycosuria, determination of specific gravity affords an approximation to the osmolal concentration of urine. Its determination in a random sample of urine is of limited value. It is most useful as a measure of the extent to which renal tubules are capable of establishing an osmotic gradient between the blood and the urine in the collecting ducts under conditions of fluid restriction.

Diminution in the power to concentrate the urine may be due to (1) an inability to produce vasopressin in response to fluid deprivation such as occurs in diabetes insipidus; (2) failure of the renal concentrating mechanism to respond to vasopressin; this category includes patients with a wide variety of acute and chronic renal diseases (e.g. pyelonephritis) and extrarenal conditions such as hyperparathyroidism and lithium intoxication; or (3) the existence of an osmotic diuresis.

The maximal capacity of the kidneys to concentrate urine may be determined after depriving the patient of fluid for a standard time. In clinical practice the concentrating ability of the kidney is usually assessed by an eight hour fluid deprivation test. During this procedure, urinary specific gravities greater than 1022 are obtained in healthy volunteers corresponding to a urinary osmolality in excess of 800 m osmol/l. If such a result is not achieved during the test, the subsequent administration of desmopressin 2 μg intramuscularly, a vasopressin analogue, will help to distinguish between cranial and nephrogenic diabetes insipidus. Restriction of fluid can be dangerous in severe cases of diabetes insipidus and the test should be discontinued if more than 5% of bodyweight is lost during the period of fluid restriction.

Urinary pH

In health and on a normal diet, 40–80 mmol of acid is excreted daily in the urine. The greater part of this acid is excreted buffered partly in the form of dihydrogen phosphate, and partly as ammonium ions. A very small amount of free hydrogen ion is also excreted and it is this which is measured when the pH is determined. Little information is gained from the routine determination of urinary pH in random samples. The urine is normally more acid than pH 6.0. Occasionally the finding of a urine with a pH of 7.0 or above is due to the consumption of alkali or a vegetarian diet, or to infection in the urinary tract by organisms other than *Esch. coli*.

The ability of the renal tubules to excrete hydrogen ions is depressed in certain circumstances such as distal renal tubular acidosis occurring either as an inherited or acquired defect. These patients can be recognised by their inability to acidify the urine below pH 5 following the oral administration of ammonium chloride.

Proteinuria

Urine testing for protein should be part of every clinical examination. As the urine should be sufficiently concentrated, an early morning sample is best for analysis. During a febrile illness and in cardiac failure, proteinuria may be a transient finding. Occasionally in young adults, proteinuria is present only when upright (postural proteinuria). This condition may occur in the absence of glomerular disease and can be diagnosed by comparing samples obtained fully recumbent and while up and about. Laboratory testing for micro-albuminurea is a useful method of screening for diabetic nephropathy at an early stage.

Once proteinuria has been confirmed, a quantitative measurement should be performed. A result greater than 150 mgm per day is abnormal; one in excess of 2 gms daily indicates glomerular disease. Urine microscopy should be undertaken on all patients with significant proteinuria.

Test strips. A reagent strip such as Albustix or the Albym test is the most convenient method for detecting proteinuria. The strips, which are impregnated with buffered tetrabromophenol blue, are dipped momentarily into the urine. The test end of the strip should not be touched nor should the strip be left in the urine or passed through a urine stream. Protein, if present, is absorbed on to the strip and produces a greenish-blue colour, which should be compared immediately with the appropriate colour chart. It is best to read the strip in daylight.

False positive results may occur in patients receiving large doses of phenothiazine drugs, if the urine has become very alkaline or if it has been contaminated with detergents or antiseptics. False negative results may be obtained from urine which has been acidified for purposes of preservation.

Bence Jones proteins. These are rarely found in urine but are important because their presence is practically diagnostic of multiple myeloma, though they are detected in less than 25% of such cases. The Albustix test will detect Bence Jones proteins only at concentrations above 150 mg/dl. A sensitive test is to mix five parts of urine with one part of 50% acetic acid and three parts of saturated sodium chloride solution. Bence Jones proteins are precipitated at once at room temperature, dissolve on boiling and reappear on cooling. Other urinary proteins are precipitated by these reagents but do not disappear on boiling.

Glycosuria

Qualitative test for glycosuria (*Clinistix, Diastix, Glukotest* and others). The presence of glucose in the urine is best detected using a reagent strip impregnated with glucose oxidase, a peroxidase and a KI chromogen. When dipped into urine containing glucose and withdrawn, the glucose is oxidised by atmospheric oxygen in the presence of glucose oxidase to form gluconic acid and hydrogen peroxide. The latter reacts with the chromogen in the presence of the peroxidase to produce colours which range from green to brown. The colour change is observed in exactly 10 seconds. For all practical purposes the reaction in the test strip is specific for glucose, and is sensitive to quantities greater than 100 mg/dl. The reaction is affected by such factors as temperature, pH and the amount of ascorbic acid present and, for this reason, the test is not quantitative. False positive reactions can occur if the urine container has been contaminated with hydrogen peroxide, hypochlorite (e.g. household bleach) or detergents containing sodium perchlorate.

This enzyme test might lead to failure to recognise the rare condition of congenital galactosaemia, for which early diagnosis is essential. For this reason the less specific quantitative test for glucose described below is recommended for infants as screening procedure. In older children and in adults the simple specific enzyme test is adequate since failure to detect rare abnormalities such as pentosuria or fructosuria is not likely to have serious consequences.

Quantitative test for glycosuria (Clinitest). Semi-quantitative tests for glycosuria in urine utilize the reducing properties of glucose in its reaction with an alkaline solution of a copper salt. The test is not specific and positive results may be obtained from other reducing substances including fructose, lactose, galactose, glucuronides and phenolic drugs such as salicylates. In very concentrated specimens reduction may also occur with creatinine or uric acid. Ascorbic acid in high concentrations may give a positive reaction and the urine of patients with alcaptonuria has reducing properties. The test is available as self-heating tablets which are very hygroscopic and must be kept in a tightly sealed container. Any tablets which become discoloured should be discarded.

The test is carried out as follows: with the special dropper provided, 5 drops of urine are placed in a clean dry test-tube. The dropper is rinsed and 10 drops of water are added. One Clinitest tablet is then dropped into the test-tube. The reaction should be observed as the mixture effervesces. The tube should not be shaken during this period and the effervescence should be allowed to settle. Fifteen seconds after the effervescence has subsided the tube should be shaken gently and the colour produced compared with the chart provided, which ranges from blue (no glucose) to orange (2 g/dl glucose). If, while the reaction is taking place, an orange colour appears, even for a moment, and then changes to greenish brown, more than 2 g/dl of sugar are present. Failure to watch the reaction and to note the 'orange flash' may give a misleading result.

The different sensitivities of Clinistix and Clinitest occasionally result in a urine being found to be positive for Clinistix and negative for Clinitest. This result means that glucose is present in the urine in concentrations of between 100 mg/dl and 250 mg/dl.

The determination of blood glucose

Test strips such as Glucostix 1-44, Visidex II or B.M. test which, like Clinistix or Diastix, contain glucose oxidase, are specific for the presence of glucose in the blood. Read visually they provide an approximate assessment of the concentration of blood glucose. The method is increasingly being used by patients to monitor their insulin requirements. It is also particularly helpful in an emergency or at night in detecting values outside the lower and upper ranges of normal, or in suggesting that the blood glucose may be sufficiently low to account for the occurrence of coma. Confirmation of an abnormal result observed with a test strip should be obtained as soon as possible by more accurate biochemical methods.

Capillary or venous blood may be used, but blood samples to which sodium fluoride has been added must be avoided as the enzyme in the test strip may be inactivated. Using Glucostix a large drop of blood is spread over the printed side of the test area of the reagent strip; smears of blood must not be used. After exactly one minute the strip is held vertically and the blood is washed off with a fine jet of cold water conveniently kept in a plastic wash bottle and applied for no longer than two seconds. The colour of the strip is compared immediately with the chart provided. If too short a time is allowed for the reaction, the result will tend to be low; if the timing is greater than one minute the result will be too high. Over and under washing lead to similar errors.

The test strips should be kept in their original container and protected from exposure to heat, light and moisture. They should be stored in a cool place (not in a refrigerator). The bottle should be recapped immediately and tightly after use. Any strips with a brown discoloration should not be used.

Ketonuria

The detection and semi-quantitative assessment of

ketonuria may be of importance in patients with diabetes mellitus and in those suffering from starvation or persistent vomiting. In these conditions acetoacetic acid, acetone and β-hydroxybutyric acid appear in the urine as a result of their increased production. There is no satisfactory method for the urinary detection of β-hydroxybutyric acid and in ketosis acetoacetic acid is present in concentrations about ten times more than that of acetone. For practical purposes only acetoacetic acid is detected by the tests described. Acetoacetic acid is liable to decomposition to acetone especially in the presence of bacteria. Refrigeration is the best way of preserving the specimens if analysis is delayed.

Rothera's nitroprusside test. This has been modified and incorporated into reagent strips (*Ketostix* and *Keturtest*) and a standardised tablet test (*Acetest*). The strips are easier to use but Acetest easier to interpret. Both are reliable for qualitative purposes but are unsatisfactory when used semi-quantitatively because some observers find difficulty in differentiating the colours induced by ketosis of varying severity. Atypical colours are also produced if the patient is taking levodopa.

Bilirubin in the urine

Conjugated bilirubin is water soluble, and appears in the urine whenever there is interference with the excretion of bilirubin glucuronide in the bile, i.e. in extrahepatic biliary obstruction and some cases of hepatocellular disease. In these circumstances bilirubin can be detected in the urine before jaundice can be recognised clinically. Large quantities of bile pigment in the urine make it brownish in colour and a stable yellow froth is easily produced on shaking.

A test for bilirubin is incorporated in some reagent strips (Multistix and Bili-Labstix). *Ictotest* tablets provide a more specific and a more sensitive test which can detect very small amounts of bilirubin in the urine and which can be used if there is any difficulty in interpreting the reagent strip test.

Urobilinogen and porphobilinogen in the urine

These two compounds appear in the urine in en-

tirely different disorders; they are described together because they both give a colour reaction with Ehrlich's aldehyde reagent.

Urobilinogen is present in excess in haemolytic disease and in the early and recovery stages of hepatocellular disease. It is detectable in abnormal amounts in heart failure and often in infectious mononucleosis. Urinary urobilinogen is absent in complete obstruction of the biliary ducts when, of course, bilirubin is detectable in the urine.

Porphobilinogen can be detected in acute intermittent porphyria, in variegate porphyria, and in certain drug induced porphyrinurias.

Ehrlich's aldehyde test. Two ml of the reagent (2% dimethylaminobenzaldehyde in HCl 7 mol/l) is added to 5 ml of fresh urine. Urobilinogen and porphobilinogen both give a pink colour within five minutes. To distinguish between these substances add 1 ml saturated sodium acetate solution and 2 ml chloroform. Stopper the tube and shake for one minute. Allow the chloroform and aqueous layers to settle. If the pink colour is due to urobilinogen it will be extracted into the chloroform (lower) layer, but if it is due to porphobilinogen it remains in the aqueous (upper) layer. Several substances interfere with the detection of urobilinogen and porphobilinogen. Positives occur with patients receiving sulphonamides and in the presence of acetone or during treatment with para-aminosalicylic acid.

Urobilistix and *Multistix* also detect urobilinogen but not porphobilinogen with reliability. The strip is dipped into fresh urine for 5 seconds and read in exactly 45 seconds. Results are expressed in Ehrlich units, one unit being equivalent to 1 mg urobilinogen/dl and the scale rises to 12 units. Commonly a trace (1 mg/dl) is present.

Phenylketonuria

Phenylketonuria is a rare genetically determined defect in the metabolism of phenylalanine which, if untreated, may lead to mental deficiency. Its early detection in infants is extremely important if the severity of the mental defect is to be minimised. In classical phenylketonuria, phenylpyruvic acid is elevated in the blood; its derivatives are excreted in urine and can be detected by using

Phenistix. Unfortunately screening of infants using Phenistix is unreliable and microbiological assay on blood obtained by heel prick is usually employed, i.e. the *Guthrie test*. Phenistix gives a reddish brown colour if salicylates are present in the urine. This reaction may be used as an aid to diagnosis in cases of coma or to ascertain whether patients advised to take para-aminosalicylic acid are really doing so.

Blood and haemoglobin in the urine

Red blood cells may be detected in urine by microscopic examination. Chemical methods of detection are sensitive and are positive in the presence of haemoglobin which may have been released from cells when the urine is hypotonic or has been standing for some time or in haemoglobinuria. Chemical determination depends upon the peroxidase-like action of haemoglobin. In the presence of a peroxide, haemoglobin and its derivatives bring about the oxidation of a variety of substances including otolidine. The method is conveniently carried out using *Haemostix* reagent strips, the test end of which is dipped into urine and removed immediately. The colour of the strip is then compared with the appropriate chart after 30 seconds. A positive test goes blue within this period of time.

In health, urine will give a negative result with this method which is capable of detecting as little as 50–100 red blood cells per mm^3 or 15 μg haemoglobin/dl urine. Significant degrees of haematuria below this level are extremely rare. Falsely positive results may be obtained if the urine contains iodide in high concentrations as may occur if, for example, the patient is being given potassium iodide.

Miscroscopic examination of the urine

Microscopic examination of the centrifuged deposit of a fresh specimen is the only reliable method of detecting the presence of red blood cells, pus and casts. These structures rapidly disintegrate if the urine is allowed to stand and the microscopic appearances become further confused by the formation of various crystals as the pH alters and as the urine cools. Patients with significant bacteriuria almost always show bacilli or other organisms.

Microscopy is indicated when certain conditions are under consideration, such as urinary tract infections, infective endocarditis, glomerulonephritis or proteinuria. In appropriate geographical areas, microscopic examination of the last few drops of urine passed is the standard method for the discovery of the ova of *Schistosoma haematobium* in bilharziasis (Fig. 12.1) *Trichomonas vaginalis*, may also be recognised in both males and females.

About 15 ml of urine should be centrifuged in a clean tube for two minutes at 3000 r/min. The supernatant urine is then discarded by decanting, leaving about 0.5 ml in the centrifuge tube. Any sediment is then mixed by gentle shaking and a drop of this is placed on a clean microscope slide and a cover slip added. The specimen is examined at first with reduced illumination under low-power magnification. It is common in health to detect in each low power field one or two red cells and an occasional hyaline cast, epithelial cell and white blood cells. In many pathological states these cellular constituents are present in larger numbers and their nature should be confirmed by examination under higher magnification.

Cells. Cells seen in the urinary deposit are illustrated in Figure 12.1 *Red blood cells* are recognised as round, refractile, non-nucleated discs. Shrunken crenated cells occur in concentrated urine. Enlarged cell 'ghosts' may be seen in hypotonic urine. *Epithelial cells* are two to four times larger than red cells and are nucleated. *Pus cells* are easily distinguished by their roundness, the refractile granularity of their cytoplasm and by the presence of lobed nuclei. Pus cells very often appear in clumps or groups and are slightly larger than red cells. These features may be rendered more prominent if a 10% solution of acetic acid is run under the cover slip.

Urinary casts. These are best seen in subdued light with the microscope condenser at its lowest adjustment and are illustrated in Figure 12.1. Casts are cylindrical bodies of coagulated protein, so called because their shape represents a cast of the renal tubular lumen. Their presence in the urine therefore indicates that the proteinuria has its origin in the kidney. Hyaline casts are transparent, homogeneous structures. Although an

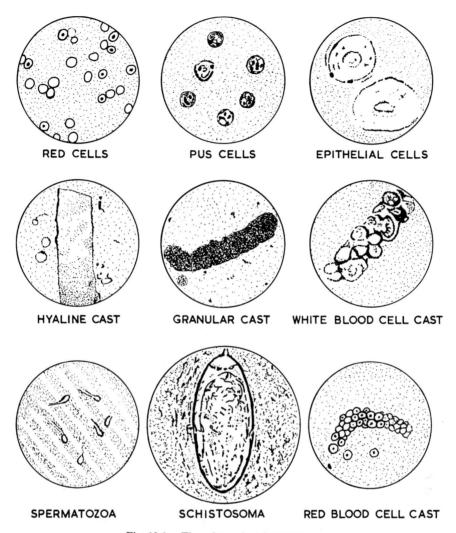

RED CELLS   PUS CELLS   EPITHELIAL CELLS

HYALINE CAST   GRANULAR CAST   WHITE BLOOD CELL CAST

SPERMATOZOA   SCHISTOSOMA   RED BLOOD CELL CAST

Fig. 12.1   The urinary deposit ($\times 375$)

occasional hyaline cast may be found in healthy persons, their numbers rise significantly as proteinuria increases. Tubular cells in varying stages of degeneration subsequently adhere to their surface to form epithelial and granular casts. These indicate the presence of tubular damage and desquamation such as occurs in pyelonephritis. Red blood cells casts are composed of masses of conglutinated red cells which give them an orange or brown colour. Leucocyte casts are formed in a similar way. Red blood cells casts always reflect glomerular disease, as in acute proliferative glomerulonephritis.

Crystals. A variety of crystals may be visible on microscopic examination of the urine but individual identification is seldom of value. An exception to this is the rare condition of cystinuria, in which hexagonal crystals of cystine are found. While the diagnosis may be suspected on the basis of the microscopic appearance of the crystals, it should always be confirmed by chemical analysis. Patients with a history of renal colic should be asked to sieve the urine. Any calculus that is passed should be analysed chemically.

Bacteriological examination of the urine

For the detection of tubercle bacilli, three or more

early-morning or 24-hour specimens should be sent to the laboratory. For all other bacterial infections a fresh, clean-voided, midstream specimen of urine is required, and detailed attention must be paid to the technique of collection. The patient is provided with a sterile container. The specimen is collected by switching the container into the stream of urine. For the ambulant male patient, collection is usually made at a urinal. Woman should squat over a lavatory seat, separating the labia by the index and middle finger of one hand. While urine is being passed, the wide mouthed container is switched into the stream with the other hand. For ill patients of either sex, some assistance and common-sense modifications of these techniques may be required. The collection of urine from infants and children is described on page 319.

The specimens of urine should be conveyed to the laboratory at once. Some bacterial contamination is almost unavoidable, and as each organism may divide every 15 to 20 minutes, a false result may be obtained if the urine is not fresh. Furthermore, a large population of contaminant may sometimes suppress the growth of pathogens. If immediate delivery is not possible, the specimen should be quickly cooled, preserved in an insulated container at 0 to 4°C and sent to the laboratory within 15 hours.

Dip inoculation culture (e.g. Oxoid dip slide). A slide with nutrient agar on one side and MacConkey's agar on the other is dipped momentarily into a fresh specimen voided into a sterile container. Organisms are caught on the agar surfaces in numbers proportional to their concentration in the urine and the slide is returned to a securely closed sterile vial. After 16–24 hours incubation at 37°C, direct reading of the bacterial growth can be made by comparing the appearance of the slide with colony density models. Considerable experience is required if accurate results are to be obtained. No information of antibiotic sensitivity is forthcoming. In spite of these shortcomings the technique is of value if delay in sending specimens to a laboratory is unavoidable. The results can subsequently be validated by subculture of the slides. Thus the technique is of particular value in community screening tests for urinary tract infection.

Nitrite test. This is based on the ability of about 90% of urinary pathogens to reduce the nitrate, normally present in urine, to nitrite. Best results are obtained by testing urine which has been incubating in the bladder for some hours and a fresh early morning sample is preferred. The nitrite in the urine reacts with arsalanic acid in the strip to form a diazonium compound which in turn forms a pink colour with naphthyl ethylene diamine. The pink colour is not quantitatively related to the number of organisms and any degree of colouration indicates the presence of at least 10^5 organisms per ml. The nitrite test is available in the *N-Multistix* and *N-Labstix* strips.

Microstix and *miniaturised culture test* have three separate reagent areas, (1) a chemical test for nitrite, (2) a culture area for a total bacterial count and (3) a culture area to support Gram-negative growth only. The strip is immersed in fresh urine for 5 sec and the nitrite reaction is read in 30 sec. Thereafter it is inserted into the sterile pouch provided, which is squeezed to exclude air and sealed by pressure at the ends. The strip can be applied to a conventional culture plate at a convenient later time, and the organisms and their antibacterial sensitivity determined. Alternatively, it can be incubated at 35–37°C for 18–24 hours; the great majority of urinary organisms reduce the triphenyltetrozolium, with which the media is mixed, and matching of the culture areas with colours provide a semiquantitative estimate of the number of organisms present.

EXAMINATION OF THE BLOOD

Blood is the most easily biopsied tissue in the body. Its components, both cellular and fluid, can be accurately measured and provide invaluable information in a wide range of clinical conditions.

Blood samples

Venepuncture. This is the best method of obtaining blood for blood counts. Modern counting equipment generally requires volumes of blood that can be collected only in this way. Under certain circumstances, smaller volumes can be used and may be collected by skin puncture techniques.

If a tourniquet is required it should be applied for as short a time as possible to keep haemoconcentration distal to the site of the tourniquet to a minimum. A clean venepuncture is essential, otherwise tissue fluid may contaminate the needle and cause platelet aggregation which will interfere with platelet counting. For blood counts the blood should be transferred immediately to a tube containing potassium EDTA anticoagulant and gently but thoroughly mixed by repeated inversion.

Skin puncture. If blood cannot be obtained by venepuncture, puncture of the skin may be used. Suitable sites are the pulp of the finger, the ear lobe or, in infants the heel. A disposable sterile stilette should be used. Always discard the first drop of blood obtained by skin puncture.

Storage. Changes in leucocyte morphology occur quickly in vitro but are slowed if the blood is kept in a refrigerator until examined. It is best to make blood films within one hour but reasonable results can be obtained for up to eight hours. Haemoglobin estimation, reticulocyte and platelet counting can be undertaken satisfactorily for up to 24 hours after anticoagulation. The erythrocyte sedimentation rate should be measured within 8 hours.

Haemoglobin

Many methods have been devised for the determination of haemoglobin. The majority are based on measurement of the extinction of light at wave length 540 or 525 nm by a lysate of red cells. Most laboratories now use automated electronic equipment but cruder estimations can be obtained from the use of the Gray Wedge photometer or the Sahli haemoglobinometer.

In healthy adults the haemoglobin ranges between 135 and 180 g/l in males and 115 and 160 g/l in females. At birth the haemoglobin level is very high, ranging between 160 and 250 g/l but this rapidly falls in the first three months of life to between 90 and 120 g/l. During childhood the haemoglobin gradually rises until adult levels are achieved following puberty.

Measurements of the red blood cells

A number of measurements of the red blood cells can now be made very accurately with electronic counting equipment. These include the mean cell volume, the mean corpuscular haemoglobin con-

centration, the mean cell haemoglobin and red cell diameter. Of these the mean cell volume is probably the most useful. The normal range is from 76 to 98 fl. Below 76 the cells are microcytic and above 98 macrocytic.

Haematocrit (Packed cell volume, PCV). The haematocrit expresses the percentage volume of red cells in whole blood and is useful as a screening test for anaemia where it can be used as an alternative to the haemoglobin estimation. It can be measured either by centrifugation of the blood to achieve tight packing of the red cells or alternatively be calculated indirectly from other estimations as is done in electronic techniques.

Blood films

The blood film provides a great deal of invaluable information about the cellular components of the blood. Blood smears are also useful for the recognition of certain human parasites such as in malaria and trypanosomiasis.

A chemically clean slide, free from dust, is polished with a grease-free cloth. A small drop of the patient's blood is placed towards one end of the slide. The unbroken, smooth end of another slide or a specially manufactured slide spreader is used to spread the film and is placed at an angle of 45° to the slide bearing the patient's blood (Fig. 12.2). Films are generally stained with Romanowsky stains and provide preparations which last for several years.

Understanding the blood film report

The red blood cells. In health the red cell is a circular biconcave disc showing pallor of staining

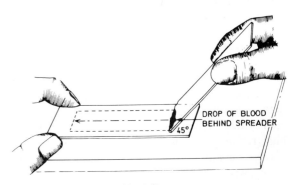

DROP OF BLOOD
BEHIND SPREADER

45°

Fig. 12.2 Spreading a blood film.

at the centre. It is described as being *normochromic* and *normocytic*. The former means that the degree of colouring of the cell is within the normal range and by inference, therefore, the haemoglobinisation of the cell is normal; the latter term indicates that the shape of the cell is also within normal limits. Some variation in size is acceptable, as is the finding of a small proportion of oval cells and occasionally slightly misshapen cells. In the first few weeks of life the number of irregularly shaped cells is greater. Cells which have a bluish tinge (basophilia) and which are slightly larger than average are usually young red cells (reticulocytes). The presence of many basophilic cells in a blood film produces a multi-coloured effect known as polychromasia and usually indicates a raised reticulocyte count. A reticulocyte count requires a special preparation in which the red cells are supravitally stained. In health the result is usually less than 1% ($10-100 \times 10^9/1$).

Pathological changes in the red cells. Failure of haemoglobin synthesis (usually iron deficiency) leads first to a reduction in the size of cells (*microcytosis*) and when more severe, to thinner red cells which have a reduced concentration of haemoglobin and appear to have an unusual degree of pallor in the centre (*hypochromia*). There may be variation in size (*anisocytosis*) and increased numbers of elliptical cells are almost always seen. The presence of target cells and punctate basophilia should suggest β thalassaemia minor.

Deficiency of vitamin B12 and/or folate leads to increase in the average red cell size (*macrocytosis*) and to both anisocytosis and considerable variation in shape (*poikilocytosis*). The oval macrocyte is a most useful cell in drawing attention to the possibility of megaloblastic change as it appears before other forms of poikilocytosis. Because the red cells are larger, they may give the impression of being more deeply stained but the cells contain a normal concentration of haemoglobin, unless there is co-existing deficiency of iron, leading to a 'dimorphic' picture.

Macrocytosis may be evident in disorders other than megaloblastic blood formation. It may be seen where there is brisk marrow activity with a high reticulocyte count, in hypothyroidism, liver disease, invasive disease in the marrow, in association with cytotoxic chemotherapy, excessive alcohol intake and occasionally for no apparent reason.

The *microspherocyte* is found classically in hereditary spherocytosis but also with some acquired haemolytic anaemias, particularly those due to auto- and iso-immune processes, in malaria, in association with extensive burns and indeed any process which traumatises the red cell and results in membrane loss.

Fragmentation of the red cells *schistocytes* together with spherocytes is seen when the red cells are traumatised in the circulation as in the presence of prosthetic heart valves, disseminated intravascular coagulation and the administration of drugs such as sulphasalazine and dapsone. Target cells (cells with a central dot of staining) suggest liver disease, the presence of an abnormal haemoglobin or thalassaemia when associated with a microcytic hypochromic picture, if iron deficiency has been excluded. The combined presence of target cells and red cells containing nuclear fragments known as *Howell Jolly bodies* and iron containing inclusions (*Pappenheimer bodies*) suggest previous splenectomy or reduced splenic function. Punctate basophilia is seen in lead poisoning, β thalassaemia and other toxic states.

Large numbers of elliptical or oval red cells usually indicate hereditary *elliptocytosis*. This disorder is benign in over 90% of patients and in the other 10% only mild reductions in red cell survival occur which are seldom clinically important.

Rouleaux are reported when the *red* cells pile up together in long strings as opposed to clumps. Their presence usually indicates abnormalities in the plasma protein and is associated with a raised ESR. Red cell agglutination reflects either anti-red cell antibodies or red cell damage from severe infection such as B Welch's septicaemia.

The white blood cells. White blood cells or leucocytes are present in blood as they migrate from bone marrow to the tissues. Their absolute and relative numbers vary considerably, generally within fairly clearly defined limits. They divide into two groups; the granulocyte:monocyte group and the lymphocytes. The first group are 'end' cells which never return to the circulation and have short lives. The monocytes are the precursors of the tissue macrophages. The life span of lymphocytes varies, some being short whilst on the other hand others are very long lived.

The differential white cell count provides a means of establishing the relative proportions of the white cells in the blood and is particularly useful in assessing the causes of leucocytosis and leucopenia but may also define abnormalities when the leucocyte count is within normal limits ($4-11 \times 10^9/1$).

In neonates and infants the number of lymphocytes is considerably greater than in the adult and they form the majority of the total white cell count. Furthermore a lymphocytosis may result from infections which would produce a neutrophil leucocytosis in the adult. The absolute numbers of neutrophils in the young child is very similar to that in the adult.

At all ages a neutrophilia may reflect a pyogenic infection but may also occur in the early stages of viral infections although these very often eventually produce a neutropenia. Eosinophils are increased in many hypersensitivity reactions and helminth infections. Eosinophilia may also be found in polyarteritis and in some cases of Hodgkin's lymphoma.

If serious errors are to be avoided in interpreting the meaning of differential white cell counts it is essential to relate the percentage to the absolute leucocyte count.

The normal differential count (adults)

Neutrophil granulocytes 40–75% ($2.0-7.5 \times 10^9/1$)
Esosinophil granulocytes 1–6% ($0.04-0.4 \times 10^9/1$)
Basophil granulocytes less than 1% ($0.01-0.1 \times 10^9/1$)
Lymphocytes 20–45% ($1.5-4.0 \times 10^9/1$)
Monocytes 2–10% ($0.2-0.8 \times 10^9/1$)

The numbers in brackets are the absolute figures for white cell counts within the normal range of $4.0-11.0 \times 10^9/1$.

Abnormal nucleated cells

Nucleated red cell precursors, usually normoblasts, may be seen circulating in the marrow. This may simply reflect very brisk marrow activity after haemorrhage or when there is severe haemolytic disease. Alternatively it may reflect the infiltration

of the marrow by leukaemia, fibrosis or secondary carcinoma. These conditions are often also associated with the appearances of precursor white cells in the blood and the film is said to show a leucoerythroblastic blood picture. When red cell production in the marrow is megaloblastic the circulating red cell precursors will be megaloblasts.

Primitive white cells of all types and stages of maturation are seen in leukaemias. In chronic leukaemia the total white count tends to be higher than in acute leukaemia and frequently exceeds 100 $\times 10^9/1$ in untreated cases. Generally the count is higher in chronic granulocytic leukaemia than in chronic lymphocytic leukaemia. Both these leukaemias are recognised by the presence of fairly large numbers of 'mature' cells of the appropriate series, although there may also be varying numbers of more primitive cells, particularly in the granulocytic variety.

Acute leukaemias are divided into acute lymphoblastic and acute non-lymphoblastic (myeloblastic or myelomonocytic). They are characterised by the predominance of primitive cells known as blast cells, which are morphologically very similar to the most primitive recognisable marrow elements. Their presence in large numbers reflects the fact that these primitive cells do not mature. At an early stage the cells are found only in the bone marrow and there may be very few or no abnormal cells in the peripheral blood. The total leucocyte count may be reduced. This is known as subleukaemic or aleukaemic leukaemia. Later blast cells spill into the blood and the leucocyte count rises.

The platelet count is often helpful in differentiating between acute and chronic leukaemias, usually being profoundly depressed in the former and either raised, normal, or only slightly depressed in the latter.

Plasma cells are seldom found in the blood of adults, but are not uncommon in children, particularly during febrile illnesses such as measles. They are usually found in association with 'Turk' cells or proplasmacytes and reflect an immunological reaction. Myeloma cells may be found circulating and constitute plasma cell leukaemia.

Large atypical mononuclear cells are frequently found in infectious mononucleosis and some other viral infections such as cytomegalovirus

(CMV). They are thought to be transforming T lymphocytes.

Platelets. A crude assessment of the platelet count can be made from a blood film and also morphological variations can be detected. Clumping of the platelets will indicate that the platelet count is almost certainly erroneous.

Tropical diseases. The parasites of malaria, filariasis, trypanosomiasis, kala azar and other forms of leishmaniasis may be seen in the blood as may be the spirochaete of relapsing fever.

Erythrocyte sedimentation rate (ESR)

The ESR is a very simple test in which anticoagulated blood is allowed to stand in a 200 mm graduated glass or disposable plastic Westergren tube of 2 mm internal diameter, held or suspended vertically. The extent to which the red cells fall in the first hour is read from the graduations on the tube. In health the ESR is usually less than 15 mm is the first hour and on average is lower in males. Above the age of 60, the normal values rise until over 80 years when levels of up to 50 mm may not necessarily indicate an abnormality.

Inflammatory disease is by far the commonest cause of a raised ESR. However, the measurement of C-reactive protein is a more sensitive index of acute inflammation. Reduction in haemoglobin level causes a raised ESR but this tends to be minimal in iron deficiency anaemia. Correction for anaemia is unrewarding because different types of anaemia affect the result to a varying extent.

A very high ESR may be found in multiple myeloma, but less than 10% of patients over the age of 40 with an ESR above 100 mm in the first hour have this disorder. A normal ESR may be reassuring but should not encourage complacency. Patients in cardiac failure and those with polycythaemia tend to have low readings.

Examination of the bone marrow

Bone marrow aspiration. Inspection of the bone marrow may be a vital investigation of haematological disorders and other conditions which may affect this tissue.

The preferred sites in the adult are the posterior and anterior iliac crest. Occasionally the sternum

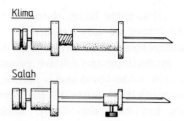

Fig. 12.3   Needles for aspiration of bone marrow

and, more rarely, the vertebral spine is used. In infants the upper end of the tibia is used.

Two types of needle are available; the Salah and the Klima (Fig. 12.3). Both have a guard. The distance from the guard to the tip of the needle can be varied, or the guard can be removed. The guard is essential if the sternum is the site. It may be necessary to dispense with the guard for iliac crest marrows unless a much longer needle is available. Marrow slide preparations are stained in the same way as peripheral blood films and a very detailed analysis of the cytology can be obtained. A crude estimate of the marrow iron stores can also be made.

Trephine biopsy of bone marrow. This provides invaluable material for histological sectioning, and is particularly useful for assessing marrow cellularity, fibrosis and in demonstrating invasion by foreign tissue such as tumour. Individual cell morphology is much less satisfactory than with aspirate. A different bone marrow needle is used for this minor operation; the Jamshidi being probably the most widely used.

Sickle cell haemoglobin

Haemoglobin S, the cause of sickling of red cells, is the most common abnormal haemoglobin. The vast majority of cases are found in African blacks, and the incidence of the abnormality is high in West, Central and East Africa, and the distribution corresponds to the areas in which falciparum malaria is rife. It is common elsewhere among people of African black extraction but is also seen among peoples from the Middle East and India. Haemoglobin S is found in the carrier state (heterozygote) where it provides approximately 30% of the total adult haemoglobin in each red cell. Sickle cell trait is a benign disorder usually associated with normal health, a normal haemoglobin level and no distinctive blood film abnormality. The patient, who inherits the abnormality from both parents (homozygote), suffers from sickle cell anaemia, and all the red cells contain approximately 98% haemoglobin S. In other patients, the inheritance of haemoglobin S is associated with that of haemoglobin C to give rise to haemoglobin SC disease, a less severe form of sickle cell disease. The problems associated with haemoglobin S have now become important in those countries where there is a large immigrant community of African extraction.

Sickling tests. A positive sickling test indicates only that haemoglobin S is present. It is positive in sickle cell anaemia, sickle cell trait, haemoglobin SC disease and sickle cell/thalassaemia. Sickle cell anaemia can, in the majority of cases, be recognised from a stained blood film where the sickle cell forms, resembling the blade of a sickle, are seen and are virtually diagnostic. The additional presence of target cells, polychromasia, and nucleated red cells indicates a fairly severe and sustained haemolytic process. Haemoglobin SC disease may be suspected by the holly-leaf pattern of sickling, but requires haemoglobin electrophoresis for confirmation.

Patients of African black extraction should be screened for haemoglobin S before general anaesthesia and before undertaking dry field surgery in which a limb is exanguinated and the circulation stopped during an operation. Failure to do so could result in an infarcted limb.

Tests in haemorrhagic disease

The great majority of bleeding disorders require specialised laboratory investigation. When a bleeding problem arises a coagulation screen should be undertaken. Normally this would include a platelet count, a prothrombin time and an activated partial thromboplastin time (APTT). In some cases, particularly where fibrinolysis is suspected as in DIC, fibrinogen level and fibrin degradation product should also be measured. The prothrombin time monitors the final common pathway of blood coagulation and the extrinsic coagulation mechanism. The APTT will detect abnormalities in the intrinsic system in which Factor VIII and Factor IX play a key role and will also detect the presence of inhibitors. A thrombin time which in some places is also part of the basic screen will reflect low levels of fibrinogen and heparin-like activity in the plasma. Fibrin degradation products will give a clue to the degree of fibrinolytic activity in the blood. Where abnormalities are detected the problem can be investigated further in greater detail and specific abnormalities identified. Where the patient shows signs of purpuric bleeding, a bleeding time is an essential part of the haemostatic screen.

Where the patient's problem is thrombotic rather than haemorrhagic antithrombin III and protein C estimations should be undertaken and the patient's ability to mount a normal fibrinolytic response should be evaluated with venous occlusion techniques.

Screening the haemostatic mechanism does not always detect a localised abnormality. Severe bleeding can occur because of local fibrinolysis such as in the prostatic bed, in the lung and the brain. In such situations there are no specific laboratory tests that will delineate the problem accurately. Clinical judgement and experience may allow the judicious use of anti-fibrinolytic agents.

Special problems of massive haemorrhage may sometimes arise when the fibrinogen level has been severely lowered by intravascular coagulation and fibrinolysis. In the vast majority of cases, intravascular coagulation initiates overactivation of the fibrinolytic system with the production of the fibrinolytic enzyme, plasmin, to remove the deposited fibrin. Plasmin does not distinguish between fibrin and fibrinogen and the latter is also digested, producing severe deficiency. This problem may be seen in relation to childbirth, particularly with antepartum haemorrhage and intrauterine death of the fetus but also after incompatible blood transfusion, in carcinomatosis, and in septicaemia. Management of such a condition, which is often associated with other deficiencies (e.g. thrombocytopenia) requires intensive skilled laboratory suppport.

REFERENCES

Baughan A S J, Patterson K G, Linch D C, Tillyer L,
   Treleaven J G, Machin S J 1986 Manual of haematology.
   Churchill Livinstone, Edinburgh
Ford M J, Robertson C E, Munro J F 1987 Manual of
   Medical Procedures. Churchill Livingstone, Edinburgh

13. Appendix

Contents

1. STAGES IN THE DEVELOPMENT OF INFANTS AND CHILDREN

4 weeks
Prone position — pelvis high, knees under abdomen.
Almost complete head lag on pulling into sitting position.
Grasp reflex present.

6 weeks
Head held momentarily in same plane as rest of body on ventral suspension.
Prone — pelvis high, knees no longer under abdomen.
Considerable, but not complete, head lag on pulling into sitting position.
Grasp reflex may be lost.
Smiles at mother.
Follows objects with eyes.

3 months
Head held beyond plane of rest of body on ventral suspension.
Prone — pelvis flat on couch.
Only slight head lag on pulling to sit.
Momentary grasping when object placed in hand.
Squeals of pleasure.
'Hand regard' evident, i.e. visual study of own hands.
Turns head to sound.

6 months
Sits supported by own hands.
Supine — spontaneously lifts head off couch.
Bounces when held standing.
Feeds self with biscuit.
Transfers object from one hand to other.
Responds to name.

9 months
Crawls by pulling forward with hands.
Can achieve sitting position.
Sits steadily without overbalancing.
Can stand holding on to furniture.
Can release grasped objects.
Waves 'bye-bye'.

1 Year
Walks supported by one hand.
Beginning to throw objects to floor.
May understand simple phrases.
Uses two or three words with meaning.

18 months
Walks up stairs with support.
Seats self on chair.
Builds 3 to 4 cubes on top of each other.
Takes off socks, gloves.
Scribbles with pencil.
Points to parts of body.

2 years
Goes up and down stairs.
Runs.
Turns door knob.
Kicks ball.
Puts on socks, etc.
Turns pages of book singly.
Asks for things.

3 years
Jumps off a step.
Rides tricycle.
Dresses and undresses.
Copies circle with pencil.
Knows nursery rhymes.
Can count, e.g. up to 10.

5 years
Skips on both feet.
Ties shoelaces.
Gives age when asked.
Can name four colours.

Table 13.1 Average head circumference

Age	cm	inches	Age	cm	inches
Birth	35.0	13.8	6 years	51.2	20.2
3 months	40.4	15.9	7 years	51.7	20.3
6 months	43.4	17.1	8 years	52.0	20.4
9 months	45.2	17.8	9 years	52.2	20.6
1 year	46.4	18.3	10 years	52.5	20.7
1½ years	47.7	18.8	11 years	52.9	20.8
2 years	49.0	19.3	12 years	53.4	21.0
3 years	49.6	19.5	13 years	53.8	21.2
4 years	50.0	19.7	14 years	54.1	21.3
5 years	50.7	20.0	15 years	54.8	21.6

One standard deviation from these means is approximately $\pm 2\frac{1}{2}\%$.

Table 13.2 Average times of eruption of teeth in primary and secondary dentitions

Deciduous teeth	Date of eruption	Permanent dentition	Date of eruption
Central incisors	8th month	First molars	6th– 7th year
Lateral incisors	10th month	Central incisors	6th– 7th year
First molars	12th month	Lateral incisors	7th– 9th year
Canines	18th month	First premolars	10th–11th year
Second molars	24th month	Canines	10th–12th year
		Second premolars	10th–12th year
		Second molars	12th year
		Third molars	17th–25th year

years

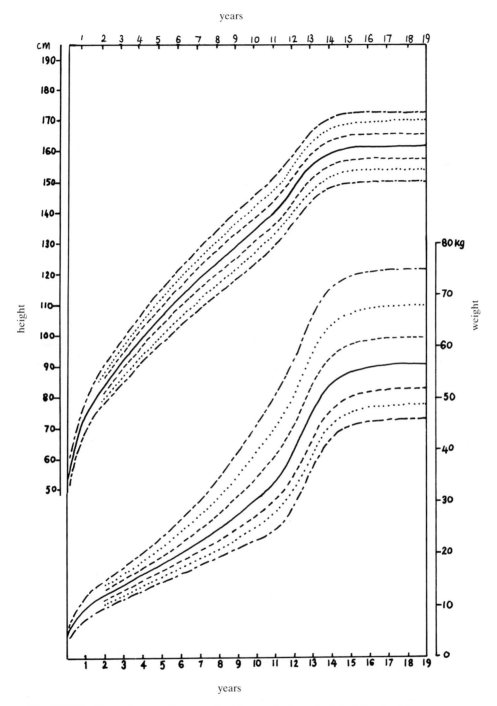

Fig. 13.1(A)   Charts for recording growth with mean and standard deviation in girls.

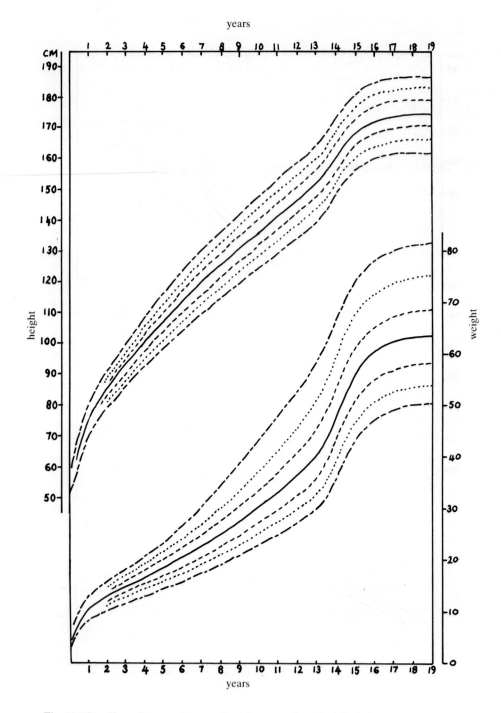

Fig. 13.1(B)   Charts for recording growth with mean and standard deviation in boys.

Table 13.3 Physical sexual development: centile distribution of the ages at which the stages of puberty occur (2+ indicating that Stage 2 is reached but not yet Stage 3). The centile values are the reverse of what might be expected. Thus the 97th centile represents the early age limit at which only 3% of children will show this feature and 97% remain to do so; conversely the 3rd centile indicates the late end of the normal age range.

Boys: genital development

Stage 1 Preadolescent: the testes (<3 ml), scrotum and penis are of about the same size and proportions as in early childhood.

Stage 2 Enlargement of the scrotum and testes (>5 ml). Skin of scrotum reddens and changes in texture. Little or no enlargement of penis.

Stage 3 Lengthening of the penis. Further growth of the testes and scrotum.

Stage 4 Increase in breadth of the penis and development of the glans. The testes and scrotum are larger; the scrotum darkens.

Stage 5 Adult.

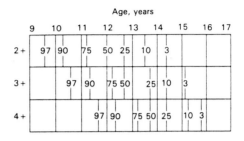

Boys: pubic hair

Stage 1 Preadolescent.

Stage 2 Sparse growth of slightly pigmented downy hair chiefly at the base of the penis.

Stag 3 Hair darker, coarser and more curled, spreading sparsely over junction of pubes.

Stage 4 Hair adult in type, but covering a considerably smaller area than in the adult. No spread to the medial surface of the thighs.

Stage 5 Adult.

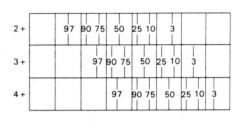

Girls: breast development

Stage 1 Preadolescent: elevation of papilla only.

Stage 2 Breast bud stage. Elevation of the breast and papilla as a small mound. Enlargement of the areola diameter.

Stage 3 Further enlargement and elevation of the breast and areola, with no separation of their contours.

Stage 4 Projection of the areola and papilla above the level of the breast.

Stage 5 Mature stage, projection of the papilla alone due to recession of the areola.

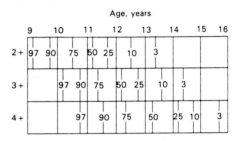

Girls: pubic hair

Stage 1 Preadolescent.

Stage 2 Sparse growth of slightly pigmented downy hair chiefly along the labia.

Stage 3 Hair darker, coarser and more curled, spreading sparsely over junction of pubes.

Stage 4 Hair adult in type, but covering a considerably smaller area than in the adult. No spread to the medial surface of the thighs.

Stage 5 Adult.

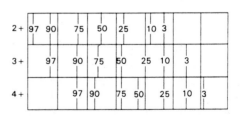

Menarche

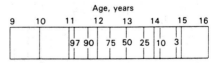

2. DESIRABLE WEIGHTS OF ADULTS

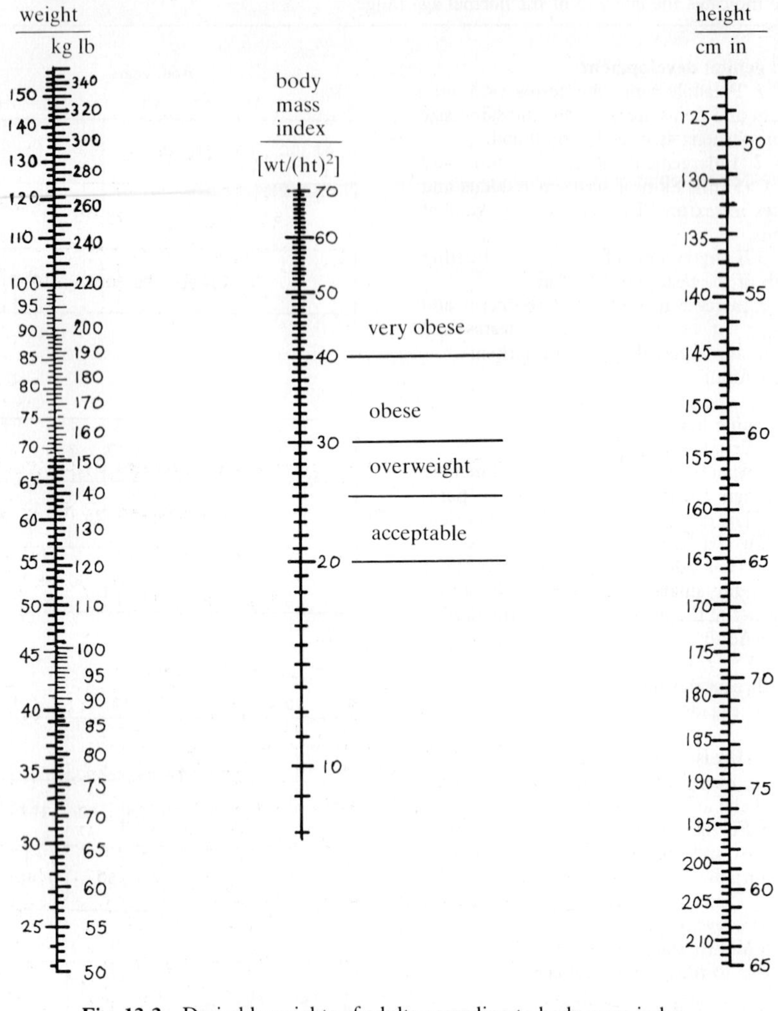

Fig. 13.2 Desirable weights of adults according to body mass index.

Body mass index (BMI) is derived from the weight in kgs divided by the square of the height in metres (Kgm/m^2). The 'normal' range is 20–25. Grade I obesity is >25–30, grade II >30–40 and grade III >40.

To use the nomogram, place a ruler or straight edge between the body weight in kg (indoor clothes) and the height in cm (without shoes). The body mass index is read from the middle of the scale.

3. THE GLASGOW COMA SCALE

In the examination of a patient with altered consciousness from whatever cause, it is important to have an easily applied, reproducible method of assessment and evaluation. This renders previously used ill-defined and confusing terms such as semi-comatose or stuperose obsolete. The Glasgow

Coma Scale is the most widely used method of assessing consciousness in such patients. Although initially instituted and applied to patients with head injury, it is also useful in the assessment of patients with altered consciousness from medical as well as surgical causes.

The Scale uses three clinically determined parameters: the *eye opening* response, the *best verbal* response, and the *best motor* response to painful stimulus. For each of the three categories, a score is given and the three scores are then summated. Any total score of between 3 and 15 is therefore possible. The patient's conscious level can then be expressed as a numerical value e.g. GCS 8/15.

A numerical fall in the Glasgow Coma Scale indicates a deterioration in conscious level and, by implication, represents either primary neurological deterioration or impairment of other vital processes such as circulation and respiration essential to normal neurological function. Repeated performance and documentation of the scale in an individual patient are important and, combined with other vital signs, are essential to assess responses to therapy or to detect early deterioration in the patient's neurological condition.

When used in this way, the Glasgow Coma Scale is an important tool in the assessment of consciousness, allowing both the direct evaluation of an individual and a recognised means of communication with other clinicians. Its application does, however, require a degree of commonsense. Thus, the estimation of the best verbal response in young children will be dependant upon the age and normal developmental state of the child. Similarly, patients who have an endotracheal tube in place for whatever reason will be unable to verbalise, although if conscious, may be able to show their understanding in other ways. Finally, local trauma to the face or limb may render the eye opening and motor responses difficult or impossible to assess.

The Glasgow Coma Scale

Eye-opening response:	Score
spontaneous	4
to speech	3
to painful stimulus	2
none	1

Best motor response (in upper limbs):	
obeys commands	6
localises	5
withdraws	4
flexes abnormally } to painful stimulus	3
extends	2
none	1

Best verbal response:	
orientated	5
confused conversation	4
inappropriate words	3
incomprehensible sounds	2
none	1

GCS total =

4. THE USE OF QUESTIONNAIRES

With particular reference to sexual problems in the male

In a literate society questionnaires constitute an efficient and time-saving method of obtaining information. They can be used in health reviews and as a data base in problem orientated case notes (p. 361). Questionnaires can also provide detailed information in special situations. They are particularly useful in assessing sexual problems, for example infertility, because the questions can be posed without the embarrassment of an interview and the sexual partner can help to answer them.

In sexual problems in the male the questionnaire consists of two parts. In the first the patient provides details about his past and present health, with appropriate reference to
1. conditions such as sexually transmitted disease, mumps and tuberculosis which may affect the testes,
2. his marital status including offspring,
3. current and previous cigarette and alcohol consumption,
4. medication and drug abuse, and
5. nature of employment and previous occupations.
The second part of the questionnaire contains

explicit questions about sexual activities. First a general sexual history is obtained and then more specific information is sought, as, for example, about problems with erection or ejaculation. In all cases psychological factors are also assessed. Examples of such questions are given below.

Sexual problems questionnaire for men (Part 2)

Sexual history
1. How often on average do you try to have intercourse?
2. Does shift work or absence from home interfere with opportunities to have sex?
3. Do you have any physical difficulties with the sex act that would prevent conception, e.g. pain during intercourse sufficient to prevent penetration?

If the answer to any of the above questions is *yes*, please give details.

Partner
1. Does your partner experience pain during sexual intercourse?
2. If *yes*, is the pain sufficient to make you stop having intercourse on occasions?
3. Has your partner had a sterilisation operation?
4. Has your partner had a hysterectomy?

Problems with erection
Do you get satisfactory erections of the penis for sexual purposes?
If not please answer the following questions:
1. Which is the situation that most closely resembles your own?
   (i) No erection of any sort at any time.
   (ii) Incomplete erections occasionally but the penis is not firm enough to allow penetration.
   (iii) Firm erections at first allowing penetration but not lasting long enough for completion of sexual intercourse.
   (iv) Firm erections in the morning or during wet dreams but unable to have erections when trying to have intercourse with partner.
   (v) Firm erections but the penis is bent when erect making sexual intercourse impossible.
2. When was the last time you had a normal erection firm enough to allow normal sexual intercourse or masturbation?
3. Do you get morning erections?

Problems with ejaculation
Do you get satisfactory ejaculation of sperm?
If not please answer the following questions:
1. Do you think you ejaculate —
   (i) normally when having sex with your wife/partner,
   (ii) normally when masturbating,
   (iii) sometimes when asleep during dreams?
2. During ejaculation do you feel that —
   (i) the sperm goes the wrong way,
   (ii) ejaculation occurs too quickly,

   (iii) there is no ejaculation?
3. If you ejaculate too quickly, does ejaculation occur —
   (i) before there has been any penetration of the penis,
   (ii) very soon after penetration?
4. If you do not ejaculate at all, do you —
   (i) have no sex because you have no erections,
   (ii) have normal erections but despite much stimulation cannot ejaculate?

Psychological Problems
Do you think that your problem is caused by emotional or psychological difficulties?
If *yes* please try to tell me what these are.

Scrutiny of the answers to the questionnaire quickly identifies the main problem which the clinician can then clarify at an interview with the patient. It must be borne in mind, however, that no questionnaire is complete and that the patient must be given the opportunity to speak about any other related matters.

5. A SYSTEM OF CASE RECORDING

Name: Age: Sex: Status:
Address: Telephone No:
Occupation: Provide that of patient and of
               partner. In the case of a child give
               the parent's occupations.
Family doctor:
Date of admission to hospital:
Date of examination:
Source of history (e.g. patient, close relative etc).

HISTORY

Present illness. Begin by naming the presenting or principal symptoms and the duration of each. Proceed with a chronological account of the mode of onset and course of the patient's illness up to the day of the examination.

Systemic Enquiry. Record the presence or absence of cardinal symptoms such as cough, breathlessness, digestive or urinary troubles, pain, insomnia or change in weight. Note any *drugs* taken and any *allergy*.

Previous health. Illness, operations, accidents, and their dates. Note any travel abroad, prophylactic medication, vaccination and immunisation. Date and result of any previous medical examination (e.g. for life insurance) or radiological examination. History of birth in the case of infants and children.

Family history. Note age, health, or cause of death of parents, siblings, spouse and children (Fig. 1.1, p. 6).

Social and personal history. Record the relevant information about occupation, housing, and personal habits regarding recreation, physical exercise, alcohol and tobacco, and in the case of children, about school and family relationships. In the elderly, describe the level of self-dependence and the available support such as Home Help services.

PHYSICAL EXAMINATION

General assessment

In an introductory statement comment on the patient's *demeanour* and *general condition*, i.e. physique, nutrition, state of hydration, posture, gait, personality and mental state. Record height and weight. Note any abnormality not recorded under a systemic heading, e.g.:

Hands and arms. Note any information of diagnostic value obtained from inspection of hands and nails. Epitrochlear and axillary lymph nodes.

Head, face and neck. Describe in detail any abnormality such as goitre or enlarged lymph nodes.

Skin. Colour; pallor, cyanosis, pigmentation, jaundice, etc. Specific lesions.

Subcutaneous tissues. Nodules; vascular abnormalities; oedema.

Breasts. Note findings on palpation.

Cardiovascular system

Arterial pulse and pressure. Rate, rhythm, wave form and volume of radial pulse. Blood pressure.

Jugular venous pulse and pressure. Note form of the jugular pulse wave and height of the jugular venous pressure.

Heart.
Inspection. Pulsations and deformity of anterior chest wall.
Palpation. Position of apex beat, character of apical impulse and other pulsations; thrills.
Auscultation. First and second heart sounds; added sounds; murmurs.

Peripheral circulation.
Arterial. Pulsation of limb arteries; skin temperature and colour; local nutrition; bruits.
Venous. Abnormal vessels; signs of inflammation or occlusion.

Respiratory system

Note cough, character and quantity of sputum, wheeze or other respiratory difficulty.

Upper respiratory tract. Nose; tonsils; pharynx.
Chest.
Inspection. Shape and lesions of chest wall; respiration rate and depth; chest expansion; mode of breathing.
Palpation. Range of movement; position of trachea.
Percussion. Anterior, lateral and posterior chest wall; hepatic dullness.
Auscultation. Breath sounds, vocal resonance and added sounds.

Alimentary and genitourinary systems

Mouth. Lips, tongue, teeth, gums and other mucosae. Character and quantity of any vomitus.
Abdomen.
Inspection. Scars; veins; hair. Abdominal wall: shape, general and local changes, e.g. hernias and movement of respiratory, peristaltic, vascular or fetal origin.
Palpation. Tenderness; guarding; individual organs and abnormal masses; hernial orifices; inguinal lymph nodes.
Percussion. Fluid, gas, and individual organs.
Auscultation. Frequency and character of bowel sounds; vascular bruits.
Genitalia.
Inspection.
Palpation. Penis, testes, epididymes and vasa deferens. Vaginal examination in special circumstances only.
Rectum. Inspection of the anus and examination of rectum if indicated; inspection of and testing of faeces for occult blood, if indicated.
Urine. Volume, colour, opacity, odour, reaction, specific gravity; microscopy; chemical tests for protein, glucose and other substances as indicated.

Nervous system

Speech. Language function, articulation, phonation.

Cranial nerves.
First. Sense of smell (if indicated, p. 193).

Second. Visual acuity; visual fields; ophthalmoscopic examination.

Third, fourth and sixth. Eyelids, ptosis, palpebral fissures; pupils, size, shape, symmetry and reflexes; eye movements, diplopia and nystagmus.

Fifth. Facial sensation; muscles of mastication, corneal reflex and jaw jerk.

Seventh. Movements of facial muscles; taste on the anterior two thirds of the tongue.

Eighth. Auriscopic examination; estimation of auditory acuity; tuning fork tests; positional nystagmus.

Ninth. Sensation of pharynx and of the posterior third of the tongue; palatal and pharyngeal reflexes.

Tenth. Phonation; movements of palate and posterior pharyngeal wall; palatal and pharyngeal reflexes (if indicated, p. 212).

Eleventh. Sternomastoid and upper trapezius muscles.

Twelfth. Inspection of tongue and its movements.

Motor system. Inspection of musculature; involuntary movements including fasciculation; tone; clonus; power; coordination; fine movements; dyspraxia.

Sensory system. Touch, pain and temperature; position and vibration sense; cortical sensory function, e.g. two point discrimination, stereognosis.

Reflexes. Tendon reflexes; abdominal and plantar responses.

Supplementary tests. Bruits audible in the neck or skull. Meningeal or nerve root irritation. Tetany.

Locomotor system

Describe any abnormality of gait.

Spine. Shape and movement of neck and trunk.

Joints of limbs. Movements, deformity, swelling, tenderness, temperature.

Muscles. Atrophy, contractures, swelling, tenderness.

Bones. Deformity, tenderness.

Psychiatric examination

The mental state.
1. General appearance and behaviour.
2. Thought processes. Sample of talk.
3. Mood.
4. Delusions.
5. Hallucinations.
6. Obsessions.
7. Evidence of intellectual defect.
   a. Orientation.
   b. Memory.
   c. Attention and concentration.
   d. General information.
   e. Intelligence.
8. Insight and judgement.

Personality diagnosis.

CLINICAL DIAGNOSIS

Record the differential diagnosis in order of probability.

FURTHER INVESTIGATIONS

It is helpful to outline a plan of any further investigations considered necessary at this stage.

TREATMENT AND PROGRESS NOTES

These should be entered from day to day.

FINAL DIAGNOSIS

SUMMARY

It is advisable to conclude the case recording with a brief summary incorporating the principal symptoms, the main abnormalities on physical examination, the significant findings on further investigation, the diagnosis, the therapeutic measures employed and the decisions regarding further management. Alternatively the summary can take the form of a 'problem list' as described below.

6. PROBLEM-ORIENTATED MEDICAL RECORDS

The traditional method of case recording has been adapted in some centres to incorporate the problem-orientated medical record developed by Weed and his colleagues (1968). Basic information is collected by the methods described in this book but its recording is orientated around the patient's problems. Weed's system is structured into four main components, the data base, the problem list, the initial plan and the progress notes.

1. Data base. This consists of:

a. The principal complaint
b. Relevant social data and the 'profile'; the latter is a description of how the patient spends an average day. Therapeutic goals can be related to this profile
c. The history
d. The physical examination
e. Laboratory and other basic investigations, such as haemoglobin, urea and electrolytes and chest radiography.

2. Problem list. All the patient's problems, past and present, are named and numbered on a *provisional problem list*. Physical problems may comprise a symptom, such as weight loss, a sign such as cervical lymphadenopathy or a pathological condition, such as chronic bronchitis. Other problems may be social, for example cigarette smoking, or psychological such as a grief reaction from a recent bereavement. As the clinical situation is clarified, these problems are transposed to a *master problem list* which is displayed prominently in the front of the case notes. Problems are classified as either active or resolved. The former category includes not only those which have been diagnosed but also any unexplained or ambiguous findings. In the case of hospital patients the master problem list is best prepared about one or two days after admission. It is open ended and is modified as the situation changes. New problems are added as they are recognised. The master problem list serves as a guide to the case notes and provides a summary which helps not only the medical staff but also nurses, physiotherapists, social workers and others to assess the position. An example of a master problem list is given in Figure 13.2.

3. Initial plan. For each active problem an initial plan is organised from three aspects:

a. The collection of further data to clarify the situation
b. Therapy
c. Education of the patient in active participation in the management of the disease.

4. Progress notes. The records are kept up to date by entering all additional relevant information, as it is obtained, under the named and numbered title of the problem to which it pertains. The notes are further structured by sub-headings:

a. Subjective data; prominence is given first to the patient's reactions
b. Objective data
c. Interpretation; this includes both decisions and impressions
d. Therapy; this includes education of the patient
e. Immediate plans.

These notes are supplemented by *'flow sheets'* when dealing with fast moving situations such as diabetic ketoacidosis, shock or acute ventilatory failure. Then the inter-relationships of data and therapy are crucial; time, serial measurements, therapy and comment are recorded side by side and repeated as frequently as the situation demands.

Master Problem List (1.5.85)
Mrs A.B.C. (Date of birth 1.5.38)

Active	Inactive
1. Acute abdominal pain acute cholecystitis (2.5.85) cholecystectomy (10.5.85)	
2. Obesity	
3. Varicose veins	
4. Hysterical psychoneurosis	
5. Psoriasis	
6. Left facial pain secondary to 4 (4.5.85)	
7. Social deprivation (divorced; 4 children; 2 rooms)	
	8. Penicillin allergy (1972)
	9. Duodenal ulcer (1979)
10. Pulmonary embolism (16.5.85)	

Finally a *discharge report* is prepared summarising each numbered problem on the list; particular attention is paid to any problems which may not have been fully elucidated or which may recur.

Conclusion

Weed's original work should be consulted for further information about problem-orientated medical records, including illustrations of these methods in practice and the philosophy on which they are based.

The system presents data in structured ways readily amenable to assessment and audit by others. The methods, however, are initially time consuming and this has been a barrier to acceptance in their entirety. Many clinicians have found the master problem list useful, particularly in the outpatient follow up of complicated problems, as a flexible, intelligible and up-to-date summary which allows an immediate grasp of the medical and social situation and reduces errors of omission and commission in treatment.

REFERENCES

Weed L L 1968 Medical records that guide and teach. New England Journal of Medicine 278: 593 and 652
Weed L L 1970 Medical records, medical education and patient care — The problem-orientated record as a basic tool. Press of Case Western Reserve University, Cleveland, Ohio

7. KEEPING CASE RECORDS

The system of case note recording and of problem orientated medical records outlined above can, when appropriately used, give a well-structured and easy to follow assessment of a patient's situation including the working diagnosis, and the resulting investigation and treatment plan.

The importance of accurate, legible and structured case notes containing a record of examination, treatment prescribed, consent to procedures and any instructions given to the patient cannot be overemphasised. Remember that other clinicians may require to take over the patient's care at any time because of a sudden deterioration in their condition or because of cross-cover arrangements. The legibility of doctors' handwriting has in the past been a source of much humour. However, scrupulous attention to legibility is vital to ensure the patient's safety. Remember also that although a patient's case records are confidential, they may at any time in the future require to be examined either by the patient, other medical practitioners, or be exhibited as evidence in a court of law. Illegibility, humorous or flip comments neither help the management of the patient, nor the clinician required to give evidence in the witness box, months or years later.

Follow-up clinical notes should be entered on a regular basis and include the performance of investigations and their results, any change in therapy or other aspects relating directly to the patient's care. It is particularly important that concise notes are made as soon as practicable after any emergency treatment such as a cardiac arrest.

Finally, every single note entry in the case record should be signed together with the date and time that the record was completed.

8. CONTINUING MEDICAL EDUCATION

Medical audit and self-assessment

It has been suggested that the true aim of education is an understanding of method rather than a knowledge of fact. Once the student has learned how to learn, the accumulation of knowledge must continue, particularly in a discipline like medicine where scientific advances are continuous and often rapid. In clinical practice the acquisition of reliable methods of examination is the essential prerequisite and these must be kept under constant review. Medical students have their skills scrutinised and constructively criticised by their tutors. When clinical methods have become established they can be tested by medical audit and self-assessment.

Medical audit has become particularly important in the current climate of complaint and litigation. Many complaints and subsequent distressing medico-legal actions are the result of poor communication between doctor and patient or their relatives, or between doctors involved in the management of a single patient. Where a patient or close relative feels that an aspect of clinical management has been mishandled, or where an actual error has occurred the actions and behaviour of the clinician can do much to allay and defuse a difficult, and occasionally threatening, situation.

Medical audit has become national policy in the United States to evaluate standards of clinical practice; it will no doubt play an increasing part in Britain and other countries. Audit is most effective when criteria are agreed beforehand and where the aim is educational; it is potentially abrasive and counter-productive when it is conducted by an independent body and where it carries a punitive threat.

Self-audit involves a conscious effort of appraising one's own clinical practice; it should be an integral part of medical care. A practical example of audit by others in the clinical field is when two or more clinical teams (firms, cliniques, etc.) take part. Notes are chosen at random from among patients recently discharged from hospital and these are subjected to scrutiny by the other team. They may be studied from the point of view of errors of omission or commission in the clinical record and they may bring to light lack of information, for example about smoking habits, or faulty judgements such as decision to treat 'hypertension' on the basis of a single estimation of blood pressure. Such activity conducted in a friendly atmosphere and in good faith can provide an excellent climate for learning and lead to a general improvement in performance.

The use or abuse of ancillary services can also be assessed by audit. It has demonstrated, for example, the limited value of routine chest radiographs in patients under 40 years of age without pulmonary symptoms. Furthermore medical audit can evaluate the safety and efficiency of new drugs and the optimum use of limited resources in relation to new, and often costly, techniques.

It would however be incorrect to suggest that audit by others is ever totally without threat, that it is yet generally accepted, or that there is agreement as to whether clinical judgement, for example, is capable of being assessed.

Self assessment is another aspect of continuing education. One simple method involves a written diagnostic analysis of each patient at the time of initial interview, followed by a critical reappraisal once the results of investigations are available. There are now many self assessment programmes (SAPs) which attempt to assess both factual knowledge — a relatively easy task — and judgement, and such programmes are becoming available. Skills can also be tested by multiple choice questions (MCQs) and this textbook is supplemented by various publications specifically designed to perform such a task.

Conclusion. The critical scrutiny of both practice and records by one's peers and by oneself provided by medical audit and self assessment will be welcomed by those interested in ensuring that their professional standards have kept up with progress in medical skills and knowledge. These methods are logical developments in a scientifically orientated discipline; they constitute a responsibility and a challenge in the continuing study of medicine.

REFERENCES

Fleming P R et al 1980 1200 MCQs in medicine. Churchill Livingstone, Edinburgh

Flynn M D, Ashford R F U, Venables P J W 1987 100 Data Interpretation Questions for the MRCP, 2nd edn. Churchill Livingstone, Edinburgh

Ford M J, Nicol F 1987 MCQS for MRCP Part 1. Churchill Livingstone, Edinburgh

Index